ADVANCES IN THE BIOSCIENCES

Volume 32

GASTRIC CANCER

ADVANCES IN THE BIOSCIENCES

Latest volumes in the series:

GASTRIC CANCER

Proceedings of the International Symposium on
Gastric Cancer, Birmingham, 22-23 September 1980

Editors:

J. W. L. FIELDING
C. E. NEWMAN
C. H. J. FORD
B. G. JONES

The Queen Elizabeth Hospital, Birmingham

PERGAMON PRESS

OXFORD · NEW YORK · TORONTO · SYDNEY · PARIS · FRANKFURT

U.K.	Pergamon Press Ltd., Headington Hill Hall, Oxford OX3 0BW, England
U.S.A.	Pergamon Press Inc., Maxwell House, Fairview Park, Elmsford, New York 10523, U.S.A.
CANADA	Pergamon Press Canada Ltd., Suite 104, 150 Consumers Rd., Willowdale, Ontario M2J 1P9, Canada
AUSTRALIA	Pergamon Press (Aust.) Pty. Ltd., P.O. Box 544, Potts Point, N.S.W. 2011, Australia
FRANCE	Pergamon Press SARL, 24 rue des Ecoles, 75240 Paris, Cedex 05, France
FEDERAL REPUBLIC OF GERMANY	Pergamon Press GmbH, 6242 Kronberg-Taunus, Hammerweg 6, Federal Republic of Germany

First edition 1981

British Library Cataloguing in Publication Data

International Symposium on Gastric Cancer
(*1980 Birmingham*)
Gastric cancer. - (Advances in the biosciences;
v.32)
1. Stomach - Cancer - Congresses
I. Title   II. Fielding, J. W. L.
III. Series
616.99'4'33   RC280.S8
ISBN 0-08-026398-4

Library of Congress Catalog Card no. 81-81229

In order to make this volume available as economically and as rapidly as possible the authors' typescripts have been reproduced in their original forms. This method unfortunately has its typographical limitations but it is hoped that they in no way distract the reader.

Printed in Great Britain by A. Wheaton & Co. Ltd., Exeter

CONTENTS

Contents

PREFACE

Information collected by the Birmingham Cancer Registry regarding cases of cancer of the stomach occurring in the West Midlands Region of England, from 1935 onwards, was analysed by a small group of us between 1960 and 1972. The results generally conformed with national statistics and showed that stomach cancer was the fourth commonest of all malignancies, that the overall 5-year cure rate was approximately 5%, and that during the period of study the cure rate was not improving.

As a preliminary step in efforts to try and improve the treatment of the condition, a small group of clinicians and statisticians (later calling itself the Birmingham Stomach Cancer Group) undertook a double blind trial to evaluate the possible value of chemotherapy in inoperable stomach cancer. During the 2-year study the group joined with workers from other centres and eventually a British Stomach Cancer Group was evolved. Following publication of that first study, a further large project to investigate the value of adjuvant chemotherapy in operable stomach cancer was undertaken, and the results of this will be published in the near future. In addition to information regarding cure rates, these studies produced much information regarding the incidence and natural history of the disease, factors affecting prognosis, and problems of treatment regimens.

Whilst our own results had not shown any great improvement, other centres, notably in Japan, had published significantly better results in early diagnosis and treatment. Other advances such as histological grading and tumour markers had been reported by other workers. In early 1980 the Birmingham Group felt that there would be considerable value in holding an International Symposium and gathering today's leading authorities in the investigation and treatment of stomach cancer to present and argue their views. This meeting was held in Birmingham on September 22 and 23, 1980.

We are grateful to the experts who travelled from a number of countries to take part in that Symposium. The total of their individual contributions was much enhanced by the stimulating discussions that followed the papers, and in which so many of the prime speakers were involved.

The group felt that the material presented in the papers and in the discussion afterwards would be of interest to many more than those who were able to attend the meeting. For this purpose this book is being published, and our thanks are due to those who took part for allowing us to present their work. We would also express our gratitude to the commercial organisations whose financial aid did much to make the Symposium and the publication possible, and to the Special Trustees of the Central Birmingham District Endowment Fund for underwriting the costs of the meeting.

Finally, it must be recognised that much of the credit for the success of the venture was due to the enthusiasm and hard work of the organising committee of J. W. L. Fielding, B. G. Jones and C. E. Newman.

V. S. Brookes.

ACKNOWLEDGEMENTS

We wish to express our sincere thanks to the University of Birmingham for providing us with the facilities for the symposium and to Professor G. Slaney, Barling Professor of Surgery for his support and encouragement. We also thank the other members of the Stomach Cancer Group for their interest and support during the organisation of the conference.

This Symposium would not have been possible without the generous financial support we have received from Smith, Kline and French, Imperial Chemical Industries, Lundbeck Ltd., Bayer UK Ltd., the Upjohn Company, West Midlands Regional Health Authority, University of Birmingham and in particular the Special Trustees of the Queen Elizabeth Hospital.

We are indebted to Margot Morris, the Conference Coordinator, for her invaluable help with the organisation and running of the Symposium and with the editing of the book. Also to Mr. J.A. Griffin for recording the discussions and to our dedicated staff especially Joan Sharpe and Amanda Dorrell for their assistance during the meeting. Editing has been kept to a minimum to preserve the original style of the papers and atmosphere of the discussions and in order to expedite publication.

Finally, it is a pleasure to thank the publishers, Pergamon Press, for their help with the preparation of the book.

> J.W.L. Fielding.
> C.E. Newman.
> C.H.J. Ford.
> B.G. Jones.

Changing Patterns in the Incidence of Gastric Cancer

T. Hirayama

Epidemiology Division, National Cancer Center
Research Institute, Tokyo, Japan

ABSTRACT

The gastric cancer death rates and incidence rates are still higher
than any country in the world in Japan although both are on the
steady decline in recent years. Calendar year effect was observed
to be stronger than cohort effect in this tendency to decline. The
reason for the recent decline in gastric cancer mortality in Japan is
interpreted as a reflection of rather sudden dietary improvement in
Japan, just as in other developed countries. Frequent intake of
green-yellow vegetables, for instance, was noted to lower the
gastric cancer risk both in smokers and non smokers. Cessation of
smoking is recommended together with dietary improvement, in
particular increased intake of vitamin A.

KEYWORDS

Gastric cancer; trend; green-yellow vegetables; cigarette smoking;
Japan.

INTRODUCTION

In Japan, just as in most of other developed countries, the pattern
of cancer has been changing rapidly in recent years. Cancer of the
stomach and cervix have shown a steep downward trend, whereas
cancers of the lung, pancreas, intestine, prostate, ovary, breast,
urinary organs, and leukemia have been increasing steadily. One of
the most impressive changes has been the decrease in gastric cancer
mortality. Factors possibly related to the changing trend are
reviewed.

MATERIALS AND METHODS

Vital statistics in Japan from 1955 to 1978 and results of the
National Nutritional Survey from 1949 to 1978 provided the data for
this presentation. Standard methods of both descriptive and analytic

epidemiology were fully utilized in analyzing the data.

OBSERVATION AND DISCUSSION

1) International comparison:

Gastric cancer incidence rates are higher in Japan than any of cancer registries in the world. Japanese in Hawaii showed significantly lower incidence rate.(Fig. 1)

Fig. 1

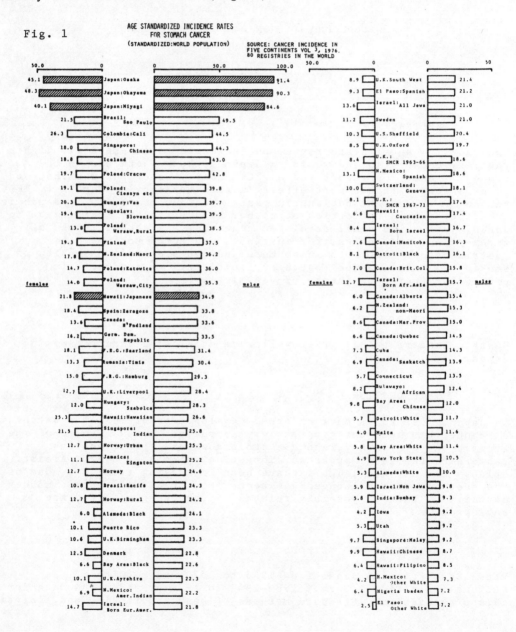

AGE STANDARDIZED INCIDENCE RATES
FOR STOMACH CANCER
(STANDARDIZED:WORLD POPULATION)

SOURCE: CANCER INCIDENCE IN
FIVE CONTINENTS VOL 3, 1976.
80 REGISTRIES IN THE WORLD

When compared with age specific incidence rates in USA, 10-20 fold
increaseswere noted in younger age groups in Japan. The ratio
became smaller with the advance of the age.

2) Trend in age adjusted death rates:

The age-adjusted death rates (adjusted to 1935 census population in
Japan) for cancer of stomach show dramatic decrease both in males
and in females in the last two decades. The steep decrease was also
noted for cervical cancer. On the other hand, a sharp increase was
observed for cancers of the lung, pancreas, prostate, urinary
organs, colon-rectum, liver, breast, ovary, and leukemia.(Fig. 2)

Fig. 2

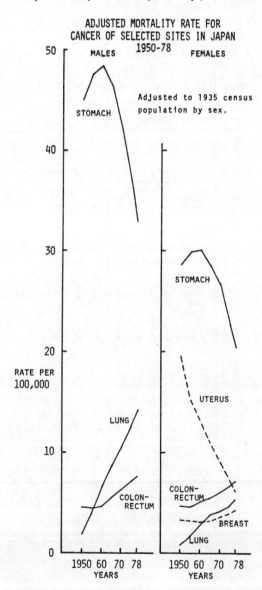

ADJUSTED MORTALITY RATE FOR
CANCER OF SELECTED SITES IN JAPAN
1950-78

3) Trend in age adjusted incidence rates:

Similar trends have been observed in incidence rates in selected cancer registries. As shown in Table 1, 2 and 3, the slope of decline in mortality rates for gastric cancer in Osaka is slightly steeper than that in incidence rates in the same area.

Table 1

AGE-ADJUSTED INCIDENCE RATE
BY SELECTED PRIMARY SITE, SEX, AND SURVEY PERIOD
(/100,000 POPULATION, OSAKA)

	SURVEY PERIOD	ALL SITES (140-209)	ESOPHAGUS (150)	STOMACH (151)	COLON (153)	RECTUM (154)	LIVER (155)	PANCREAS (157)	LUNG (162)	BREAST (174)	UTERUS (180-182)	BLADDER (188)	LEUKEMIA (204-207)
M	1963-65	216.1	10.9	109.2	4.3	7.1	17.1	4.6	19.1	-	-	-	-
	1966-68	211.1	9.8	101.2	5.4	6.1	16.1	5.6	20.6	-	-	5.2	3.6
	1969-71	204.7	9.1	92.0	6.1	6.9	15.4	5.5	22.8	-	-	5.1	4.0
	1972-74	200.3	9.0	82.7	6.3	7.2	18.0	5.6	26.0	-	-	5.2	3.9
	1975	205.3	8.8	78.8	8.1	7.3	20.6	5.5	31.9	-	-	4.7	4.6
	1976	210.9	8.6	79.8	8.6	8.4	21.2	6.3	29.2	-	-	5.2	4.4
F	1963-65	160.1	3.5	52.8	3.5	4.7	9.0	2.4	6.3	11.0	39.8	-	-
	1966-68	152.1	3.5	49.9	4.6	4.8	7.2	2.8	6.4	11.0	33.0	2.0	2.6
	1969-71	144.2	3.0	45.8	5.1	4.6	6.9	3.1	6.8	11.9	27.9	1.5	3.1
	1972-74	140.1	2.4	41.6	5.8	4.2	6.9	3.2	8.1	13.3	25.1	1.6	3.0
	1975	130.2	2.2	39.1	5.4	4.3	6.3	3.5	7.9	11.7	25.5	1.5	3.8
	1976	133.9	1.9	39.0	6.2	5.0	6.9	3.1	8.9	11.9	25.8	1.3	3.4

Table 2

AGE-ADJUSTED MORTALITY RATES
BY SELECTED PRIMARY SITE, SEX, AND SURVEY PERIOD
(/100,000 POPULATION, OSAKA)

	SURVEY PERIOD	ALL SITES (140-209)	ESOPHAGUS (150)	STOMACH (151)	COLON (153)	RECTUM (154)	LIVER (155)	PANCREAS (157)	LUNG (162)	BREAST (174)	UTERUS (180-182)	BLADDER (188)	LEUKEMIA (204-207)
M	1963-65	162.5	9.4	82.6	3.3	5.3	-	4.2	15.0	-		3.0	2.9
	1966-68	160.3	8.2	74.0	3.6	4.5	-	5.0	17.2	-		2.3	3.3
	1969-71	154.8	8.3	69.6	4.7	5.0	14.3	4.9	18.6	-		2.4	3.5
	1972-74	157.3	8.1	65.4	4.3	5.6	16.0	5.1	22.0	-		2.9	3.4
	1975	159.3	7.8	60.1	5.6	5.6	18.0	5.0	26.6	-		2.6	4.2
	1976	158.7	8.3	58.0	5.5	5.8	19.0	5.5	25.0	-		2.4	3.9
F	1963-65	103.4	2.9	41.3	2.7	3.6	-	2.0	5.0	3.7	17.0	1.1	2.6
	1966-68	102.0	3.0	36.8	3.1	3.5	-	2.4	5.5	5.6	15.7	0.8	2.5
	1969-71	98.0	2.6	35.6	3.7	3.5	6.1	2.8	5.7	4.7	13.6	1.0	2.7
	1972-74	99.4	2.2	34.0	4.2	3.3	6.4	3.0	7.0	5.7	12.7	1.0	2.6
	1975	92.3	1.7	30.6	3.9	3.6	5.9	3.4	6.0	5.1	12.0	0.9	3.3
	1976	92.2	1.8	28.5	4.8	3.6	6.3	2.9	7.1	5.8	11.4	0.7	2.8

Table 3

PERCENTAGE CHANGE OF CANCER INCIDENCE AND MORTALITY RATES
BY SELECTED SITE AND SEX, OSAKA

PERCENT CHANGE OF RATES	ALL SITES (140-209)	ESOPHAGUS (150)	STOMACH (151)	COLON (153)	RECTUM (154)	LIVER (155)	PANCREAS (157)	LUNG (162)	BREAST (174)	UTERUS (180-182)	BLADDER (188)	LEUKEMIA (204-207)
M)												
INCIDENCE	- 2.4	- 21.1	- 26.9	100.0	18.3	24.0	37.0	52.9	-		-	-
MORTALITY	- 2.3	- 11.7	- 29.8	66.7	9.4	-	31.0	66.7	-		- 20.0	34.5
F)												
INCIDENCE	- 16.4	- 45.7	- 26.1	77.1	6.4	- 23.3	29.2	41.3	8.2	- 35.2	-	-
MORTALITY	- 10.8	- 37.9	- 31.0	77.8	0	-	45.0	42.0	56.8	- 32.9	- 36.4	7.7

$$\text{PERCENT CHANGE OF INCIDENCE AND MORTALITY RATES} = \frac{\text{RATE FOR 1976} - \text{RATE FOR 1963-65}}{\text{RATE FOR 1963-65}} \times 100$$

4) Trends in age specific death rates:

The age-specific death rate for gastric cancer has been declining since 1955.(Fig. 3)

Fig. 3

ANNUAL TREND OF AGE SPECIFIC DEATH RATE
FOR STOMACH CANCER IN JAPAN (1955-1979)

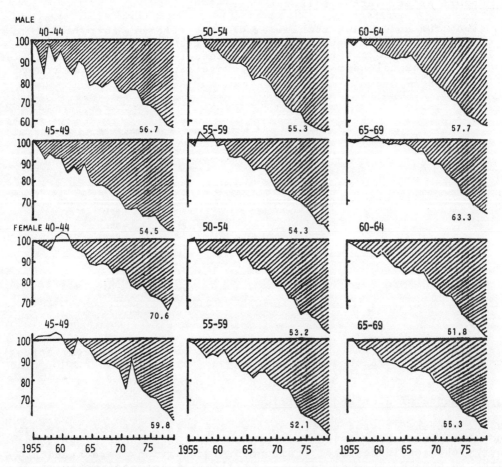

Among males, the death rate in 1978 in the 40-44 age groups was 43% lower than it was in 1955. The proportion of decline was 46%, 45%, 46%, 42%, and 37% for the age groups 45-49, 50-54, 55-59, 60-64, and 65-69, respectively. In females, the proportion decline was 29%, 40%, 47%, 48%, 48%, and 45% for the age groups 40-44, 45-49, 50-54, 55-59, 60-64, and 65-69, respectively.

5) Selected features of recent decrease:

The decline was most striking for cancer of the pylorus, percentage decrease in age adjusted death rate from 1958 to 1978 being 62% in males and 56% in females and far less for cancer of the cardia, percentage decrease from 1958 to 1978 being 33% in males and 31% in females; furthermore, it was most striking in metropolitan areas, next in other cities, and least in counties. The decline was observed for most occupational groups except for sales workers.

6) Cohort effect versus calendar-year effect:

To study the underlying mechanism of the decrease, correlation coefficients of the death rates for selected age groups were calculated between cohort pairs and calendar-year pairs. In case of gastric cancer calendar-year effects were far stronger than cohort effects.(Table 4)

Table 4

Simple and Partial Correlation Coefficients between Gastric Cancer Death Rates for Selected Age Group. Japan 1950–1975

Type of correlation	Sex	Pairs	Correlation between age group, 40–44, and other age groups:			
			45–49	50–54	55–59	60–64
Simple correlation	Male	Cohort pairs	0.85	0.78	0.27	−0.25
		Calendar year pairs	0.93*	0.91*	0.72*	0.77*
	Female	Cohort pairs	0.63	0.06	−0.64	−0.02
		Calendar year pairs	0.91*	0.92*	0.92*	0.86*
Partial correlation	Male	Cohort pairs	0.45	0.55	0.31	−0.09
		Calendar year pairs	0.80*	0.84*	0.73*	0.75*
	Female	Cohort pairs	0.38	0.10	−0.52	0.37
		Calendar year pairs	0.87*	0.92*	0.90*	0.87*

* Correlation coefficient higher.

A similar tendency was observed for breast cancer. However, strong cohort effects were observed for lung and cervical cancer.

7) Influence of diet and nutrition:

As the decrease in the gastric cancer death rate was considered as due mostly to calendar-year effects rather than cohort effects, yearly changes in selected environmental conditions were studied. Although considerable differences still exist between the nutritional intake of the Japanese people as compared to people in the United States, there has been a striking change as demonstrated by the National Nutritional Survey. The consumption of milk and milk products increased by 28-fold from 1949 to 1978. The ratios of the increases in consumption of other food items are as follows; meat, 12.8; eggs, 13.0; oil, 10.2; fruits, 6.6(Fig. 4). The decreasing ratio in the age adjusted death rates for gastric cancer in 12 districts in Japan was noted to be correlated closely with fat and vitamin A intake. The decreasing ratio showed high association with amount of intake of vitamin A and dietary fat.(Fig. 5)

Fig. 4

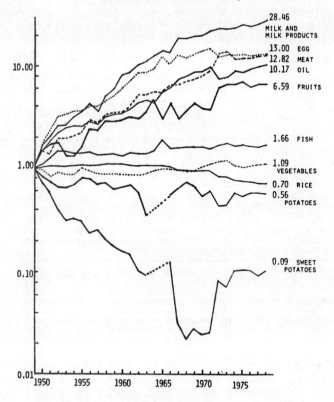

CHANGE IN AMOUNT OF INTAKE OF SELECTED FOOD IN JAPAN 1949-1978

(RATIO TO AMOUNT OF INTAKE IN 1949)

Fig. 5

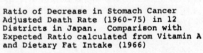

Ratio of Decrease in Stomach Cancer
Adjusted Death Rate (1960-75) in 12
Districts in Japan. Comparison with
Expected Ratio calculated from Vitamin A
and Dietary Fat Intake (1966)

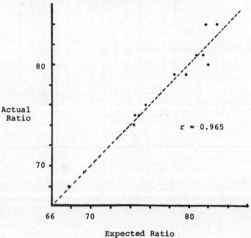

T. Hirayama

This is in line with the results of our ongoing prospective studies
(1966-78), for 265,118 adults aged 40 years and above, 95% of 1965
census population, in 29 Health Center Districts in Japan on risk
factors of gastric cancer. The results clearly showed a significant inverse trend with the frequency of green-yellow vegetables
intake both in males and females.(Fig. 6)

Fig. 6

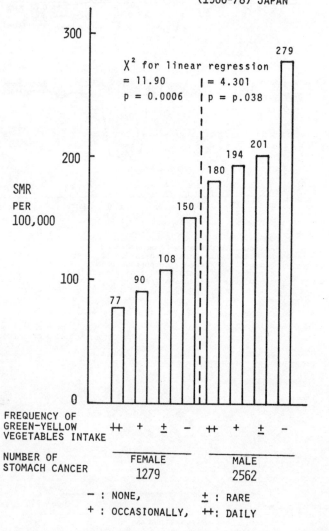

STANDARDIZED MORTALITY RATE
FOR STOMACH CANCER BY SEX AND
BY FREQUENCY OF GREEN-YELLOW VEGETABLES INTAKE
PROSPECTIVE STUDY
(1966-78) JAPAN

X^2 for linear regression
= 11.90 | = 4.301
p = 0.0006 | p = p.038

SMR
PER
100,000

300

279

201
194
200   180
             150
108
90
77
100

0

FREQUENCY OF
GREEN-YELLOW   ++ + ± - ++ + ± -
VEGETABLES INTAKE

NUMBER OF   FEMALE   MALE
STOMACH CANCER   1279   2562

- : NONE,   ± : RARE
+ : OCCASIONALLY, ++: DAILY

8) Influence of cigarette smoking:

The relative risk of stomach cancer in daily smokers compared to non-smokers was 1.47 in males and 1.25 in females. Although this was much lower than the risk of lung cancer(4.13 in males and 2.10 in females), the absolute magnitude of excess deaths per 100,000 among daily cigarette smokers for gastric cancer was similar to that for lung cancer, 64.2 and 64.8 in males and 19.6 and 17.4 in females respectively. The attributable risk percent related to daily cigarette smoking was 26.3% for gastric cancer, whereas it was 69.4% for lung cancer in males. It is noteworthy that the influence of age at start of smoking is more striking than daily amount of smoking in case of gastric cancer. Daily cigarette smoking is thus important as one of the risk factors for gastric cancer and of particular significance in explaining the reason for the consistent preponderance of males in the mumber of reported gastric cancer cases. The relative risk is similar to those found in prospective studies reported in the literature: 1.45 in seven studies (USDHEW 1964). That daily cigarette smoking is a risk factor in gastric cancer is also significant in that it provides human evidence that the intake of selected extrinsic chemical carcinogens, initiator and/or promoter, can surely increase the risk of gastric cancer, and an intensive search must be undertaken for such carcinogens in our daily environment of life-style, particularly in our food. Thus if people were to stop smoking cigarettes, the risk for gastric cancer would surely go down further, and the slope of the decline in Japan would become even steeper. The much lower decreasing ratio of the mortality rate for cancer of the cardia of the stomach can be explained by the fact that the promoting effect of cigarette smoking is strongest for cancer of the cardia, the relative risk being 1.86 in cardia and 1.23 in pylorus. The dose-response relationship is clearer in former. However, neither the inter-country variation nor the decreasing trend in the gastric cancer death rate in general appears to be explained by the smoking factor. The difference or change in dietary pattern must be far more important in explaining such geographic variation and the overall downward trend in gastric cancer mortality.

9) Interaction of smoking and diet:

The risk lowering effect of green-yellow vegetable intake was observed both in daily cigarette smokers and in non smokers.(Fig. 7) The extent of risk elevation due to cigarette smoking is much more striking in males than in females reflecting a higher amount of smoking and earlier age at start of smoking in males. However, the risk lowering effect by green-yellow vegetables intake was observed in an almost similar extent in males and females. Since 50-60% of the vitamin A intake of Japanese is derived from daily intake of green-yellow vegetables, these results probably indicate, 'promoter inhibiter' effect of vitamin A.

10) Suggested preventive measures:

Cessation of cigarette smoking and improvement of diet must be key elements of gastric cancer prevention. Frequent intake of highly salted food, such as salted pickles and fishes, should be avoided.

Fig. 7

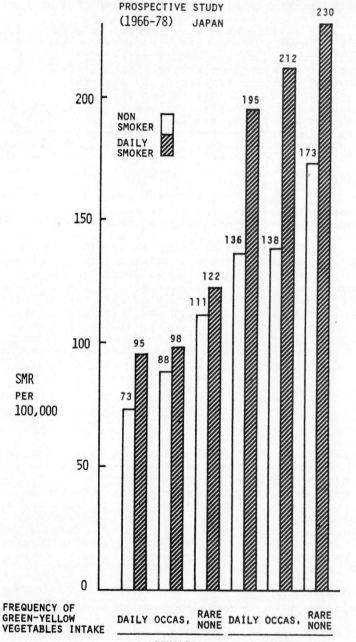

STANDARDIZED MORTALITY RATE
FOR STOMACH CANCER BY SEX, BY SMOKING HABIT
AND BY FREQUENCY OF GREEN-YELLOW VEGETABLES INTAKE

Increased intake of green-yellow vegetables and dairy products should
be encouraged as these are the sources of vitamin A. Frequent
intake of vegetables and fruits is also recommended as it provides
vitamin C. As these measures are quite simple and carry no risk,
an intensive health education should be concentrated toward the
direction.

REFERENCES

Hirayama, T. (1963). Bul. Inst. Public Health, 12, 85.
Hirayama, T. (1968). Gann Monogr., 3, 15-27.
Hirayama, T. (1971). Gann Monogr., 11, 3-19.
Hirayama, T. (1975). Proc. XI Int. Cancer Congress., American
   Elsevier.
Hirayama, T. (1975). Cancer Res., 35, 3460-3463.
Hirayama, T. (1979). Gastric Cancer, C.J. Pfeiffer, Gerhard Wizst-
   rock Publishing House, Inc., New York.

DISCUSSION

G. Slaney. As the incidence of stomach cancer is coming down, it looks as though the incidence of carcinoma of the colon and rectum is going up. Do those things in the diet which you have identified correlate with the increasing incidence of colo-rectal cancer? In other words, if you change the diet to protect the stomach, are we just pushing the incidence of the cancer lower down the gut?

T. Hirayama. The first candidate I thought of was meat intake and to my surprise a very large intake of meat reduced the risk of colon cancer. A significantly lower rate of colon cancer was observed in people who had a daily intake of meat. So meat is the one thing which, at least as far as Japan is concerned, is considered to be lower down the list of significant factors in carcinoma of the colon and carcinoma of the stomach. Probably vegetables, fibre rich foods, could reduce the frequency of colon cancer and the same diet could be beneficial in gastric cancer, for different reasons. Perhaps because of vitamins A and C. I think we know some common foods which reduce the incidence of both diseases and this is one of the specific targets of our research. We already know that excess fat intake increases the risk of breast and pancreatic cancer. We are trying to avoid eating excess fat and we would like to report the results of this in the future.

W. Longmire. Your incidence is decreasing more rapidly than mortality in stomach cancer. Can you infer from this that the virulence of the disease may be decreasing?

T. Hirayama. Well, I once thought that but the most recent data which I showed today from the Osaka Cancer Registry showed that the mortality rate is coming down and is slightly steeper than the incidence rate. I think that the incidence rate decline is definitely influenced by the diet. That is my conviction, but in addition, there might be some effect of better detection which we will discuss this afternoon. So, in my opinion, the mortality decline is a combination of dietary improvement and better detection.

W. Longmire. Pursuing the salt factor first. What is it in the salt that seems to provoke cancer?

T. Hirayama. There are a lot of hypotheses but I think osmotic pressure itself could explain certain effects. If you keep taking such highly salted food, gastric juice must be secreted and this can lead to chronic gastritis. Some people consider that hypersecretion of gastric juice could be the start of this whole story. This is one explanation. But as you said, some specific chemical components connected with salt intake might also be involved. This is still a hypothesis.

E. Deutch. It has been indicated that the drop in U.S. regional gastric cancer is due to the presence of anti-oxidants in our breakfast cereals. Can you make some comment? Have you any experience in breakfast cereals particularly those commercial brands that have or do not have anti-oxidants in them?

T. Hirayama. I am interested in the hypothesis but I have no special comment.

V. Brookes. You mentioned the difference between male and female incidences, we found, in our studies, that the operability rates and the survival rates in similar cases in women were much better than in men, as if women are particularly favoured in this disease. Did you find the same effect?

T. Hirayama. I have no specific answer to your question.

C. Walters. Is it usual for the salt to contain nitrate?

T. Hirayama. Yes, I think so.

E. Deutch. You do not sound as though you think it is a very important question.
Do you think it is?

T. Hirayama. I think Professor Crespi will answer this question.

M. Crespi. You show the very interesting fact that refrigerators are associated
with the decline in stomach cancer. Do you have a plot of any figures about car
ownership, plastic containers and stomach cancer because it could be that
refrigeration has something to do with the decrease of stomach cancer but it could
also be that it reflects a rise in the socio-economic ladder?

T. Hirayama. I am thankful that you did not mention television. We do not trust
this kind of correlation study only. We must have evidence for individual risk
for individual follow-up. This is just in addition to the individual risk of the
patient. Nothing else.

Regional Variations and Established Prognostic Factors in Gastric Cancer

J.A.H. Waterhouse

University of Birmingham, Queen Elizabeth Medical Centre,
Birmingham B15 2TH, U.K.

ABSTRACT

Stomach cancer shows wide variations in incidence around the world, and certain
areas, such as Japan, South America, and Eastern Europe, show very high rates.
On a smaller scale there is also variation within the country, instanced by
England and Wales, and changes over time periods. Almost everywhere the
incidence rate is diminishing.

Survival rates in general are poor, except for very early cases. Prognosis
is examined in relation to duration of symptoms, histology, spread and disease,
and localisation of the growth within the stomach.

KEYWORDS

Epidemiology, Incidence, Prognosis, Gastric cancer; regional variation.

INTRODUCTION

A discussion of regional variations in stomach cancer is of relevance in the
context of this Symposium only in so far as it may provide some pointers to the
elucidation, either of the aetiology of the disease, or of its treatment, and
of its subsequent survival patterns. If it cannot suggest the formulation of
hypotheses, together with methods of investigating and testing them, then it
is of no more than anecdotal value, as describing a situation of apparently
fortuitous occurrence. When differences exist, however, and when they are
often large in size, it is not difficult to propose explanations which may be
tenable, though there is no certainty that they may be correct. It is then
in devising appropriate ways of testing their feasibility that interest
becomes focused , as well as in the usefulness of the relationship to reduce
the incidence of the disease or to improve its survival.

REGIONAL VARIATIONS

Where should we look for such information in the case of stomach cancer? In
many parts of the world today, new cases of the disease are reported to cancer
registries. If those registries belong to the variety known as "population-

17

based", and their registration efficiency is high - of the order of 90% or more -
they can provide reliable data on the incidence of the disease in the population
they monitor. Few - if any - registries can justifiably claim 100% efficiency of
registration, but many can legitimately claim more than 90% and, moreover, can
substantiate that claim. The majority of such registries contribute their data
to the successive quinquennial volumes of the book *Cancer Incidence in Five
Continents*, from the third volume of which Fig. 1 is taken. It shows the
distribution around the world of the registries which are included in the volume:
a distribution which is by no means as widespread as would be desirable but which,
nevertheless, does include some representation from each of the continents.

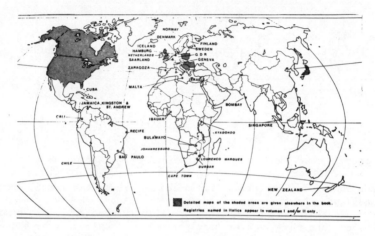

Figure 1

Figure 2, based on an earlier volume, indicates the relative incidence of stomach
cancer as determined by cancer registries, and as adjusted for the very different
age characteristics of the base populations. It shows the very high incidence
in Japan, South America, Iceland and Eastern Europe. It is misleading and over-
ambitious however in suggesting by its shading that the situation is equally wellknown for the whole of Australia, including New Zealand and Tasmania, or that the
whole of the USA is divided into two zones by a curiously straight diagonal line.
Not withstanding that, my purpose in showing this map is adequately served by two
outstanding features: first, the wide variation in incidence across the world;
and secondly, the location of the high-spots, which continue to hold their positions.
It is clear therefore that regional variations exist on a world scale, in ratios
exceeding thirty times. Can we find variations in a more confined area, where the
extremes of possible differences out of which to generate explanatory hypotheses are
less widely separated?

For stomach cancer, the pattern of survival in general is, outside Japan, unhappily
rather poor. In these circumstances, the use of mortality experience, rather than
that of morbidity, will convey very much the same picture. I draw my next
example therefore from the mortality data for England and Wales. First I show
the mortality from all causes, for males, Fig. 3, as a basis of comparison. There
is relatively little variation in the SMR - the standardised mortality ratio -
over the country: the highest rates are found in Liverpool and South Wales, and
the lowest in the Isle of Ely. Figure 4 shows the incidence of stomach cancer
mortality for males, displaying a much wider range of variation. The standardised
mortality ratio (SMR) is constructed in such a way as to compensate for the
changes in age distribution and to represent, by the figure 100, the rate for the
whole country. An SMR of less than 60, at the lower end of the range, is

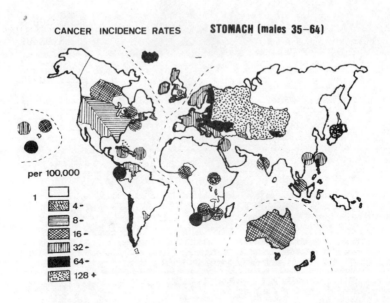

Figure 2

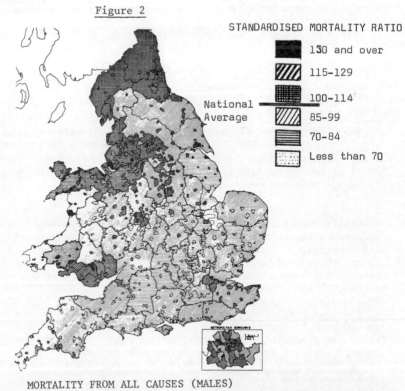

MORTALITY FROM ALL CAUSES (MALES)

Figure 3

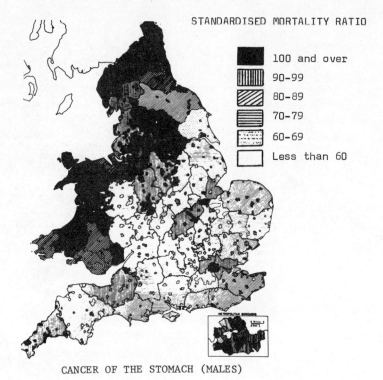

CANCER OF THE STOMACH (MALES)

Figure 4

therefore about half the average rate for the country, and at the upper end, the
SMR of 160 and over is more than one-and-a-half times the average rate. These
high rates are found predominantly in North Wales, but also in Stoke-on-Trent.
Turning to female rates, Fig. 5 depicts the mortality from all causes, showing
slightly more variation than for males, with the highest rates in the North and
West. Figure 6 shows the impact of stomach cancer for females, again with a wide
range of variation, and concentrated in Wales and in the North-East, but again in
Stoke-on-Trent and some other parts of Staffordshire.

I have taken these illustrations from Melvyn Howe's National Atlas of Disease
Mortality in the United Kingdom. They have been drawn to show the pattern of
disease in the various local government areas of this country for which figures
were available. They did not indicate the sizes of the base populations of those
areas, which would give a measure of the reliability of the findings. Medical
geographers have adopted various devices for this purpose, which inevitably
carry with them unfamiliar patterns of representation. Figure 7 shows Professor
Howe's style for depicting the mortality among males from all causes. The size
of the square or diamond relates to the population, in accordance with the key
at the base; squares refer to urban areas and diamonds to rural; and the shading
shows the gradations of the SMR, according to the scale at the top right. The
overall range is smaller than in the previous map for all causes, and so it is
for stomach cancer in the map (Fig. 8) compared with its predecessor. There is
similar grouping of high spots, however, in the North-West and South Wales, and
again in Stoke-on-Trent. Next are the corresponding maps for females: first
(Fig 9) for all causes showing a range of about 10% above or below the average SMR
of 100; and secondly for stomach cancer (Fig. 10), ranging about 30% either side

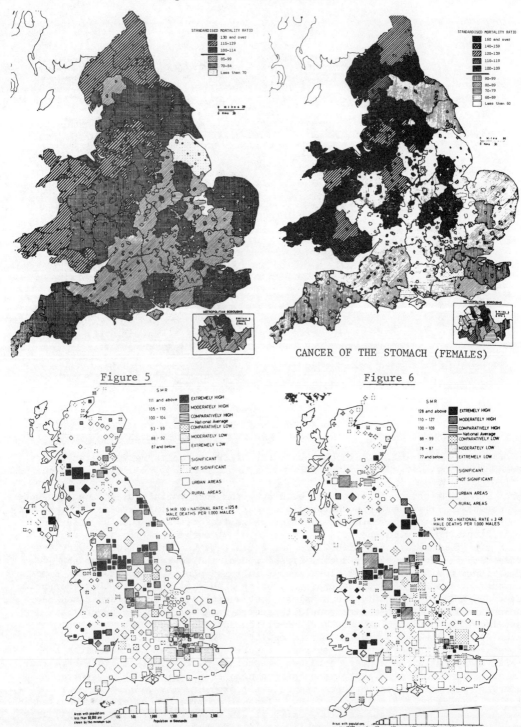

Figure 5

Figure 6

CANCER OF THE STOMACH (FEMALES)

MORTALITY FROM ALL CAUSES (MALES)

Figure 7

Figure 8

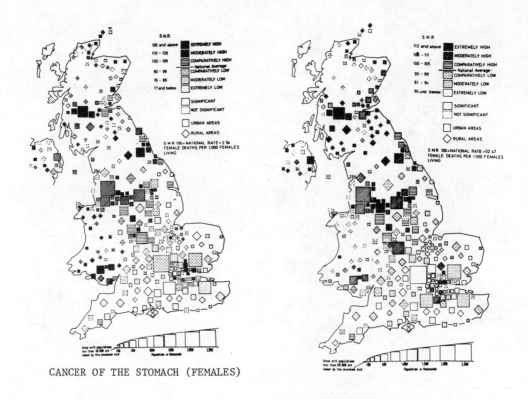

CANCER OF THE STOMACH (FEMALES)

Figure 9   Figure 10

of the average of 100. Again, however, the distribution is very similar to its predecessor.

What are the kinds of inference to be drawn from such variations in the incidence of disease? It is unlikely that aetiologically active agents are to be found only in the geographical differences, whether of soil or climate, though it is true that Stocks and Davies showed a higher rate of stomach cancer in soils with a high zinc content or high zinc to copper ratio. We know that high stomach cancer rates are found among lower social class groups, and we know also that the distribution of lower social class groups in this country is in many ways similar to that of the high SMRs, the frequency being higher in the North-West, North-East and Wales, especially South Wales. But social class grades are based on occupational groupings and we should therefore look for specific occupations showing a relationship to gastric cancer. In addition to direct, we should consider the indirect, involuntary or unwitting ingestion of atmospheric constituents, whether gaseous, vaporous or particulate. We have ourselves been able to demonstrate a higher incidence of stomach cancer in factories where there is exposure to oil mist. Hirayama has shown an association with cigarette smoking. An occupation in which the relevant exposure may well be to particulate matter is that of coal-mining. Some colleagues of mine are at present engaged in a study of the high rates in Stoke-on-Trent, in this region, where there is a good deal of coal-mining, and where there is also the centre of the British pottery industry - another source of several atmospheric pollutants. Whatever their eventual findings, however, such studies form the natural and essential follow-up to the demonstration of the existence of regional or other variations of incidence, in order to discover the identity of the agent ultimately responsible.

PROGNOSTIC FACTORS

From a brief exploration of the use of variations in the impact of the disease to seek aetiological factors, let me turn now to another area of the epidemiological study of associated factors, this time in relation to prognosis.

What is the pattern of survival of patients with gastric cancer? Figure 11 shows the percentage, by sex, remaining alive up to 15 years from diagnosis.

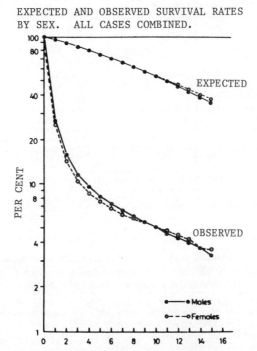

EXPECTED AND OBSERVED SURVIVAL RATES
BY SEX.   ALL CASES COMBINED.

Figure 11

It shows also, for the same period of time, the percentage, by sex, "expected" to survive. These latter curves are taken from the national Life Tables, for a group made up in the same way by age, for each sex, as those with gastric cancer, but exposed only to the mortality risks of the general population. Towards the end of the fifteen year period the two sets of curves are very nearly parallel. Since the vertical scale is a logarithmic one, this means that they are dying at about the same rate, which can be taken to imply that after about ten to a dozen years of survival the mortality risk for the survivors is no different from others in the population who are of the same age and sex. This figure is from the Cancer Registry of Norway and is based on more than 20,000 cases. Figure 12 is a later group of patients, also from Norway, for whom it is only possible to show survival up to five years. As in the former graph, the behaviour of the two sexes

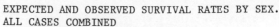

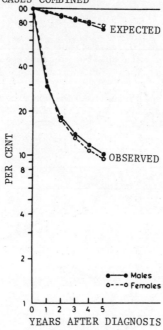

EXPECTED AND OBSERVED SURVIVAL RATES BY SEX.
ALL CASES COMBINED

Figure 12

is closely similar. The curves, shown as "expected" and "observed", are not yet parallel in slope, however, so that the cancer patients are still at a disadvantage compared with their contemporaries in the general population.

It is possible to make use of standard Life Tables in a similar way in order to adjust, or compensate, for the sometimes rather haphazard effect that the age composition of a group of patients can exert. Since the so-called natural mortality increases so sharply with age, it is useful to have an accepted technique which can make allowance for its distortions, and thereby provide an adjusted or "corrected" survival rate - sometimes also called a "relative" survival rate. Figure 13 shows the effect of such corrections on 5-year survival rates by age. These are from local figures and show some irregularity: the increased effect of the correction at older ages is clearly apparent, though it does not quite, in the radically treated group, amount to a flat rate of age-adjusted survival.

Has survival improved with the passage of time? Figure 14 shows the experience of Norway for three successive periods of time. Though the curves are close together, they do show a consistent improvement in the males, which is not quite so clear in the females. More recent Norwegian experience is shown in Fig. 15 where both sexes show slight but consistent improvement. By selecting out just the five-year survival rates, corrected to avoid the distorting effects of changes in age distributions, we can see (Fig. 16) a clearer picture, for Norway, of improving rates in the male, but rather less marked in the female.

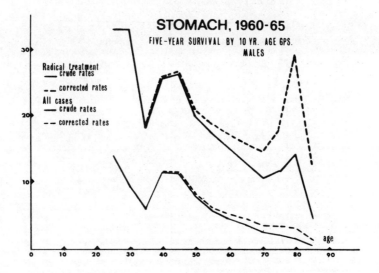

Figure 13

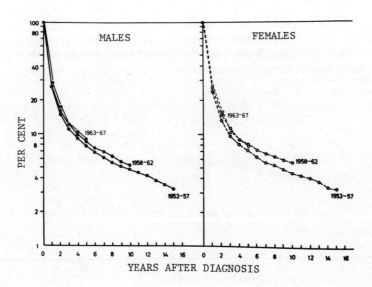

Figure 14

J. A. H. Waterhouse

OBSERVED SURVIVAL RATES BY PERIOD OF DIAGNOSIS

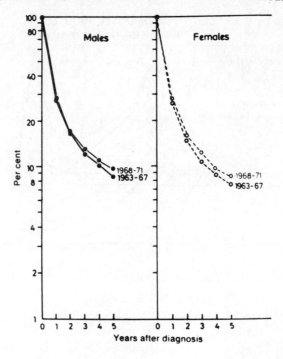

Figure 15

Five-year relative survival rates by sex and period of diagnosis. All cases combined.

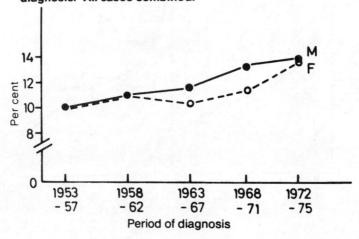

Figure 16

We have looked at our local figures by ten-year age groups, in successive periods
of time, to see if there has been an improvement (Fig. 17). Our numbers are
rather small when broken down in this way, but there seems to be some evidence
for it, even if not entirely consistent.

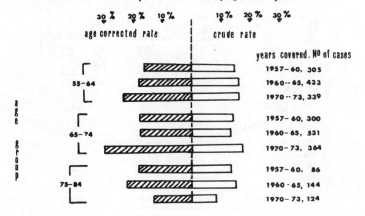

Figure 17

From American data we can compare the survival of patients by race and period of
diagnosis. In Fig. 18 are the relative (age-adjusted) survival curves for Whites,
for five successive periods.

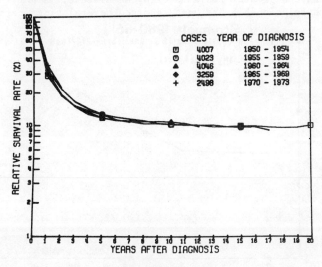

Figure 18

J. A. H. Waterhouse

The curves clearly are so close together that they effectively overlie each other.
Figure 19 shows survival for Blacks, which is much more variable, but does show
clear improvement except for the second period.

BLACK PATIENTS

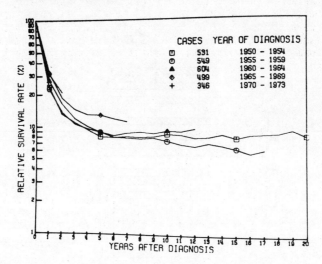

Figure 19

Turning now to features more directly related to the disease itself and its
manifestation in the patient, we have in Fig. 20 the relationship, for radically
treated cases, of 5-year survival rate to the duration of symptoms. Whether the
explanation is that a slow-growing tumour is more amenable to treatment, or that
some patients have a greater resistance to the disease, is not known, although
the fact of the relationship has been reported several times before.

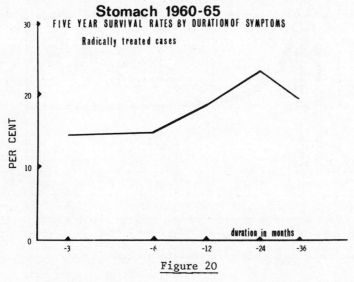

Figure 20

Histology certainly has an important bearing on survival, but about 70% of all
stomach tumours are adenocarcinomas with a five-year survival rate of 10%. Mucoid
carcinomas have very much the same survival rate while anaplastic have rather less
(7%). Malignant lymphomas, thought they may closely simulate carcinomas, have
a survival rate (18%) nearly twice that of the adenocarcinomas.

Survival in relation to the spread of the disease at the time of diagnosis shows
very much what might be expected. In Fig. 21 are some graphs for three age-groups,
for patients with tumours that were localised, or showed regional spread, or had
distant metastases. Except for the oldest age group (75+) where the local and
regional are close together, the three stages of disease are well separated in their
survival pattern.

OBSERVED SURVIVAL RATES BY SEX, AGE AND STAGE

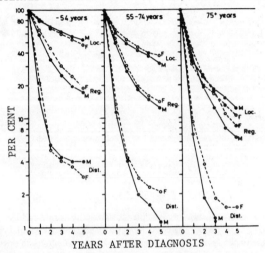

YEARS AFTER DIAGNOSIS

Figure 21

We have recently examined (Fielding et al., 1980) our own records of more than
13,000 cases of gastric cancer seen in the ten year period 1960-69 for examples
of "early" cases. Defining such cases as limited to invasion only of the submucosa of the stomach, we found 90 cases (0.7%). Their crude five-year survival
rate was 57.8%, which when age-adjusted became 70.4% - almost comparable to the
high rates now achieved in Japan for early cases. Less than one in five had lost
weight, but nearly all had had symptoms referable to the gastrointestinal tract.
A substantial improvement in prognosis would thus result from earlier detection
of the disease.

Figure 22 shows the influence on survival of the site of the primary growth within the stomach. The percentage figures for each site are the five-year survival
rates for all forms of treatment, while that for radical treatment is given in
parentheses. The commonest site is the pyloric antrum followed by the lesser
curvature; these two sites have similar rates, but the next in order of frequency,
the body, has the worst prognosis. The redically treated cases shown in this
diagram formed about three-quarters of all radically treated cases. The remainder
(24%) lacking detailed site of primary, had a very similar survival. Of the other
group, however, those with site detail amounted to only 43%, and the poor survival
of the remaining 57% reduced the figure to about half its size. These figures

MALIGNANT TUMOURS OF THE STOMACH 1960-1965

FIVE YEAR SURVIVAL RATES BY SITE OF PRIMARY
(Rates for radically treated cases in parentheses)

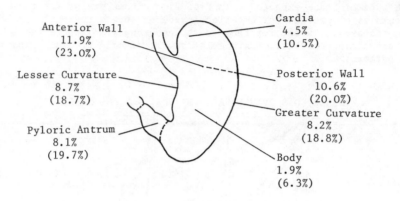

Anterior Wall
11.9%
(23.0%)

Cardia
4.5%
(10.5%)

Lesser Curvature
8.7%
(18.7%)

Posterior Wall
10.6%
(20.0%)

Greater Curvature
8.2%
(18.8%)

Pyloric Antrum
8.1%
(19.7%)

Body
1.9%
(6.3%)

Based on:

3,459 cases with site detail - all treatments
1,277 cases with site detail - radically treated

Figure 22

serve only to reflect of course the fact that, of the radically treated cases those
lacking site detail had either failed to include that information where notified
to the Registry or were more extensive and not limited to a single subsite. In
the other group there would be a much larger fraction who received no surgery, nor
were endoscoped or autopsied - a group whose prognosis would naturally be much
worse and for whom no data on site of origin would be available.

In this review of factors influencing prognosis it has only been possible to show
their separate effects rather than to present them in combination. When our own
more detailed data become available for analysis, we hope to be able to
investigate inter-relationships between a greater number of potential indices, and
thence to provide a better guide to the estimation of prognosis.

REFERENCES

Cancer Incidence in Five Continents
          Vol. 1 (1966) Ed: Doll, R., Payne, P., and Waterhouse, J.
          Springer-Verlag, Berlin.

          Vol. 2 (1970) Ed: Doll, R., Muir, C., and Waterhouse, J.
          Springer-Verlag, Berlin.

          Vol. 3 (1976) Ed: Waterhouse, J., Muir, C., Correa, P., and Powell, J.
          IARC, Lyon

National Atlas of Disease Mortality in the United Kingdom
          G. Melvyn Howe (1970) Nelson, London.

Survival of Cancer Patients: Cases diagnosed 1953-67.
          The Cancer Registry of Norway (1975): Oslo.

Survival of Cancer Patients: Cases diagnosed 1968-75.
          The Cancer Registry of Norway (1980): Oslo.

Cancer Patient Survival: Report No. 5 (1976)
          Ed: Axtell, L.M., Asire, A.J., and Myers, M.H.
          U.S. Dept., of Health, Education and Welfare, Bethesda, Maryland.

Waterhouse, J.A.H.: Cutting Oils and Cancer.
          Ann. Occup. Hyg., 14, 161;170, (1971)

Fielding, J.W.L., Ellis, D.J., Jones, B.G., Paterson, J., Powell, D.J., Waterhouse,
J.A.H., and Brookes, V.S.: Natural history of "early" gastric cancer: results
of a 10-year regional survey.
          Brit. med. J., 281, 965-966, (1980)

Stocks, P., and Davies, R.I., Zinc and copper content of soils associated with the
incidence of cancer of the stomach and other organs.
          Brit. J. Cancer, 18, 14-24, (1964)

DISCUSSION

<u>P. Wrigley</u>. In view of the multi-racial nature of our society have you any pointers as to the incidence of carcinoma of the stomach in the different populations and their outlook?

<u>J. Waterhouse.</u> Well, I wish I had. Unhappily not. We have virtually no information on racial origin. The question that we ask is place of birth because that is the question that relates to the census and then we can get our base populations for rates and so on. It is not always filled in. Sometimes you get race put in, West Indian or Pakistani but not regularly. I think this is a very important matter to consider especially, as you say, in areas like this where there are quite a number of immigrants. It would be very useful to be able to see in what way the rates are different and in what way the prognosis may be different. But I am sorry to say that we have remarkably little information.

<u>S. Glick</u>. You noticed an increased incidence in the Midlands, for example, at Stoke-on-Trent. Is it related to stability of populations or is it related to the environment?

<u>J. Waterhouse</u>. I do not know how to answer that because in terms of stability of population the higher rate in Stoke-on-Trent has been present for 20-30 years at least both in incidence and in mortality. We hope that the present investigation that is underway there will help to indicate the factors that people living in Stoke-on-Trent are exposed to which may enhance the stomach cancer rate. Among those I did mention are coal-mining and the pottery industry which are the obvious things to look for, particularly when coal-mining is known to be associated with a higher incidence.

<u>J. Elder</u>. Do you have any information on alcohol consumption and regional variation? Certainly in the West of Scotland where the incidences are similar to North and South Wales, there is a very high incidence of consumption of spirits. I wonder if your figures here confirm or refute that?

<u>J. Waterhouse</u>. I do not have any figures on alcohol consumption that I can relate in quite the same way. In fact I am not sure where I would look for them, other that to do a special study. I do not know whether there are sales figures on these. I would imagine that in Scotland it relates more to spirits than to beer.

<u>T. Hirayama</u>. The title of your paper is 'Regional Variation and Established Prognostic Factors'. I would like to ask you what is established and what is not extablished?

<u>J. Waterhouse</u>. I wish I could answer that precisely. I don't think I can give a useful answer to that.

<u>J. Alexander-Williams</u>. This is a serious answer to Mr. Elder's question, suggesting that it might be possible to see if you could relate it to convictions for drunkeness because there must be some good statistics for that and they must be very high in the West of Scotland.

<u>V. Brookes</u>. Is the incidence of carcinoma of the stomach related to convictions for drunkeness, rather than alcoholism?

<u>J. Waterhouse</u>. Well again, I suppose one gets such information from either the police or the local County Courts and one would have to go back into the records for quite a long time. There are some countries, Scandinavian countries eg. Finland, where they keep a register of alcoholics and where there is a fairly good definition, and this would be perhaps a richer field to look at. The other is, of course, Dr. Hirayama's own prospective study, where he has got alcohol

consumption data over a long period of time.

R. Pichlmayr. You did show some improvement of the survival rates in the follow-up periods. As a surgeon one would be happy to think that this was a consequence of surgery - better surgery - but I think it might be more a consequence of the earlier detection of gastric cancer. Do you have any figures on the proportion of early gastric cancers in this period?

J. Waterhouse. The simple answer to that is no. We do know from a study made by Mr. Fielding, who has looked into very early cancer in this region, that there are remarkably few that are really caught in the earliest stages. I think under 1% was his own finding. I agree it would be an interesting study to undertake to try and distinguish the effects of early detection from improvements in therapy.

R. Pichlmayr. Do you think that this proportion may alter the survival rates at this moment?

J. Waterhouse. I mentioned the small proportion because if it is of the order of 1% even if it does improve, it will still make little impact on the survival until it gets to 5 - 10%

C. Veys. Stoke-on-Trent is the black spot. I would like to ask one question and to make a further comment. Are there any other high spots in the Birmingham region apart from that country borough which you showed so clearly on the maps? Secondly, we do have one or two early results in the Stoke-on-Trent study, which from looking at the regression curves show that there is not the same fall for Stoke-on-Trent when compared with the national figures, nor for Stoke-on-Trent versus Stoke-on-Trent over the last 15 years, as we might have expected if we were continuing national trends. Something is keeping the Stoke-on-Trent rate very high. Our study is not finished and we are particularly looking at the occupational hazards, coal mining, the leather industry, the pottery industry, the iron and steel industry. In the case of the field study over three years about 200 matched sets on a 4:1 basis are now under analysis.

J. Waterhouse. We are looking forward to the results of this study. It is true from other data, I did not make it clear from these maps, that the decline in the Stoke-on-Trent rate of stomach cancer has been much less than in the general population, so clearly there are factors which are delaying the fall. You asked whether there were any other similar places in this region, well West Bromwich is one of them. I think it has another name now, Sandwell, and that is a high incidence area but it has declined more in keeping with the general population than has Stoke-on-Trent.

V. Brookes. In fact when we talk of black spots, the urban areas were greater than the expected incidence level and the rural areas less than the expected level.

J. Waterhouse. That is perfectly true. There must be some urban factor.

Nitrates and Bacteriology. Are these Important Etiological Factors in Gastric Carcinogenesis?

M. Hill

Bacterial Metabolism Research Laboratory,
Central Public Health Laboratory, Colindale Avenue,
London NW9, U.K.

ABSTRACT

Because N-nitroso compounds are such potent carcinogens in animals their role in
human carcinogenesis has been the cause of much speculation. They are formed from
nitrite and a suitable nitrogen compound either at acid pH or, in the presence of
suitable bacteria, at more neutral pH values. Since most nitrite in the body is
derived from dietary nitrate there is a possible double role for bacteria - the
production of nitrite substrate and the catalysis of N-nitrosation reaction. The
pharmacology of nitrate and nitrite are described and the conditions under which
N-nitroso compounds are formed in vivo are described.

My conclusion is that bacteria and nitrite are important etiological agents in
gastric carcinogenesis only in persons who have already developed the precurser
lesion of atrophic gastritis.

KEYWORDS

Gastric cancer; bacteria; nitrite; N-nitroso compounds.

INTRODUCTION

The stomach is the first resting place for all ingested carcinogens and so it is
almost certain that gastric cancer has a multifactorial etiology. Under different
circumstances different agents will be of major importance in the causation of
gastric malignancy. Thus in studies of an etiological agent we must first decide
whether the agent can cause gastric cancer under any circumstances and, if so, we
must then determine the circumstances under which the agent will be of importance.

Nitrites and bacteriology are potentially of importance in human carcinogenesis
because they are two of the reactants in the formation of N-nitroso compounds. I
will first briefly review N-nitroso compounds as carcinogens. I will then discuss
the circumstances favouring the formation of N-nitroso compounds in the body.
Finally, I will present the data indicating that bacteria and nitrite might be
etiological factors in gastric carcinogenesis and discuss the circumstances in
which they might be important etiological factors.

N-NITROSO COMPOUNDS AS CARCINOGENS

The chemistry of N-nitroso compounds has been reviewed by Magee and Barnes (1967) and by Magee (1977). They are formed by the action of nitrite on a suitable nitrogen compound; secondary amines give N-nitrosamines, amides give N-nitrosamides ureas give N-nitrosoureas etc. The N-nitrosation is catalysed at acid pH and by a range of anions; it can also proceed at more neutral pH values in the presence of bacteria. The N-nitroso compounds are probably the most widely studied family of carcinogens and their carcinogenicity has been reviewed by Magee and Barnes (1967). Most N-nitrosamines are organotropic carcinogens, the target organs in the rat including the bladder (dibutylnitrosamine), the kidney (dimethylnitrosamine), the liver (diethylnitrosamine), the lung (N-nitrosomorpholine) and the oesophagus (N-nitrosopiperidine). The target organ may vary between test animals as well as between N-nitrosamines; for example, N-nitrosomorpholine gives lung tumours in the rat but oesophageal carcinomas in the hamster. Since the target organ of a given N-nitrosamine varies from rodent to rodent, no deduction can be made from animal studies concerning the target organ of any N-nitrosamine in the human. Nevertheless all animal species tested are susceptible to N-nitrosamine carcinogenesis and there are no grounds for believing that humans are uniquely resistant.

In contrast to N-nitrosamines, N-nitrosamides and N-nitrosoureas are direct acting carcinogens giving tumours at the site of application. These direct acting carcinogens are also direct acting mutagens, whereas the N-nitrosamines are not mutagenic until they have been activated (usually in the laboratory by using rat liver microsomal enzymes). The characteristics of these various classes of N-nitroso compunds are summarised in Table 1.

TABLE 1   Characteristics of Various Groups of N-nitroso
Compounds

	N-nitrosamines	N-nitrosamides	N-nitrosoureas
Site of action	Organotropic; target organ depends on the species of animal and on the alkyl substituents on the molecule	Local at site of application	Local at site of application
Mutagenicity	Requires microsomal activation	Direct acting	Direct acting
pH optimum of formation	2	3	2
Alkali sensitivity	No	Destroyed by alkali	Destroyed by alkali

The N-nitrosation reaction is acid catalysed, the pH optimum varying from 1.5 to

3 depending on the nature of the nitrogen compound being nitrosated. The reaction is also catalysed by a range of anions and these can affect the pH optimum of the reaction. The acid-catalysed nitrosation reaction has been reviewed excellently by Mirvish (1972). In the human body the only site at which the acid-catalysed reaction could occur is the stomach, and the formation of N-nitroso compounds in the normal acidified human stomach has been demonstrated in vivo (Sander et al, 1968; Fine et al, 1977).

In addition to the above mechanism, the N-nitrosation reaction can also be catalysed at more neutral pH values by the presence of bacteria. The nature of the catalysis has to be determined but it is unlikely to be enzymic. This is of interest because there are many more sites in the body favourable to bacterially catalysed N-nitrosation than there are sites favouring the acid-catalysed reaction. In addition, many of the bacteria which catalyse the reaction also produce nitrite from nitrate; the importance of this will be described later.

In order to assess the chance of bacterially catalysed N-nitrosation occurring in the body, we need to determine the pharmacology of nitrite and the distribution of bacteria in the body. From this data we can deduce the sites at which N-nitrosation could take place by this mechanism.

THE PHARMACOLOGY OF NITRITE

Nitrite either enters the body preformed as part of the diet or is formed from nitrate by bacterial action; the latter is by far the most important source. Nitrite is a food additive which is used to inhibit the growth and toxin produced by Clostridium botulinum in hams, cured meats, continental sausage etc. It is also used for cosmetic reasons - it makes bacon and ham an attractive pink colour. There are limits on the amount of nitrite to which food stuffs can be exposed; further, nitrite is a highly reactive anion which reacts with many components of the food to which it is added. Consequently, the amount of nitrite detectable in food is much less than the amount added and, for this reason, the amount of nitrite in the diet is relatively small when compared with the amount of nitrate (White, 1975). Unlike nitrite, nitrate is a normal component of vegetables and is present in large amounts in, for example, salad components, spinach, kale etc. Since it is present in sea salt it is also present in salted foods; it is also added to cured meat products as a source of nitrite. It has been suggested that nitrite might be endogenously synthesised in the lower small intestine (Tannenbaum et al, 1978) and many groups (including my laboratory) have found that persons consuming a virtually nitrate-free diet excrete nitrate in the urine (Tannenbaum et al, 1978; Bartholomew et al, 1980). However, the reports that ileostomy fluid contains large amounts of nitrite (Tannenbaum et al, 1978) have not been confirmed (Bartholomew et al, 1980) and I believe that endogenous synthesis has still to be confirmed. For the purposes of this communication it will be assumed that all nitrite is of dietary origin and is ingested as either nitrite or nitrate.

The pharmacology of dietary nitrate has been summarised recently (Tannenbaum et al, 1977; Hill, 1980a). A small but undetermined proportion of the nitrate is reduced by bacteria to nitrite during the first passage through the mouth before passing to the stomach and then the small intestine. A very high proportion (about 98%) of the nitrate is absorbed rapidly from the upper small intestine and is secreted in saliva (and also tears, sweat, gastric juices etc) then ultimately excreted in the urine. The concentration reaches a maximum value in secretions about 1 hour after ingestion of the original dose of nitrate and returns to its baseline value within 5 hours; the urinary concentration reaches a maximum 3 - 5 hours after ingestion and returns to the control value within 24 hours. Since nitrate is present in all of the secretions tested (tears, sweat, saliva, gastric secretion) and since there is also evidence that it is present in vaginal secretion (since N-nitroso compounds have been reported from that site) it is likely that it is present in other secretions not yet tested (eg colonic secretion). In saliva a proportion of the nitrate is reduced to nitrite by bacterial action; the proportion varies between persons (Tannenbaum et al, 1977; Hill, 1980a) and probably with diet.

Because the amount of dietary nitrite is quite small, the overwhelming proportion of nitrite in the upper gastrointestinal tract of humans is of salivary bacterial origin, but nitrite is a reactive anion (especially at Ph2) and so it has a short half-life in the normal stomach and normal resting gastric nitrite levels are very low. Nitrite will, however, be produced wherever nitrate and bacteria co-exist since nitrate reductase is produced by a very wide range of species of bacteria; these sites include the infected urinary bladder, the achlorhydric stomach, the colon and lower ileum etc.

The factors controlling the nitrite concentration vary between sites. In the mouth the major factor is the amount of dietary nitrate, but other variables include the rate of secretion in saliva (the maximum salivary nitrate + nitrite concentration in response to a standard dose of dietary nitrate varied in 6 persons by a factor of 2), the composition of the oral flora (the proportion of nitrate reduced to nitrite varied in 6 persons from 2% to 55%) and the diet (a soluble defined diet is readily utilisable by oral bacteria and results in a much more profuse oral flora than does a "normal" diet rich in high molecular weight nutrients). In the stomach the nitrite concentration depends on the rate of entry of nitrite into the stomach from the mouth, the rate of formation of nitrite in situ in the stomach from nitrate by bacterial nitrate reductase, and the mean survival time of the nitrite ions. Thus, in the stomach the major factors are the amount of dietary nitrate, the amount of nitrite swallowed as saliva, the half-life of the nitrite (dependent on gastric pH), the concentration of bacteria in the gastric juice (dependent on pH) and the activity of bacterial nitrate reductase (dependent on pH). In the urinary bladder the major factors are the urinary nitrate concentration (dependent on the amount of dietary nitrate), the infecting organism (some urinary tract infections are caused by bacteria which do not produce nitrate reductase) and the number of infecting organisms (the infection secondary to bilharzia is caused by a mixture of organisms whereas most uncomplicated infections have a single causative organism; the nitrate reductase of a mixed infection is much more active than that of a single species).

In summary, because nitrate is present in a wide range of secretions it is likely to be present in a wide range of sites in the body and so nitrite will be formed whenever this nitrate comes into contact with bacteria.

DISTRIBUTION OF BACTERIA IN THE BODY IN RELATION TO IN VIVO
N-NITROSATION

It can be assumed that wherever there is dying tissue there will be a bacterial flora scavenging on the dead cells; it can also be assumed that wherever there is a body surface there will be dead tissues. Consequently bacteria grow on all body surfaces, but the composition of the flora depends on the particular conditions at the surface in question; this has been reviewed recently (Skinner and Carr, 1974; Drasar and Hill, 1974).

From the point of view of N-nitrosation, many of the body surfaces are normally unimportant. For example, the skin is normally only thinly populated and with organisms which rarely produce nitrate reductase. In contrast, some regions of the gastrointestinal tract have a permanent flora rich in nitrate-reducing bacteria. Nitrate reductase is only produced under anaerobic conditions in the bacteria investigated to date (this is reasonable since it is an electron transport mechanism which would be redundant in the presence of oxygen), but this is not an important factor in determining the sites of nitrite production since the micro environment inhabited by the bacteria appears normally to be anoxic and the bacterial flora of the mouth, for example, which might be thought to be bathed in a stream of air, is in fact largely anaerobic. The bacteria live as an aqueous suspension in the crypts and crevices of the surface in mixed populations in which aerobic organisms utilise and so remove the dissolved oxygen leaving an anoxic environment for the rest of the flora.

Normal saliva contains about 10^7 organisms/ml, about 50 - 80% of which are anaerobic and about 30% of which produce nitrate reductase. The normal acid stomach is virtually sterile; bacteria can often be recovered from gastric juice but at pH values below 4 they do not proliferate and are metabolically inactive. With increasing gastric anacidity at pH values between 4 and 5 only the acid resistant organisms (streptococci and lactobacilli) grow and they do not reduce nitrate. Above pH5 a mixed flora containing a high proportion of nitrate-reducing organisms proliferates.

Normally the upper small intestine is virtually sterile, because the gastric contents entering the duodenum contains very few live organisms and because the large volume of secretory fluid flushes out the mucosal crypts and prevents colonisation. Thus the small intestine is only colonised when either the gastric juice is colonised or when there are small intestinal diverticulae or blind loops.

In the ileum, by contrast, the rate of transit of the gut contents is much slower allowing time for bacterial proliferation. There is relatively little secretion and so bacteria are able to establish themselves in the mucosal crypts and continuously inoculate the luminal contents.

The large intestine, an area of considerable stasis and where there is net absorption of fluid rather than of secretion, bacteria are free to proliferate to the limit of the available nutrients. Normal large bowel contents contain 10^{11} bacteria per gram, and more than 50% of the faecal mass is bacterial.

In addition to the gastrointestinal tract, the urinary tract may also be heavily infected at times. Asymptomatic urinary tract infections are common; in a study in rural general practice it was found that 20% of the population had a urinary tract infection at some time during a year. Most urinary tract infections in western persons involve a single organism, usually Escherichia coli or Proteus species and the bacterial concentration reaches 10^8 per ml. Under these conditions more than 50% of the urinary nitrate may be reduced to nitrite. In patients with bilharzia the cystic infection of the bladder wall provides a focus for infection and so infections of the bladder lumen which would normally be asymptomatic and would "wash out" after a short time are able to establish at these foci; repeated infection will be addative and give rise to a mixed bacterial infection which is capable of more efficient nitrate reduction.

In summary, bacteria are normally present in large numbers in the oral cavity and in the lower intestine and may also be present in large numbers in the urinary bladder or the stomach, and more rarely in the small intestine. It should be noted that when the small intestine is heavily colonised the possible formation of N-nitroso compounds is a relatively minor problem (since the effects are relatively long term).

IN VIVO INTERACTION BETWEEN BACTERIA, NITRITE AND NITROSATABLE COMPOUNDS

There is a wide range of nitrosatable nitrogen compounds produced endogenously in amounts considerably in excess of those from exogenous sources. Walters et al (1978) have assayed the total amount of nitrosatable compound in body fluids by the simple expedient of drastic nitrosation followed by assay of the N-nitroso compound formed. In this way he has shown that there are large amounts of suitable nitrosatable compounds in most body fluids; these are likely to be of endogenous origin and secreted into saliva, gastric juice etc, or excreted in the urine. Thus N-nitroso compounds could be formed at many sites in the body (Table 2) and their formation has been demonstrated in the saliva, the normal acid stomach, the achlorhydric stomach, the colon, the urinary bladder, the vagina and in the colon of persons with a ureterosigmoidostomy (Table 3).

TABLE 2 Nitrate, Nitrite and Bacteria at Various Sites in the Digestive Tract.

Site	Bacterial concentration (organisms/ml)	Nitrate concentration (ug/ml)	Nitrate concentration (ug/ml)
Mouth (saliva)	10^7	2-200	2-100
Stomach - normal	$< 10^2$	10	1
- achlorhydric	10^6	10	0-10
Duodenum	10^2	?	?
Lower ileum	10^8	0-.002	0-.002
Faeces	10^{11}	0-.001	0-.001
Urinary bladder - normal	0	20 to 150	0
- infected	10^8	20-100	10-70

It has been shown that the acid catalysed nitrosation of nitrogen compounds has a reaction rate proportional to the square of the nitrite concentration but to only the first order of the amine concentration; it is likely that the bacterial catalysed reaction has similar kinetics with the additional complication that the numbers and types of bacteria will be of importance. However, in vivo the amount of nitrosatable nitrogen compound at a site is not really a variable; these compounds are largely of endogenous origin and result either from essential metabolic reactions in the liver or from inevitable microbial reactions in the large bowel and the amounts produced are unlikely to vary greatly with diet or with disease except during treatment with nitrosatable drugs. The amount of nitrite at a site will depend mainly on the amount of dietary nitrate but also on the bacterial flora at the site considered; it will also depend, in the colon, saliva, vagina etc on the rate of secretion of nitrate which may vary between persons. The bacterial flora at a site will play a double role in determining the amount of N-nitrosation since it will affect both the amount of nitrite formed and also the rate of N-nitrosation.

TABLE 3   Sites Where N-nitrosation Has Been Demonstrated
in vivo

Site	Reference*
Mouth – (saliva)	Tannenbaum et al
Stomach – (normal acidified)	Fine et al
– (achlorhydric)	Walters et al
Colon – (faeces)	Varghese et al
– (urine of patients with uretero-sigmoidostomy)	Stewart et al
Urinary bladder – (urinary tract infection)	Brooks et al
– (bilharzial infection)	Hicks et al
Vagina – (trichomonas infection)	Alsobrook et al

*For full references see review by Hill (1979) or Hill, (1980b)

Having demonstrated the production of N-nitroso compounds in vivo, the next problem is to determine the relevance of this to human carcinogenesis. Of the N-nitroso compounds, the volatile N-nitrosamines are the only ones readily measureable but are also the only ones not to be locally-acting carcinogens. Thus the demonstration of N-nitrosamines in the urine of persons with bladder infections does not indicate that such persons are at risk of developing bladder cancer (indeed, we know from epidemiology that uncomplicated bladder infection does not predispose to bladder carcinogenesis), but it suggests that they might be at risk of developing carcinoma at another site which happens to be the target of the N-nitrosamine formed. We do not, of course, know the target organ of any N-nitrosamine in humans. Only a few studies have been reported in which non-volatile N-nitroso compounds have been assayed, and none of these report assays of N-nitrosamides or N-nitrosoureas. There are very good reasons for this lack of data, because the analytical problems are only exceeded by the difficulties in obtaining specimens and transporting them to the analytical laboratory without generating or destroying the compounds to be assayed. Consequently, our measure of the relevance of N-nitroso compound formation comes from epidemiology and is only supported by analytical data which is incomplete.

If N-nitroso compounds are formed endogenously and if they are locally acting and cause carcinomas, then the incidence of carcinomas should be related to (a) the nitrite concentration at the site of N-nitrosation, which is related to the nitrite intake, and (b) to the extent of bacterial colonisation at that site (both in terms of numbers of organisms and numbers of species of bacteria). The questions we need to ask concerning the role of N-nitroso compounds in gastric

carcinogenesis are (i) is there any evidence that N-nitroso compounds can cause
cancers in humans at all, and (ii) if so, is there any evidence that they can
cause gastric cancer.

Role of N-nitroso Compounds in Human Carcinogenesis

There is a little evidence that N-nitroso compounds can cause cancer in humans.
In the human the greatest density of bacteria is to be found in the colon, where
the density of organisms is more than 10^{11} per gram, and where many hundreds of
species of bacteria are to be found in the same sample of colonic contents
(Drasar and Hill, 1974). Normally the amount of nitrate and nitrite in the colon
is very small. In contrast, the amount of nitrate in normal human urine is large
since this is the major route of nitrate excretion; the urine is also the major
route of excretion of nitrosatable compounds such as secondary amines, alkylureas
and basic compounds such as spermidine. When urine is mixed with faeces, the
ideal conditions for N-nitrosation are generated, and this occurs when patients
are treated for severe bladder disease by ureterosigmoidostomy. In pilot studies
we have been able to demonstrate the presence of N-nitroso compounds and also
mutagens in the "urine" of such patients; these patients have a risk of colon
cancer at the anastamotic site which exceeds that of normal persons by a factor of
500-1000 (Stewart et al, 1980) and it has been postulated that this enormous risk
of carcinogenesis is due to the formation and local activation of N-nitroso
compounds.

A similar situation in which the urine is exposed to mixed bacterial populations
of high density is patients with bacterial infection of the urinary bladder
secondary to bilharzia and these patients, too, have a very high risk of bladder
cancer; the bladder carcinogenesis in these patients has been postulated as being
due to the N-nitroso compounds (Hicks et al, 1977).

Thus, there is some evidence that in situations in which N-nitroso compounds are
likely to be formed in large amounts the incidence of carcinoma at the site of
N-nitrosation is also very high.

N-nitroso Compounds and Gastric Cancer

The relationship between nitrate exposure and gastric cancer has been reviewed
elsewhere (Hill, 1979; 1980a; 1980b; Tannenbaum, 1977). The epidemiological
evidence that high exposure to nitrite and gastric bacteria is summarised in
Table 4. In studies in Colombia and Chile where gastric cancer is very common the
incidence of gastric achlorhydria in young adults is also very high (Tannenbaum
et al, 1977), possibly due to the high salt content of the diet of the Andean
peoples (Joossens, 1980). In Japan, where the incidence of achlorhydria in young
adults is also high (Joossens, 1980) the nitrate intake is higher than that in
western peoples by a factor of 3 (Kawabata et al, 1980) and the incidence of
gastric cancer is very high. In studies correlating nitrate intake to gastric
cancer incidence in Worksop and in Hungary there are no data on the incidences
of gastric achlorhydria. It is possible that in these populations the nitrate
exposure increases the risk of carcinogenesis only in the proportion of the
population who have achlorhydria. In patients with gastric achlorhydria
associated with pernicious anaemia or with surgery there is a high risk of gastric
cancer, even though the nitrate exposure is not high; here, however, the whole of
the study group has the risk of N-nitroso compound formation experienced in the
normal population only by that fraction which is achlorhydric.

TABLE 4 The Relationship Between Gastric Achlorhydria,
Bacteria, Nitrate and Gastric Carcinogenesis.

	Profuse gastric	High exposure to nitrate (and therefore nitrite)	Increased incidence of gastric cancer
Narino (Colombia)	++	++	++
Japan	++	++	++
Chile	++	++	++
Worksop	?	+	+
Hungary	?	+	+
Gastric achlorhydria	++	?	+
Partial gastrectomy	++	?	+

CONCLUSIONS

Correa et al (1977) have postulated a mechanism for gastric carcinogenesis in
which the first stage is gastric atrophy which progresses to intestinal metaplasia,
dysplasia and finally carcinoma as a result of the action of N-nitroso compounds.
This is an attractive hypothesis formulated to explain the high incidence of
gastric cancer in Narino, Colombia. It can be generalised to take account of the
fact that gastric cancer undoubtedly has a multifactorial etiology; Joossens
(1980) has argued persuasively that the first stage, the causation of gastric
atrophy which allows bacterial proliferation, is due to high salt intake. If
N-nitroso compounds are one of the causes of gastric carcinogenesis, they can
only induce malignancy in achlorhydric persons (because they are only formed in
adequate amounts under these conditions).

My current belief is that nitrate and bacteria are important etiological agents in
gastric carcinogenesis in those persons who are achlorhydric due to surgery, to
genetic factors (as in pernicious anaemia) or to exposure to environmental agents
which are at present unidentified but which probably include salt.

ACKNOWLEDGEMENTS

The work from my laboratory described here was financially supported by the
Department of the Environment and by the Cancer Research Campaign.

REFERENCES

Bartholomew, B., Butt, A., Caygill, C. and Hill, M.J. (1980) Proc. Nut. Soc. (in
    the press).
Correa, P., Haenszel, W., Cuello, C., Tannenbaum, S. and Archer, M. (1977) Lancet,
    ii, 58-60.
Drasar, B.S. and Hill, M.J. (1974) Human Intestinal Flora. Academic Press, London.

44 M. Hill

Fine, D.H., Ross, R., Rounbehler, D.P., Silvergleid, A. and Song, L. (1977) Nature, 265, 753-755.
Hicks, R.M., Walters, C.L., Elsebai, I., El Aasser, A.B., El Merzabani, M. and Gough, T.A. (1977) Proc. R. Soc. Med. 70, 413-417.
Hill, M.J. (1979) J. Human Nutr. 33, 416-426.
Hill, M.J. (1980a) In "Naturally occurring carcinogens-mutagens and modulators of carcinogenesis" (eds E.C. Miller et al) J. Sci. Soc. Press, Tokyo, p229-240.
Hill, M.J. (1980b) Br. Med. Bull., 36, 89-94.
Joossens, J.V. (1980) Brit. J. Nutr. (in the press).
Kawabata, T., Ohshima, H., Uibu, J., Nakamura, M., Matsui, M. and Hamano, M. (1980) In "Naturally occurring carcinogens-mutagens and modulators of carcinogenesis" (eds E.C. Miller et al). Jap. Scientific Soc. Press, Tokyo, p195-209.
Magee, P.N. (1977) In "Origins of Human Cancer" (eds H. Hiatt, J. Watson and J. Winsten), Cold Spring Harbour Lab. Press, New York, p629-637.
Magee, P.N. and Barnes, J.M. (1967) Adv. Cancer Res., 10, 163-246.
Mirvish, S.S. (1972) J. Natl. Cancer Inst. 46, 1183-1193.
Sander, J., Schweinsburg, F. and Menz, H.P. (1968) Z. Physiol. Chem. 349, 1691-1697.
Skinner, F.A. and Carr, J.G. (1974) eds "The Normal Microbiol Flora of Man" Academic Press, London.
Stewart, M., Hill, M.J., Pugh, R.C.B. and Williams, J.P. (1980) Brit. J. Urol. (in the press).
Tannenbaum, S.R., Archer, M.C., Wishnok, J.S., Correa, P., Cuello, C. and Haenszel, W. (1977) In "Origins of Human Cancer" (eds H. Hiatt, J. Watson and J. Winsten), Cold Spring Harbour Lab. Press, New York, p1609-1629.
Tannenbaum, S.R., Fett, D., Young, V.R., Land, P.D. and Bruce, W.R. (1978) Science, 200, 1487-1488.
Walters, C.L., Ruddell, W.J. and Hill, M.J. (1978) In "Environmental Aspects of N-nitroso compounds" (eds E.A. Walker, M. Castegnaro, L. Griciute and R.E. Lyle) IARC Sci. Publication No 19, Lyon, p279-284.
White, J.W. (1975) J. Agric. Food Chem. 23, 886-896.

DISCUSSION

R. Mitchell. You mention that bacteria can catalyse nitrosation reactions. Has this been studied in any detail and if so, what is the mechanism of the reaction?

M. Hill. It has been studied by a lot of people and they have all got very confusing results. This was very fashionable back in the early '70's. Zander first showed that if you threw bacteria in with nitrates and secondary amines you got N-nitroso compounds formed, and then he left it at that. Then in 1971 we published a paper in the British Journal of Cancer, which illustrated that the reaction seemed to be very similar to the chemically catalysed reaction but it just goes at pH7. So it may be something in the bacteria which is catalysing, maybe by the same mechanism as the hydrogen ion, and the other factors which catalyse the acid catalysed reaction also catalyse the bacterially catalysed reaction. It is not an enzymic reaction in as much as you can autoclave the organisms and they still work, so it may be some heavy metal present in the bacteria, or some acid product, or something else. It is a catalysis but of unknown aetiology.

R. Mitchell. It is not enzymic then?

M. Hill. Well, it is not thought to be enzymic.

J. Topham. Could you give us any theory for the relative increase in concentration of nitrites in the stomach under normal conditions and achlorhydric conditions? Are we talking about an order of magnitude increase, or more?

M. Hill. The normal level of nitrite in the acid stomach is very low indeed, less than 5 mg/litre, whereas in the achlorhydric stomach it gets up to about 60-80 mg/litre and the highest one we have seen is about 150 mg/litre. Depending on what you take as your normal level, we are talking about a difference of one or two orders of magnitude.

R. Pichlmayr. What do we know about bacteria in the stomach? We should like to know about the superficial staining type and the 'in depth' staining type and do you have any idea of the anaerobic nature of these?

M. Hill. Yes, we have tried to do some work on this. There is not a lot of consistent data on the flora of the stomach. One of the problems is that when you take the sample, you need to neutralize it and then you really need to do your bacteriology immediately, which is usually very difficult. Alternatively, you need to have some suitable transport system for it and so there are methodological problems. But in summary, what we find is that if the pH of the stomach is less than 4 then we really don't find any evidence of bacterial metabolism in the stomach. We can often recover bacteria but there is no evidence that they are any more than just hanging on to life and that you have just fished them out in time for them to recover on the plate. Between pH 4 and 5, you can find all salivary bacteria present and obviously alive and kicking and quite acitve. The only thing is that those organisms are not very metabolically active in the reactions in which we are interested. When you get above pH5, then you start finding a resident gastric flora which is more like an intestinal flora, faecal flora. You start picking up anaerobes and in particular coliforms and such organisms, and you start finding quite large numbers of nitrate reducing organisms. There seems to be two magic pH values and I would not like to stake my life on exactly where these two values are. One of them is about pH 4, where you no longer have organisms hanging on to life but they are actually living and multiplying but they are only salivary organisms, the acid resistant organisms. Above pH 5 you can get the organisms that are metabolically active in the reaction that we are interested in. Those sort of organisms proliferate in warmth.

Iatrogenic Hypochlorhydria—is this Relevant to the Development of Gastric Cancer?

T.J. Muscroft and J. Alexander-Williams

The General Hospital, Birmingham, U.K.

ABSTRACT

There is evidence that patients whose peptic ulcers have been treated by partial gastrectomy are at an increased risk of subsequently developing carcinoma in the gastric remnant and that this increased risk is a consequence of the surgical procedure rather than the original disease. Experimental animal data support this hypothesis and suggest also that reduction in acid secretion may be responsible, at least in part, for the increased risk. Furthermore, a gastro-enteric anastomosis appears to add to the risk of developing carcinoma.

When the fasting gastric contents exceed pH 4, a rapid increase in the bacterial colonisation occurs. It has been postulated, but not yet proved, that bacterial metabolism may lead to the formation of intragastric carcinogens, such as N-nitroso compounds or deconjugated bile acids.

Until the mechanisms of carcinogenesis in these patients are established, definitive preventive measures cannot be undertaken. However, screening patients at risk may improve the present poor prognosis of remnant carcinoma.

KEY WORDS

Vagotomy; Gastrectomy; Carcinogenesis; Gastric Cancer.

INTRODUCTION

Patients with cancer of the stomach usually have achlorhydria or hypochlorhydria. However, as Sir Arthur Hurst observed in 1939, 'The achlorhydria found in 70% of cases of cancer of the stomach is not a result of the cancer but of the chronic achlorhydric gastritis of which it is a sequel'. Patients with pernicious anaemia are achlorhydric and hypochlorhydria is commonly associated with atrophic gastritis and gastric ulceration. All three conditions are possibly associated with an increased risk of gastric malignancy. Therefore, it is necessary to consider whether hypochlorhydria per se is a risk factor in the development of gastric cancer and, if so, to what extent iatrogenic hypochlorhydria is potentially harmful.

Although the term 'hypochlorhydria' may imply any degree of reduction in gastric acid concentration, for the purpose of this chapter it has been taken to indicate

a fasting intragastric pH of 4 or above, as at this level pepsinogen is not activated and metabolically active bacteria are almost always present in large numbers.

HOW DO SURGEONS AND PHYSICIANS CAUSE HYPOCHLORHYDRIA?

The object of all operations employed in the treatment of ulcers of the stomach and
duodenum is to reduce or abolish acid secretion, so allowing the ulcer to heal.
Deane and his colleagues (1979) in our unit found that after successful vagotomy
for duodenal ulcer, with or without a drainage procedure, the median pH of gastric
aspirates was 3.0. However, the range of pH values was considerable. After proximal gastric vagotomy had successfully healed the ulcer, some patients were found to
have fasting pH values greater than 5, whereas others had values as low as pH 2.
We also found that in the fasting stage after vagotomy and antrectomy the median pH
of the fasting gastric aspirates was 6.0, the same as that found in a group of 51
patients with gastric carcinoma. In the group after vagotomy and antrectomy the pH
range was also wide; some patients with no evidence of recurrent ulceration had
fasting gastric contents of pH 2. This last observation may mean that in many patients the reduction in acid secretion induced by the operation was far greater than
that necessary for ulcer healing.

The recently introduced histamine - 2 receptor antagonists are potent inhibitors of
gastric acid secretion and cimetidine is now employed extensively in the management
of patients with peptic ulceration. In fasting subjects it has been shown that
cimetidine can raise the intragastric pH to between 6 and 7 (Longstreth et al, 1976;
Deane et al, 1980; Ruddell et al, 1980). However, 24 hour studies in normal subjects (Pounder et al, 1976) and in patients with duodenal ulcer (Pounder et al,
1975) revealed that, when taking a normal diet, the intragastric pH remained below
2 for most of the 24 hours, presumably as a result of the acid-stimulating effect
of food ingestion. These authors also demonstrated that the 24 hour variation in
intragastric pH in subjects and patients taking cimetidine 1600 mg daily, in
divided doses, was similar to that seen in duodenal ulcer patients after successful treatment with vagotomy and pyloroplasty. In contrast, we have found that
many patients after gastric resection for duodenal or gastric ulcer have pentagast-
rin and insulin-fast achlorhydria. These patients, presumably, do not respond to
intake of food by acid secretion. Therefore, patients who have had a vagotomy and
antrectomy are exposed to more continuous intragastric hypochlorhydria than those
treated with cimetidine or by vagotomy without resection.

DO ULCER-CURATIVE GASTRIC OPERATIONS PREDISPOSE TO GASTRIC CANCER?

Clinical Evidence

The first recorded case of carcinoma developing in a gastric remnant was described
nearly 60 years ago (Balfour, 1922) and for many years this association was considered to be rare. However, in the last 10 years several series of such cases have
been reported (Peitsch, 1979) and it now seems likely that patients who have had a
partial gastrectomy ten or more years previously are at increased risk of developing carcinoma in the gastric remnant.

As the long time between operation and the appearance of cancer makes it difficult
to perform a prospective study, most data have been obtained by retrospective review.

Stalsberg and Taksdal (1971) found that of 630 patients with gastric cancer having
a post mortem examination, 55 had had a previous gastric operation for peptic ulceration. By comparing this group with age and sex matched controls, who died
without gastric carcinoma, they calculated that in the first 15 years after ulcer
curing operation the risk of developing gastric cancer was about half that of the
controls. The risk increased thereafter, with a relative risk factor of 5.1 after

25 years and 8.4 after 35 years.

In another retrospective study over 22 years (Papachristou, Agnanti and Fortner, 1980), 1496 patients presenting with gastric cancer were compared with a similar number of patients with a carcinoma elsewhere in the alimentary tract (pharynx, oesophagus, liver, pancreas and colon). Of the gastric cancer patients, 30 had undergone operative treatment for peptic ulceration at least 5 years before the diagnosis of malignancy, compared with 10 of the 1496 control patients. The difference was highly significant statistically. The median interval between the ulcer curative resection and the diagnosis of gastric cancer was 20 years. It is interesting to note that 34 patients from each group had been treated medically for peptic ulceration at least 5 years before the diagnosis of their malignancy.

Domellof and Janunger (1977) studied 676 patients treated by partial gastrectomy for peptic ulceration between 1952 and 1966. Of 198 patients who had died by the time of review 3 had been certified as having died of gastric remnant carcinoma. Of 336 patients who agreed to undergo gastroscopic examination, 11 were found to have carcinoma of the gastric remnant. Domellof and Janunger calculated that patients who had undergone gastric resection for benign disease more than 12 years earlier were between 2 and 3 times more likely to develop carcinoma than the general population. However, they discovered that the risk of cancer in the gastric remnant was not related to age, unlike the risk of developing gastric cancer in the general population, which increases with age. Therefore, they postulateed that patients aged 50 to 55 years, who had undergone resection for peptic ulcer disease more than 12 years previously, were 12 times more likely to develop gastric cancer than were age-matched controls.

These results, and those of other series (Saegesser and James, 1972; Morgenstern, Yamakawa and Seltzer, 1973; Nicholls, 1974; Eberlein, Lorenzo and Webster, 1978; Clemencon, 1979) indicate that patients who have had a partial gastrectomy for peptic ulceration incur a risk of developing carcinoma in the gastric remnant which is between 2 and 8 times greater than the risk in matched controls who have not underoperation. The increased incidence begins after 10 - 15 years and rises thereafter as the interval since the operation increases. The 10 - 15 post-operative interval before the increased risk is manifest seems to be relatively independent of the age of the patient, suggesting that the initiating event begins at the time of operation. These figures are more striking when it is considered that the distal portion of the stomach has been removed and it is here that a disproportionately large number of tumours arise in the intact stomach. It seems reasonable to conclude that the reduction in gastric mucosal area may account for the diminished risk of cancer during the first decade after operation.

It remains to be ascertained whether or not a partial gastrectomy for gastric ulcer is associated with a greater risk than a resection for duodenal ulcer. Nicholls (1974) considered that the risk of gastric remnant carcinoma following resection of a gastric ulcer merely reflected the risk of malignant change associated with gastric ulceration per se, whilst partial gastrectomy for duodenal ulcer was not associated with an increased risk of subsequent malignancy. Peitsch (1979) analysed the result in 857 patients treated with Billroth II gastrectomy for gastric and duodenal ulcers and concluded that although there was an increased risk of malignancy after both gastric and duodenal ulcer operations, there was a higher incidence in the former group. Other workers have not been able to show any difference in the incidence of cancer between patients who have had a resection for gastric ulcer and those who had it for duodenal ulcer (Stalsberg and Taksdal, 1971; Saegesser and James, 1972; Domellof and Janunger, 1977; Papachristou, Agnanti and Fortner, 1980). However, patients with duodenal ulcers are usually younger than those with gastric ulcers and are operated upon at a younger age; this might tend to obscure any true differences in incidence. Nevertheless, Taksdal and

Stalsberg (1973) could find no relationship between the site of the original ulcer
and the subsequent risk of malignancy and neither was there any relationship between
the histological appearance of the mucosa in the primarily resected portion of the
stomach and the later development of cancer in the remnant. They concluded that the
increased incidence of carcinoma of the gastric remnant is a result of the gastro-
enteric anastomosis alone.

Although gastric carcinoma has been reported after vagotomy and pyloroplasty (Ellis
et al, 1979) there is as yet little evidence that this procedure predisposes to
malignancy.

Experimental Evidence

Experiments in animals using chemically induced gastric carcinomas have shown that
both vagotomy and partial gastrectomy can enhance carcinogenesis. Fujita and his
colleagues (1979) performed a selective vagotomy, without a drainage procedure, on
a group of 10 dogs who were then given N-methyl-N'-nitro-N-nitrosoguanidine (MNNG),
a known gastric carcinogen, in their drinking water for 12 months. Subsequently,
42 malignant lesions were found in the stomachs of the dogs who had undergone vagotomy compared with 16 in a group of unoperated control animals. The authors postulated two explanations for this observation:- firstly, that because MNNG is rapidly
inactivated in acid, a reduction in acid secretion may retard its degradation and
secondly, that because the vagotomy may delay gastric emptying (although this was
not measured), the duration of contact between carcinogen and mucosa might be prolonged.

Similar findings were reported by Kowalewski (1973), who administered 2, 7,
diacetylaminofluorene to two groups of rats, one of which had previously had a vagotomy. Of the operated animals 18% developed gastric cancers after 46 weeks,
compared with 6% of the controls. Vagotomy in the rat causes gastric dilatation
and stasis. In addition, the study demonstrated that gastric mucosal atrophy is
common after vagotomy; perhaps the known impairment of mucosal blood flow following
vagotomy in the rat reduces the cellular resistance to carcinogens.

Morgenstern (1968) found that vagotomy in rats significantly increased the number
of tumours induced by means of threads, saturated with 20-methylcholanthrene,
implanted in the antrum. The addition of a gastroenterostomy increased the incidence of neoplasia still further; the tumours arising predominantly in the region
of the anastomosis where the greatest mucosal changes were seen. In man it is reported that the peri-anastomotic area also shows the greatest mucosal reaction
(Gough and Craven, 1975; Skinner, Heenan and Whitehead, 1975) and the majority of
carcinomas arise in this area (Schrumpf et al, 1977, Papachristou, Agnanti and
Fortner, 1980).

Deveney, Freeman and Way (1980) recently reported the effect of antrectomy on the
incidence of gastric carcinoma in rats. Antrectomy with Billroth II reconstruction
significantly increased the incidence of gastric carcinomas in rats given MNNG to
43% compared with the 13% found in the unoperated control animals. In a third group,
the divided antrum was anastomosed to the colon; this was shown to give rise to
hypergastrinaemia and the acid output of the gastric remnant in this group was similar to the intact controls. Proximal gastric tumours developed in 16% of the
animals with a retained antrum. However, adenocarcinomas occurred in 43% of the
implanted antra, suggesting that the protective effect of the retained antrum was
mediated via the continuing acid secretion rather than because of any influence of
gastrin itself on the gastric mucosa.

Dahm and his colleagues (1979) also studied the effect of MNNG in rats. One group
of animals underwent Billroth I or Billroth II resections and were then given the

carcinogen in their drinking water for 31 weeks. At this time, neoplasms had developed in 37.8% of the animals. No tumours were found in control animals with intact stomachs after 31 weeks exposure to MNNG, although 11 out of 20 control animals (55%) were found to have tumours after 41 weeks. Among a group of 33 rats in which Roux-en-Y bile diversion procedures were performed at the time of the resections, only 1 (3.1%) developed a cancer in the gastric remnant. Although this might have been the result of avoiding the damaging effect of bile reflux upon the gastric mucosa, no measurement of gastric acid secretion was made. In the absence of alkaline pancreatic secretions, the increased acid concentration in the gastric remnant may have provided the protective influence, as suggested by the study of Deveney, Freeman and Way (1980).

Finally, it is interesting to note that a 'medical vagotomy' induced by prolonged administration of propantheline to rats, increased their susceptibility to gastric neoplasia induced by 20-methylcholanthrene (Kowalewski and Kaspar, 1967). This regime was also found to produce achlorhydria and gastric mucosal atrophy in rats that had not developed tumours at the time that they were sacrificed.

WHAT ARE THE POSSIBLE MECHANISMS OF CARCINOGENESIS?

In considering the possible pathways by which hypochlorhydria can lead to cancer in patients who have had a gastric resection it is necessary to separate the effects of reduced HCL concentration alone from those due to the other consequences of ulcer curative operations; such as reflux into the stomach of bile and pancreatic secretions, alteration in the rate of gastric emptying and reduction in gastric mucosal blood flow.

Cimetidine reduces acid secretion without apparently affecting gastric emptying (Heading et al, 1977) or duodenogastric reflux (Deane et al, 1980). Twelve months continuous therapy with cimetidine (400 mg bd) in 6 duodenal ulcer patients produced no detectable change in gastric mucosal histology (Bank et al, 1980). Therefore, H-2 receptor blockade with cimetidine or similar drugs may represent a model of 'pure' hypochlorhydria. In a group of 29 patients with duodenal ulcers treated by proximal gastric vagotomy, generally considered to produce the least alteration in gastric function of all ulcer curative operations, the number of patients with atrophic gastritis increased from 3 (10%) before operation to 11 (38%) after 3 months (Roland, Berstad and Liavag, 1975), whilst in a group of 138 patients with no pre-existing atrophic gastritis who underwent Billroth I and II partial gastrectomies for peptic ulceration, 54% were found to have atrophic gastritis after two years (Pulimood, Knudsen and Coghill, 1976). Furthermore, in the latter study, this assessment was made on a mean of only 3 biopsies per patient, obtained by unguided suction biopsy. As gastritis is most commonly found adjacent to a gastro-enteric anastomosis (Lawson, 1975; Skinner, Heenan and Whitehead, 1975; Schrumpf et al, 1977) it seems likely that directed biopsy of the peristomal region would have revealed a greater incidence of gastritis.

Various factors may combine to produce mucosal damage. The deleterious effects of partial gastrectomy combined with diminished acid secretion in rats has already been mentioned (Deveney, Freeman and Way, 1980). Lawson (1972) produced gastritis in dogs by performing a Billroth II gastrectomy and then demonstrated that the gastritis would resolve if bile were diverted from the stomach by means of a Roux-en-Y reconstruction. However, as a vagotomy had not been performed in these animals, they were presumably still secreting acid. In our experience the gastritis did not resolve after bile diversion procedures for postoperative reflux gastritis or bile vomiting, in which a vagotomy had already been performed or was added to prevent stomal ulceration. It may be that both the absence of acid and presence of bile induce or maintain the gastritis.

Gastritis in both the fundic and antral regions is related to an increase in cellu-

lar proliferation, as demonstrated by Hansen and his co-workers (1977), who also
found an inverse relationship between peak acid output and the rate of mucosal cell
proliferation. The increased activity of the cell may make it more vulnerable to
carcinogens; the damaging effects of which may be further enhanced by breakdown of
the gastric mucosal barrier by bile (Davenport, 1970), prolonged contact time due
to stasis and, possibly, by alterations in the stability of particular carcinogens
following the rise in pH (Fujita et al, 1979). Thus it appears that of the current
therapeutic regimes, only H-2 receptor blockade produces pure hypochlorhydria,
whilst all operative procedures seem to produce additional, potentially harmful
effects.

Hypochlorhydria allows bacterial overgrowth in the gastric juice (Ruddell et al,
1976; Gatehouse et al, 1978; Deane et al, 1979; Muscroft et al, 1980) and the concentration of bacteria is closely related to the intragastric pH. The fasting
gastric contents are usually sterile when the pH is less than 4, whilst several
species of micro-organisms, present in large numbers, are almost invariably found
when the pH is 4 or above. The bactericidal capacity of gastric secretions seems
to be due entirely to the presence of hydrogen ions (Gianella, Broitman and Zamchek,
1972).

The hypothesis that bacterial activity may promote the formation of nitrite and carcinogenic N-nitroso-compounds has been presented in the previous chapter. Our own
studies (Deane et al, 1979; Muscroft et al, 1980) indicate that the total bacterial
count and the number of species of micro-organisms are related closely to the pH of
the gastric contents, regardless of the cause of the hypochlorhydria. Organisms
capable of reducing nitrate to nitrite are found almost exclusively in gastric samples of pH 4 or above and there is a close correlation between elevated gastric
nitrite concentrations and the presence of such nitrate-reducing organisms (Ruddell
et al, 1976; Muscroft et al, 1980). We have been unable to demonstrate any relationship between nitrite concentration and the cause of the hypochlorhydria.
Detection of N-nitroso-compounds in gastric aspirates is technically difficult as
they are present in concentrations measured in parts per billion and, furthermore,
many of the N-nitroso compounds are unstable. A relationship between pH and total
N-nitroso-compound levels has been reported (Schlag et al, 1980) but the experimental method used in this study has been criticised (Ruddell and Walters, 1980) and
further studies are required.

Hill and his colleagues (1971, 1973) have proposed that bacterial degradation of
bile acids in the colon may lead to the production of carcinogens such as lithocho-
lic acid, deoxycholic acid and possibly 20-methycholanthrene. In our laboratory,
some of the implicated bacteria, such as Clostridium spp., Escherichia coli, and
Bifidobacter, have been isolated from gastric aspirates and bile is invariably
present in the stomach following a gastric resection. Therefore, carcinogens and
co-carcinogens might be produced from bile acids by bacterial activity in the hypochlorhydric stomach. Some evidence that bacterial deconjugation of bile acids may
occur in the stomach has recently been published (Domellof, Reddy and Weisburger,
1980).

CAN THE RISKS BE AVOIDED OR MINIMISED?

None of the factors outlined above has been proven to be involved in the production of human gastric cancer and therefore only tentative conclusions can be drawn.
As it appears to be the operative procedure rather than the original peptic ulcer
that predisposes to malignancy, it may be that operative treatment should be avoided wherever possible. Effective medical treatment will help to reduce the need to
resort to operation. However, if such treatment involves the induction of hypo- or
achlorhydria, then this too may involve a risk of inducing carcinoma. Perhaps the
most effective medical treatment available is H-2 receptor blockade, which produces

only hypochlorhydria and not bile reflux. Furthermore, the hypochlorhydria produced by medical therapy may be intermittent, whereas after operation it is
permanent. However, chemical carcinogenesis is a multistage process and initiation
may be brought about by only brief exposure to the initiating carcinogen (Hicks,
1980). Thus, if hypochlorhydria does indeed allow the formation of carcinogenic
compounds, then conceivably even a short period of H-2 receptor blockade could be
harmful.

As we described earlier, our findings have shown that gastric and duodenal ulcers
may heal after operations despite only a slight elevation in fasting intragastric
pH (Deane et al, 1979). Clearly, in such individuals, as their ulcers have healed,
further reduction in acid secretion is unnecessary and, from the foregoing, could
be potentially harmful. If hypochlorhydria were shown to be a risk factor in producing gastric cancer it might be reasonable to prefer a 'minimal' operative
procedure such as proximal gastric vagotomy to a 'maximal' procedure such as vagotomy and antrectomy. In the surgical management of duodenal ulcers it may be
better to adopt an operation that produces a higher recurrent ulcer rate rather
than one that has a higher predisposition to gastric remnant carcinoma.

As the loss of the antrum and pylorus with the consequent reflux of duodenal contents after partial gastrectomy, seems to be harmful, resection should be avoided
wherever possible. If it is not possible to avoid a resection, it could be worth
considering the place of a Roux-en-Y bile diversion procedure as part of the
primary reconstruction and so avoiding exposure of the mucosa to one of the possible damaging factors (Dahn et al, 1979).

We could try to prevent the intragastric formation of possible carcinogens or try
to inactivate any that are formed. Although it would seem logical to attempt to
reduce the number of bacterial species and the total viable count in the stomach
remnant, it is difficult to know how this could be achieved in practice. Long-
term antibiotic therapy would almost certainly be followed by the overgrowth of
resistant strains, antiseptics by mouth could have potential toxicity and long-
term oral administration of hydrochloric acid is unlikely to be acceptable to the
patients or their dentists.

Vitamin C acts as a nitrite scavenger in the aqueous phase (as does vitamin E in
the lipid phase) and if taken by mouth these might reduce the amount of nitrite
available for nitrosation in the stomach. There is also some evidence that unpro-
cessed bran can absorb N-nitroso-compounds. However, it is obvious that no
rational therapy can be planned until the responsible carcinogen or carcinogens
are identified and their mode of cancer induction understood.

The prospect of curing a symptomatic carcinoma of the gastric remnant is poor, as
the tumour is often locally advanced by the time it presents clinically
(Morgenstern, Yamakawa and Seltzer, 1973). Until the condition can be prevented
the mortality might be reduced by screening the population at risk. The early
mucosal lesions are often flat and inconspicuous (Schrumpf et al, 1977), so X-ray
detection is unreliable and surveillance would entail regular endoscopic examination with multiple biopsies, particularly of the peristomal region, starting
about ten years after the operation and continuing throughout the patient's life.
This would be a formidable undertaking and the return might be small. Domellof
and Janunger (1977) found tumours in only 3.2% of the patients that they examined.
Nevertheless, Clemencon (1979), while acknowledging these difficulties, recommends
annual gastroscopic examination for the following groups of patients who have had
a partial gastrectomy: (i) those under 40 years who were operated upon more than
20 years previously; (ii) those over 40 years who were operated upon more than 10
years previously; (iii) those with chronic bile reflux who were operated upon more
than ten years previously, and (iv) all patients who have been found to have severe

epithelial dysplasia.

In the absence of facilities for screening, early lesions will inevitably be missed and in these circumstances any patient who develops upper abdominal symptoms after an earlier partial gastrectomy should be regarded as having a carcinoma in the gastric remnant until the diagnosis has been excluded by endoscopic examination.

REFERENCES

Balfour, D. C. (1922). Factors influencing the life expectancy of patients operated on for gastric ulcers. Ann. Surg., 76, 405-408.
Bank, S., Barbezat, G. O., Marks, I. N. and Vinik, A. I. (1980). Gastric acid secretion, fasting and meal-stimulated serum gastrins and gastric structure 3 and 12 months after maintenance cimetidine. Presented at the XI International Congress of Gastroenterology A.S.N.E.M.G.E., Hamburg, W. Germany.
Clemencon, G. (1979). Risk of carcinoma in the gastric remnant after gastric resection for benign conditions. Gastric Cancer, Eds. Ch. Herfarth and P. Schlag, Springer-Verlag. Berlin, Heidelberg, New York, pp 129-136.
Dahm, K., Werner, W., Eichen, R. and Mitschke, H. (1979). Experimental cancer of the gastric stump. Gastric Cancer, Eds. Ch. Herfarth and P. Schlag, Springer-Verlag. Berlin, Heidelberg, New York, pp 44-59.

Davenport, H. W. (1970). Effect of lysolecithin, digitonin and phospholipase A upon the dogs gastric mucosal barrier. Gastroenterology, 59, 505-509.

Deane, S. A., Gatehouse, D., Youngs, D. J., Burdon, D. W., Alexander-Williams, J. and Keighley, M. R. B. (1979). Bacterial flora of the postoperative stomach. Gut, 20, 931-932.

Deane, S. A., Youngs, D. J., Poxon, V. A., Keighley, M. R. B., Alexander-Williams, J. and Burdon, D. W. (1980). Cimetidine and gastric microflora. Br. J. Surg. 67, 371.

Deveney, C. W., Freeman, H., Way, L. W. (1980). Experimental gastric carcinogenesis in the rat. Am. J. Surg., 139, 49-54.

Domellof, L. and Janunger, K-G. (1977). The risk of gastric carcinoma after partial gastrectomy. Ann. J. Surg., 134, 581-584.

Domellof, L., Reddy, B. S. and Weisburger, J. H. (1980). Microflora and deconjugation of bile acids in alkaline reflux after partial gastrectomy. Am. J. Surg., 140, 291-295.
Eberlein, T. J., Lorenzo, F. V. and Webster, M. W. (1978). Gastric carcinoma following operation for peptic ulcer disease. Ann. Surg., 187, 281-256.
Ellis, D. J., Kingston, R. D., Brookes, V. S. and Waterhouse, J. A. H. (1979). Gastric carcinoma and previous peptic ulceration. Br. J. Surg., 66, 117-119.
Fujita, M., Takami, M., Usugane,M.N., Wampei,S.and Taguchi, T. (1979). Enhancement of gastric carcinogenesis in dogs given N-Methyl-N' Nitro, N-Nitroso-guanidine following vagotomy. Cancer Res., 38, 811-816.
Gatehouse, D., Dimock, F., Burdon, D. W., Alexander-Williams, J. and Keighley, M. R. B. (1978). Prediction of wound sepsis following gastric operations. Br. J. Surg., 65, 551-554.
Giannella, R. A., Broitman, S. A. and Zamcheck, N. (1972). Gastric acid barrier to ingested micro-organisms: studies in vivo and in vitro. Gut, 13, 251-256.
Gough, D. C. and Craven, J. L. (1975. Is a gastrostomy a pre-malignant condition? Gut, 16, 843.
Hurst, Sir Arthur. (1970). Selected writings of Sir Arthur Hurst (1879-1944). Ed. T. Hunt. British Society of Gastroenterology, pp.88.

Hansen, O. H., Johansen, A., Larsen, J. K., Pedersen, T. and Svendsen, L. B. (1977). Relationship between gastric acid secretion, histopathology and cell proliferation kinetics in human gastric mucosa. Gastroenterology, 73, 453-456.

Heading, R. C., Logan, R. F. A., McLoughlin, G. P., Lidgard, G. and Forrest, J. A. H. (1977). Effect of the Cimetidine on gastric emptying. Cimetidine. Proceedings of the Second International Symposium on Histamine H$_2$ Receptor Antagonists. Eds. W. L. Burland and M. A. Simkins. Excerpta Medica, Amsterdam-Oxford, pp. 145-152.

Hicks, R. M. (1980). Multistage carcinogenesis in the urinary bladder. Br.Med.Bull. 36., 39-46.

Hill, M. J., Drasar, B. S., Aries, V., Crowther, J. S., Hawkesworth, G. and Williams, R. E. O. (1971). Bacteria and aetiology of cancer of the large bowel. Lancet i, 95-100.

Hill, M. J., Draser, B. S., Williams, R. E. O., Meade, T. W., Cox, A. G., Simpson, J. E.P. and Morson, B. C. (1973). Faecal bile-acids and clostridia in patients with cancer of the large bowel. Lancet i, 535-539.

Kowalewski, K. (1973). Relationship between vagotomy, peptic ulcer and gastric adenocarcinoma in rats feed 2,7-Diacetylaminofluorene. Canad. J. Surg., 16, 210-216.

Kowalewski, K. and Kaspar, T. (1967). Achlorhydria, gastric mucosal atrophy and gastric neoplastic lesions in rats, mice and hamsters treated with an anticholinergic drug, propanthelene bromide, and a carcinogen, 20-methylcholanthrene. Canad. J. Surg., 10, 99-108.

Lawson, H. H. (1972). The reversibility of postgastrectomy alkaline reflux gastritis by a Roux-en-Y loop. Br. J. Surg., 59, 13-15.

Lawson, H. H. (1975). The role of the pyloric antrum and Hofmeister valve in the development of the chronic gastric mucosal reaction. Br. J. Surg. 63, 592-595.

Longstreth, G. F., Go, V. L. W. and Malagelada, J. R. (1976). Cimetidine suppression of nocturnal gastric secretion in active duodenal ulcers. N. Engl. J. Med., 294, 801-804.

Morgenstern, L. (1968). Vagotomy, gastroenterostomy and experimental gastric cancer. Arch. Surg., 96, 920-923.

Morgenstern, L., Yamakawa, T. and Seltzer, D. (1973). Carcinoma of the gastric stump. Am. J. Surg., 125, 29-38.

Muscroft, T. J., Youngs, D. J., Poxon, V. A., Burdon, D. W. and Keighley, M. R. B. (1980). Bacteria, nitrite and N-Nitroso-compounds in gastric juice. Presented at the Surgical Research Society, Nottingham, Summer 1980.

Nicholls, J. C. (1974). Carcinoma of the stomach following partial gastrectomy for benign gastroduodenal lesions. Br. J. Surg., 61, 244-249.

Papachristou, D. N., Agnanti, N. and Fortner, J. G. (1980). Gastric carcinoma after treatment of ulcer. Am. J. Surg., 139, 193-196.

Peitsch, W. (1979). Remarks on frequency and pathogenesis of primary gastric stump cancer. Gastric Cancer. Eds. Ch. Herfarth and P. Schlag. Springer-Verlag. Berlin, Heidelberg, New York. pp 137-144.

Pounder, R. E. Williams, J. G., Milton-Thompson, G. J. and Misiewicz, J. J. (1975). Twenty-four hour control of intragastric acidity by cimetidine in duodenal ulcer patients. Lancet ii, 1069-1072.

Pounder, R. E., Williams, J. G., Milton-Thompson, G. J. and Misiewicz, J. J. (1976). Effect of cimetidine on twenty-four hour intragastric acidity in normal subjects. Gut, 17, 133-138.

Pulimood, B. M., Knudsen, A. and Coghill, N. F. (1976). Gastric mucosa after partial gastrectomy. Gut, 17, 463-470.

Roland, M., Berstad, A. and Liavag, I. (1975). A histological study of gastric mucosa before and after proximal gastric vagotomy in duodenal ulcer patients. Scand. J. Gastroent., 10, 181-186.

Ruddell, W. J. J., Bone, E. S., Hill, M. J., Blendis, L. M. and Walters, C. L. (1976). Gastric juice nitrite. A risk factor for cancer in the hypochlorhydric stomach? Lancet ii, 1037-1039.

Ruddell, W. S. J. and Walters, C. L. (1980). Nitrite and N-nitroso compounds in
    gastric juice. Lancet i, 1187.
Saegesser, F. and James, D. (1972). Cancer of the gastric stump after partial
    gastrectomy (Billroth II Principle) for ulcer. Cancer, 29, 1150-1159.
Schlag, P., Bockler, R., Ulrich, H., Peter, M., Merkle, P. and Herfarth, C. (1980).
    Are nitrite and N-nitroso-compounds in gastric juice risk factors for carcin-
    oma in the operated stomach. Lancet i, 727-729.
Schrumpf, E., Stadaas, J., Myren, J., Serck-Hanssen, A., Aune, S. and Osnes, M.
    (1977). Mucosal changes in the gastric stump 20-25 years after partial
    gastrectomy. Lancet ii, 467-469.
Skinner, J. M., Heenan, P. J. and Whitehead, R. (1975). Atrophic gastritis in
    gastrectomy specimens. Br. J. Surg., 62, 23-25.
Stalsberg, H. and Taksdal, S. (1971). Stomach cancer following gastric surgery for
    benign conditions. Lancet ii, 1175-1177.
Taksdal, S. and Stalsberg, T. (1973). Histology of gastric carcinoma occurring
    after gastric surgery for benign conditions. Cancer, 32, 162-166.

DISCUSSION

V. Brookes. Of the surgical procedures that were aetiological risks, only the Billroth II showed significant figures, but in Birmingham the incidence following vagotomy was similar and it occurred 10 years earlier.

E. Deutch. May I ask whether it is the 12-15 years post gastrectomy, or if the patient is closer to 50 years of age, that is the crucial question about the development of cancer?

J. Alexander-Williams. That is one of those questions you cannot answer. I do not know. I guess that it is the length of time from the operation that is more important. Is this not so with carcinogenesis everywhere, there is a delay period? For example the 15 year period between smoking and developing a cancer. So perhaps we are all subject to carcinogens and the risk is greater as we get older. But if we have a gastrectomy and we become achlorhydric then a bigger factor comes in and that big boost comes after 15 years. So I would guess that it is the time since the operation.

E. Deutch. But you showed two sets of figures. The ones that were 12 - 15 years, but then you also showed another group that seemed to be at a high risk of cancer if they were operated on close to 50 years of age.

T. Muscroft. People who address themselves to this problem say that the risk is related to the time since the operation rather than the age of the patient. I showed the figure of 50 - 55 years of age because at that age the risk of the general population is very small but the risk in the operated group remains constant, and the gap at that age is very wide. As they get older, the difference decreases as the risk of the general population increases to meet the risk of the operated group.

I. Häkkinen. What we have found is that in many cases the mucosa was normal and the stomach acid. It is not always necessary to have hypochlorhydria to develop a carcinoma.

J. Alexander-Williams. I think it may be true that some of these gastric remnant carcinomas occur very close to the stoma and sometimes the atrophic changes are juxtastomal and part of the fundus remains relatively healthy. I think it may be something to do with the purely mechanical effects of regurgitation of bile, and therefore in view of that evidence you might think that bile reflux may be more important than achlorhydria. I think that bile is probably very much more damaging if it is in an achlorhydric environmant rather than an acid environment. You are quite right, there are a number of cases reported in which a gastric remnant carcinoma occurs when there is still some acid. But overall, the picture is one of it occurring in an achlorhydric stomach.

P. Reid. Together with Dr. Walters we have been studying gastric nitrosamine concentrations in many different conditions and we now have data on 350 patients. What does come out of it is that this is undoubtedly pH related; that the lower the pH the lower the nitrosamine concentration; the higher the pH the higher the nitrosamine concentreation, irrespective of the underlying condition with which you are dealing. In other words you find the highest mean nitrosamine levels in patients with pernicious anaemia who have the highest pH's, and the lowest levels in normal subjects. We have 50 individuals who volunteered to have their gastric juice aspirated, who have no history of underlying gastro-intestinal conditions, and in them the mean nitrosamine level was the lowest. We can certainly confirm the data which has been produced to date. We have also shown that the incidence of the bacteria which are nitrate reductase positive increases with increasing pH. It also increases with age, as does pH, so that there is that additional factor which is very important and this again ties in with what has been said earlier today, that

57

there is an increased incidence of gastric cancer with increasing age. We have also shown that it is higher in males than in females, which again ties in with the situation we have described epidemiologically. We have also demonstrated the situation not only in the surgically induced hypo- and achlorhydric situations but also in the medically induced conditions with the H_2 blocker which is currently available on the market, ie. cimetidine.

DAY 1. SESSION 1. PANEL DISCUSSION

P. Wrigley.   In view of the familial nature of pernicious anaemia, I wonder what is known, or expected to be found, with regard to either a familial relationship or HLA relationship in gastric cancer and whether this has any major effect on the incidence of the disease in the different countries and areas that we deal with? Knowing that, for instance, pernicious anaemia itself has a varying incidence, not only in this country but internationally.

T. Hirayama.   The incidence of pernicious anaemia is far lower in Japan compared with other countries.   I believe this to be true.   If not, Dr. Takagi please correct me.   As to the familial aggregations, we did find this in gastric cancer and this is most striking when the patient is younger.   Summarising all the evidence we still do not know if there is a clear cut relationship with HLA.   As you know the only HLA relationship reported which is probably reliable is for naso-pharyngeal cancer, studied in Singapore by the I.A.R.C. group.   For other cancers we simply do not know the relationship with HLA.   We have some statistical relationship with blood group, but that is also suggestive and I do not think that this will solve the problem at all.   We know that there are families that are truly susceptible to gastric cancer.   The maximum number of patients I have found is 16 in one pedigree but that is very exceptional and usually we find 3 or 4.   As you know, one out of eight or ten people in Japan get gastric cancer eventually, so by random occurence we find three or four cases in the same family.   We therefore have to decide whether this is a true, genetically related family aggregation, or an environmentally related one or just a random reflection of the high incidence in our country.

M. Keighley.   There has been considerable emphasis this morning on the importance of hypochlorhydria and I think there is no doubt that bacteria just do not survive if the pH is low.   But don't you think that there may be more to it than merely hypochlorhydria, because we are concerned really with the metabolically active coliform organisms usually not normally resident in the stomach, nor in the saliva, and probably arising from the duodenum?   How important do you think the relative combination of bile reflux plus hypochlorhydria is if this hypothesis is correct?

M. Hill.   I would like to make a comment about the bile reflux which is related to the earlier question addressed to Dr. Williams.   Of course, if you get bile reflux into an acid stomach the bile will just precipitate, and it will not have much irritant activity.   The peak is about four or five, even of taurine conjugated bile acids.   So you would not expect very much irritant activity of bile refluxing into an acid stomach whereas you would expect quite considerable irritant activity of bile in solution refluxing into a more neutral stomach.   Now I wish I could answer the first question about what are the factors which determine the flora in the stomach, or anywhere else for that matter.   It is difficult to know where the coliforms come from, because very few people have coliforms in the mouth.   We used to do swabs of students at all sites, trying to teach them that they were living in symbiosis with their bacteria and that they should be respectful to them, trying to identify which organisms came from where.   We found on one particular day, the whole class carried large numbers of coliforms in their throat swabs and this ruined the whole point that we were trying to make.   It turned out that the Metropolitan Police had been exercising their horses down Praed Street that morning and there was a fair amount of manure about that the eager rose gardeners had not cleared up.   So that might be the source of the coliforms.   Once coliforms are into a neutral stomach then it is a matter of them competing with other organisms in a very rich environment and they would undoubtedly compete very well. I am sure there are many factors determining the flora of the stomach but the only one that we have been able to actually get to grips with is pH, and this problem of lactobacilli being more competitive once the pH is below 5.5, but less competitive above 5.5.   There is one other factor, an immune factor.   Hypogamma-globulinaemic patients have a very rich flora, much richer than patients with

59

achlorhydria but without hypogammaglobulinaemia. I do not know the role of bile reflux.

J. Alexander-Williams. I would like to ask about the possible relationship of the activation of pepsinogen to pepsin at pH 3.5. Do you think that there is any possible relationship between the presence of pepsin activated at pH 3.5 and the destruction of bacteria, or is it independent of proteolytic enzymes?

M. Hill. I think proteolytic enzymes will really speed up the destruction of bacteria but you can grow organisms in the presence of trypsin. I do not know about pepsin, but we have grown organisms in the presence of trypsin and they leak very badly but they do grow.

B. Golematis. These people suffering from duodenal ulcer, they have not received any kind of medical or surgical treatment. Are they in the low risk or high risk category of developing a gastric cancer?

V. Brookes. We have published some results on the incidence of gastric cancer following Billroth gastrectomies and vagotomy, but we also found there was a significant incidence of gastric cancer occurring in people who have a long history of duodenal ulcer, without surgery.

B. Golematis. Without medical treatment; without drugs?

V. Brookes. It would certainly be without cimetidine, because it was in the days before cimetidine and H$_2$ receptors. I presume they all would have had antacids because they all had been investigated in hospital. I think about 7% of the gastric cancer patients we saw had a previous proven history of duodenal ulcer, without surgery.

J. Alexander-Williams. The figures that we have presented of 34 patients having previous medical treatment out of 1,400 is less than the incidence that is quoted for the occurence of duodenal ulcer in the general population. These figures are in disagreement with your comments. I have always believed that there was an increased risk in gastric ulcer, which I think is generally accepted, of about ten times the normal risk, whereas this is not proven in duodenal ulcer.

V. Brookes. I suppose the answer to this question is what is the incidence of duodenal ulcer in the population?

B. Golematis. Is the incidence in the normal population more or less?

V. Brookes. I think the answer is that one does not really know what the incidence of duodenal ulcer is in the general population. I am only talking now about people with known gastric carcinoma, and what percentage of people in that group have had previous duodenal ulcers. The number who have had gastric ulcers is insignificant.

S. Glick. You said there was a high nitrate content in vegetables and is this only in vegetables which are grown in fertilized soil, or do the so-called 'naturally' grown vegetables have a lower content of nitrate? Secondly, regarding Mr. Williams' comment about cimetidine, do we need to revise our thoughts about the dosage of cimetidine? Are we giving a medical over-kill for our duodenal ulcer patients?

M. Hill. Nitrate content of vegetables is related to the amount of nitrate fertilizer that you add to the soil. As you increase the amount of fertilizer, you increase the nitrate content. It is related to the type of climate. If you have a nice dry summer then you will have a high nitrate content, but if you have an occasional wet summer then it goes down.

J. Alexander-Williams. I think the great advantage of medical hypochlorhydria is that the medicine can be discontinued and there may be theoretically some advantage in making the stomach anacid for a while, and then letting the acid recover. Tim Muscroft has some figures to support that.

T. Muscroft. Firstly, what we have shown is the worst possible situation for cimetidine. These people are taking 1 gram per day and have been fasting from midnight. They have 200 mg at 07.00 and are sampled at 09.00, which is not the way it is normally taken. In addition to that, we have tried to do longitudinal studies in people on normal diets and the pH seldom rises to that level and the bacteria correspondingly do not rise to that level. This is the worst case. I think it is important to consider what is actually happening from moment to moment rather than in abnormal situations.

V. Brookes. You have talked about the dosage of 1 gram per day. What happens, for example, to people on maintenance doses? I think you said it was an eight week course?

T. Muscroft. Yes.

V. Brookes. What happened to the people on night maintenance of just 400 mg?

T. Muscroft. As far as we can tell, that will occur after two weeks at least, as rapidly as that. People who are taking a maintenance dose of 400 mg at night will be sampled at 09.00 ie. 9 - 12 hours later. By and large they have sterile stomachs and a pH of 1-2.

W. Longmire. In some of the studies that were reported on migrant populations in New York City a number of years ago, it was suggested that environmental factors had their influence early in life and that then there was a long latent period. Have either of you gentlemen any comments with regard to this?

M. Hill. Correa (1975) put forward his hypothesis, that I showed in my last slide, to explain gastric cancer in a population where more than 50% of the people in the high incidence area were already achlorhydric at 30 years old. That is a high incidence in that age group. Now you can get similar figures in a very high incidence area in Chile, as well. That would indicate that the factors causing the initial achlorhydria were acting very early on and the rest of it followed remorselessly. I think that is the answer. Where you are looking at factors which cause the initial achlorhydria, then they act very early on. Where you are looking at exposure to things which cause the later stages then it does not matter, because if you have not had the initial exposure you still have a normal stomach and the exposure to nitrate, or anything else, will not matter.

E. Deutch.   Dr. Hirayama pointed out that there is a reduced rate of gastric cancer in patients taking lettuce. Dr. Hill points out that we have a high level of nitrates in the lettuce. How do you reconcile these two factors?

M. Hill. In the same way that I have just answered the previous question. Lettuces may be very very good in preventing achlorhydria developing. When you have got achlorhydria, then lettuce may not be so good for you.

P. Reid. I would like to raise one point made by Mr. Muscroft concerning the worst situation for cimetidine which he said was after an over-night fast after giving 200 mg of cimetidine shortly before sampling. Perhaps that is not such a bad situation considering the fact that in the normal course of events one always has breakfast when one is ingesting nitrites, and it might in fact be worse under these circumstances if you are taking cimetidine. There is therefore some debate on this. The other point is that we have looked at nitrosamine concentrations in gastric juices. In over 130 patients on cimetidine, and for quite a number of these we have serial studies, we have shown that there is a clear cut relationship between cimetidine and a pH increase and also an increase in nitrosamines, pari passu. In the same way once you discontinue the drug, the pH will drop, but interestingly enough even 8 weeks after discontinuing the drug the actual concentration of nitrosamine had not returned to its pre-treatment level. It would appear, therefore, that the post treatment fluctuations are much greater and the question does arise, "In what way has the environment been altered for a given period of time?"

J. Elder. It was shown some years ago by Browning and Mackay, who sampled the gastric juice of post truncal vagotomy patients, that significant colonization, that is greater than 10^5 micro-organisms per ml., were obtained within the first 10 days after surgery. But sequential sampling up to six months showed that this persisted in only a very few patients in their series, and I would hate people to go away with the idea that vagotomy is a cancer producing situation. After all, very few people after vagotomy do appear to get gastric cancer. But we still do not have enough data. I would like Dr. Hill's views on the sampling techniques after vagotomy. The question I want to ask Dr. Hill is, "What has happened to the theory that transnitrosating enzyme was associated with some of the bacteria that could change nitrates to nitrites?" Is that theory no longer held?

M. Hill. Well, I have never held it. I do not know about the people who held it in the first place. I remember it appeared in one paper which has never been repeated and is rarely commented on. As far as the sampling from vagotomy is concerned, I thought the evidence was that vagotomy was not associated with gastric cancer and was not associated with elevated pH. I have not done any of those studies. Mr. Williams reported those.

J. Alexander-Williams. That first slide that I showed with pH, and the one Mr. Muscroft showed with bacteria, followed each other exactly. Vagotomy alone, and vagotomy with pyloroplasty, produced a median pH of about 3. It is true that it did produce a few people that seemed to have basal achlorhydria or hypochlorhydria, but generally speaking they did not. Despite what our chairman says, I do not think that anywhere in the published figures in the world so far has there been anything to incriminate vagotomy per se as being carcinogenic in man.

J. Elder. Not even the 500 patients, reported by Ellis and his colleagues from Birmingham, with a 5.6% incidence of gastric carcinomas within 10 years?

J. Alexander-Williams. Yes, I said that was the isolated case but it has not been reported elsewhere.

P. Reid. Don't you think in this context it is the question of the drainage which is even more important than vagotomy itself? In other words, bile reflux must play a role.

J. Alexander-Williams. There is very good experimental evidence in animals that gastro-jejunostomy is dangerous but I do not think there is any evidence in man.

V. Brookes. I could have made the same comment myself. I did say vagotomy and drainage and in actural fact I also thought that the people who had simple gastroenterostomies, or even pyloroplasties without a vagotomy, also had this increased risk. But obviously the number available for study now that have operations is very small. But it probably is a drainage operation that plays a significant part.

P. Reid. Is this a combination of an operation that does increase the pH? If you
do a vagotomy, at least if you do a successful one, you are going to increase the
pH, whereas if you do a straight gastrojejunostomy, you are not going to influence
the pH.

V. Brookes. Do you think bile reflux would make any difference there?

P. Reid. It would be marginal.

M. Hill. One of the problems here is that we always do our analysis on resting
gastric juice samples and the resting gastric juice sample in even a successful
vagotomy, may well be fairly acid. The stomach is unable to respond to a meal, so
you will get a very neutral pH during meal times, and maybe that should be the time
to do the analyses in these patients.

J. Alexander-Williams. Don't you have some evidence on this Tim, about the effect of
a meal on vagotomised patients?

T. Mustcroft. No. We have done this with cimetidine. But it has been done on
vagotomised patients and the pH does not drop. According to Pounder who has done
some basic work on cimetidine, the pH on vagotomised people stayed below 2 most
of the time. This was just an aside in his paper.

Gastric Precancer States

M. Crespi* and N. Munoz**

*Regina Elena Institute for Cancer Research, Rome, Italy
**International Agency for Research on Cancer, Lyon, France

ABSTRACT

The definition of a precancerous lesion applies, for stomach cancer, to conditions such as: chronic atrophic gastritis (C.A.G.) with intestinal metaplasic (I.M.); pernicious anaemia and related gastric lesions; gastric polyps, mainly adenomatous; Menetrier' disease and, with some debate, gastric stumps more than 10 to 15 years after resection and chronic gastric ulcer. This purely positive approach, i.e. based on the prerequisite of a precise histologic lesion does not fulfil entirely the concept implied in the definition of "gastric precancer states" because many risk factors have been demonstrated to be closely related to an increased probability of developing stomach cancer. Environmental conditions play a major role, as proven beyond any doubt by a review of epidemiological data. It seems that unknown "determinants" of the disease probably act early in life and leave a permanent mark on the individual, as demonstrated by the decrease in stomach cancer as consequence of changing life style, expecially dietary habits in many countries and in migrant populations. These clearcut trends are observed also in the histological patterns with a decrease in the incidence of the "intestinal type" of gastric cancer.

The precancerous condition more significantly interrelated with the epidemiology of gastric cancer is C.A.G. with I.M., its incidence being definitely higher in populations with a higher incidence of gastric cancer and the incidence of stomach cancer in C.A.G. is higher than in controls. Furthermore, early gastric cancer arised in 84% of cases in areas of I.M. The "incomplete" type of I.M. seems closely related to development of stomach cancer as suggested by experimental evidence in animals. True precancerous changes in the gastric mucosa are the dysplastic or borderline lesions, of which a tentative classification is presented on clinical grounds. The synthesis, in vivo, of carcinogenic N-nitroso compounds from precursors widespread in the environment may represent the long searched for "natural carcinogen" responsible for the peculiar trends observed in the incidence of gastric cancer. These may also be the causative agents for C.A.G. and I.M. in their turn responsible for a further increase in the formation, in vivo, of carcinogenic N-nitroso compounds.

Preliminary data show the presence of N-nitroso diethylamine (NDEA) in the gastric juice of patients with C.A.G. but not in controls; total and volatile nitrosamines are also higher, a promising line of research.

KEYWORDS

Gastric cancer; precancerous lesions; dysplasia; nitrosamines; epidemiology;
histologic types; risk factors; intestinal metaplasia as precursor lesion;
intestinal metaplasia.

Gastric precancer states remain controversial, despite the extensive research
performed in the last twenty years. Among gastric precancer states, undoubtedly
prominent are the 'precancerous lesions' which are defined as 'histologic
alterations in which cancer may develop in a statistically significant number of
cases'. This definition corresponds closely to that of the WHO (1973) as a
'morphologically altered tissue in which cancer is more likely to occur than in its
apparently normal counterpart'.

For stomach cancer this definition applies to such lesions or conditions as:

1. Chronic atrophic gastritis (C.A.G.) with or without intestinal metaplasia (I.M.)
and pernicious anaemia with related gastric lesions, in which a 10% index of neoplastic transformation has been reported.

2. Menetrier's disease, in which the limited data suggests a 40% incidence of
cancer in long term follow-up.

3. Gastric stumps 15-20 years after gastric resection for benign conditions, in
which the risk is in the order of 2 to 5%. For this controversial issue, the
results of a 10 to 20 year follow-up of symptomatic cases after surgery for peptic
ulcer (Hoste and co-workers, 1978) are of interest; an incidence of 3.8% was found
in Billroth I against a 2.6% in Billroth II. In 1976, Domellof, Eriksson and
Janunger reported a 5.4% incidence of stump cancer in 74 patients. Dysplastic
changes in the gastric mucosa are often present after resection, as reported
(Mittelstaed, Borchard and Kieker, 1978) in 20% of patients with Billroth II and
in 5% of Billroth I. It is always difficult to compare this kind of data, which
are strictly dependent on patient selection and conclusive evidence is not
available. Animal data on rats (Dahm and Werner, 1976) confirm human evidence,
demonstrating that after Billroth I and II operations, adenocarcinomas of the
residual glandular stomach develop.

4. Adenomatous polyps are the lesions with the highest reported rates of
transformation, 40 - 70% become malignant (Ming, 1976; Nagayo, 1977). Gastric
adenomas are true neoplasms, capable of continued growth. These lesions are
frequently surrounded by atrophic mucosa and intestinal metaplasia. Considering
the different risk associated with hyperplastic type polyps, the most frequent
polypoid lesions of the stomach, it is mandatory to judge the true nature of such
lesions only on histological grounds. This is now possible by routine use of
endoscopic polypectomy. Hyperplastic polyps, which may be considered the result of
excessive regenerative hyperplasia in areas of chronic gastritis, although not
prone to become malignant, are a warning signal for the clinician due to the
reported high frequency of a coexisting carcinoma, eg. 28% of cases (Tomasuto, 1971).

5. Chronic gastric ulcer, the most discussed and debated condition, in which
endoscopy seems to have brought a final word, indicating that the rate of cancerization of a true benign chronic ulcer is actually low, in the order of 1 to 7%
(Wenger, Brandborg and Spellmann, 1971; Nagayo, 1977). But this approach, based on
the prerequisite of a specific histologic lesion, does not fulful entirely the
concept implied in the definition of 'gastric precancer states'. In fact, many
risk factors including diet, smoking, occupational hazards, (coal miners, workers
exposed to iron dust and silica), low socio-economic status and genetic influences

seem to exert a relevant influence in the 'cancer expectancy' and therefore
environmental and genetic factors are significant for gastric cancer. A review of
the established evidence on these factors seems important if we consider it worth
attempting to elucidate the natural history of gastric cancer. The incidence and
mortality of stomach cancer has been decreasing steadily in most countries and this
tendency seems, by some unknown factors, linked with changes in life style and
dietary habits brought by a sharp increase in the socio-economic status. Even in
Japan adjusted death rates have fallen from 45 in 1950 to 22.1 in 1976, which means
a decline of about 30% in the past 20 years (Hirayama, 1978). Retrospective and
prospective dietary questionnaires have demonstrated some risk factors, but also
have some protective factors (Table 1).

TABLE 1. Diet and Stomach Cancer

Risk Factors	Protective Factors	
Consumption of salty, smoked or fried foods	Consumption of green) vegetables (lettuce)) Vit. C) index	
Pickled vegetables	Fruits)	
Cereals, corn	Milk	

Studies in migrant populations bring further confirmation of the role of the
environment in the assessment of risk developing the disease. In migrants from
high risk countries for gastric cancer, like Japan, Poland and Norway, to U.S.,
it is only in the second generation that the death rates approach those of the
country of immigration (Haenszel and Segi, 1966). Similar data was obtained for
Japanese immigrants in California and recently confirmed in a study involving
mortality data for 3,065 countries in the U.S. (Hoover and co-workers, 1975). Of
striking interest for the possible relationships with the natural history and the
aetiology of the disease are the changing patterns of the histological types of
gastric cancer in countries such as Norway (Fig. 1) where a downward trend in
mortality for the disease has been observed (Munoz and Asvall, 1971). This trend
is mainly due to a lowering of the incidence of the 'intestinal type' of gastric
cancer (as defined following the Lauren-Jarvi classification), especially in
younger age groups; whilst the incidence of the 'diffuse type' (Figs. 2a and 2b)
remains constant.

This was also demonstrated in migrant populations (Correa and co-workers, 1973)
comparing the incidence rates of histologic type in the Miyagi prefecture in
Japan and in Japanese in Hawaii. The incidence of the 'diffuse type' of gastric
cancer remains constant but the 'intestinal type' is sharply decreasing amongst
Japanese migrants in Hawaii. We may conclude that the relationship between this
histological form of cancer and the trends in incidence in different countries is
well established and can also say that 'intestinal type' of stomach cancer constit-
utes the greatest proportion in high incidence areas, as demonstrated (Munoz and
Matko, 1972) by intestinal to diffuse ration in high and low risk areas (Table 2).

The evidence discussed up to now brings us back to the relationships between one
of the precancerous lesions previously listed, namely chronic atrophic gastritis,
with intestinal metaplasia and gastric cancer. In fact the incidence of this
disease, although widespread especially in older age groups, is significantly
higher in populations with high incidence of stomach cancer, as demonstrated on
postmortem specimens comparing Japan, Chile, Poland, New Zealand and U.S. (Imai,
Kubo and Watanabe, 1971); the incidence of C.A.G. and I.M. varies more than two
fold (from 40 to more than 90% depending on age) in Japanese compared to U.S. whites.

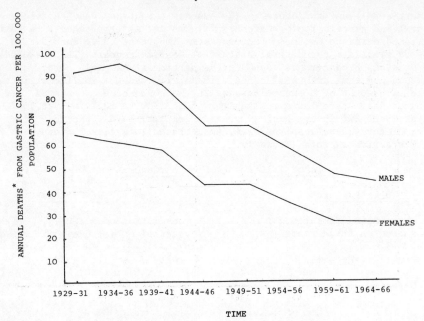

* STANDARDIZED (TO NORWEGIAN POPULATION ON JANUARY 1st 1956)

Fig. 1.   Time trends in standardized gastric cancer death rates per 100,000 in
          Norway, by sex.

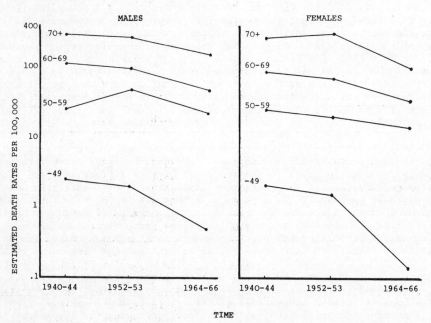

Fig. 2a.   Estimated age – and sex – specific death rates per 100,000 of 'intestinal'
           type of gastric cancer in Norway during 1940-1944, 1952-1953 and 1964-1966.

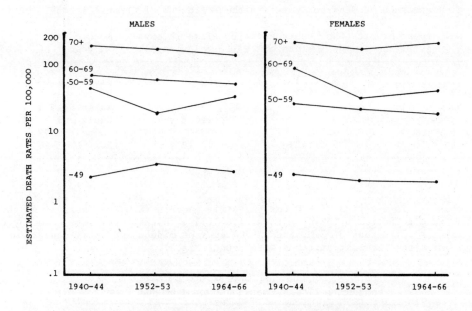

Fig. 2b. The same data as for Fig. 2a, for 'diffuse' type of gastric cancer.

TABLE 2. Histological Types of Gastric Cancer in High and Low Risk Areas.

| Geographic Areas | Total Cases | Histological Types (%) | | | Ratio Intestinal: Diffuse |
		Intestinal	Diffuse	Others	
High Risk Areas					
Cali-Colombia	191	51.8	34.0	14.1	1.52
Maribor-Yugoslavia	149	51.7	34.8	13.4	1.48
Gliwice-Poland	94	45.7	36.2	18.1	1.26
TOTAL	434	50.5	34.8	14.7	1.45
Low Risk Areas					
Cartagena-Colombia	38	28.9	55.3	15.8	0.52
Barranquilla-Colombia	13	38.5	46.1	15.4	0.83
Mexico City-Mexico	80	38.7	46.3	15.0	0.83
Koper-Yugoslavia	53	39.6	50.9	9.5	0.78
TOTAL	184	37.0	49.4	13.6	0.75

Similar findings were reported (Correa, Cuello and Duque, 1970) for populations at risk in Colombia; migrants to Cali from high incidence areas show a high prevalence of I.M., even in the younger age groups (15 years). This means that a lesion, suspected as being precancerous, is present early in life and implies that the still unknown 'determinants' or causative factors act probably in the first years of life and leave a permanent mark on the individual. Moreover, the incidence of stomach cancer in individuals with C.A.G. is, in long-term follow up studies, much higher than in controls (Table 3) and this difference is 'statistically significant'.

TABLE 3.   Incidence of Gastric Cancer in the Follow-Up of Chronic Atrophic Gastritis.

No. cases chronic gastritis	No. cases gastric cancer	Time interval (average)	Auth. and year
116	9 (9%)	10-15 y	Siurala 1966
123	9 (9%)	10 y	Hanik 1970
40	4 (10%)	9-22 y	Walker 1971
105	9 (9%)	11-18 y	Cheli 1972
278	9 (3%)	3-11 y	Munoz 1972
65	9 (14%)	10-17 y	Roesch 1980

Some recent evidence provides further data on the C.A.G. and I.M. to gastric cancer relationship. In a series of 600 early gastric cancers (E.G.C.) observed at the National Cancer Centre in Tokyo (Hirota, 1980), 551 (84.8%) were surrounded by or in continuity with areas of I.M. and in 70 cases of minute and small cancer (up to 10 mm in diameter) similar patterns were found (Fig.3).

Spatial Relation between Early Gastric Cancer and Intestinal Metaplasia Related to Histological Type.

Group	Histological Types	~ 5 mm diff.	~ 5 mm undiff.	6 ~ 10 mm diff.	6 ~ 10 mm undiff.	Total
1		17	0	29	1	47 (67.1%)
2		2	1	3	9	15 (21.4%)
3		0	2	0	0	2 (2.9%)
4		0	1	0	5	6 (8.6%)
Total		19	4	32	15	70 (100%)

T. Hirota. M.D.

Similar data are reported by Elster and Thomasko (1978): in 154 cases of E.G.C. of 'intestinal' type 70% arose in areas of I.M. and in 43% of cases, C.A.G. in the fundic region was also present.

Causes of C.A.G. and I.M. are still unknown despite extensive research work but some hypotheses point to an elevated nitrate intake or to the role of nitroso compounds. This hypothesis is quite stimulating if one considers the experimental evidence gathered in animals by administration of methyl-nitroso-guanidine and related compounds (Sugimura and Kawachi, 1973). One of these compounds, propylnitroso-guanidine (PNNG) provokes, in rats, intestinalization of the gastric mucosa and a few cancers (Sasajima and co-workers, 1979), suggesting that causative agents for both conditions could be common. We therefore can assume that C.A.G. and I.M. may represent important pathways leading to gastric malignancy, especially in high incidence areas, and this consideration gives us the opportunity to implement screening programs aimed at the early recognition of the disease (Crespi et al., 1978).   Intestinal metaplasia may also be the breeding groud for a further step towards malignancy: the appearance of a precancerous change. Its definition, i.e.

as 'histological findings indicating or suggesting that the lesion is on a course directed to the development of cancer' (Nagayo, 1977) is clear cut and quite different, in terms of clinical significance, to the one previously given for precancerous conditions. Moreover, very recent evidence points to the subdivision of I.M. into a 'complete' or 'incomplete' type, the latter being suspected to be more prone to develop malignancy (Jass and Filipe, 1979; Matsukura and co-workers, 1980). The differences between the two types are enzymatic and morphological (Table 7). This hypothesis is highly stimulating for the future possibility of an indirect enzymatic diagnosis of such a lesion.

TABLE 4. Types of Intestinal Metaplasia

Parameters	Complete (A)	Incomplete (B)
Cellular brush border	+	+
Goblet cells	+	+/-
Paneth cells	+	-
Tissue structure	regular	sometimes irregular
Sucrase	+	+
Maltase	+	+
Trehalase	+	-
Alkaline phosphatase	+	-

The precancerous changes, as previously defined, are also called 'dysplastic' for 'borderline' lesions. These are very confusing terms which are dangerously misleading to clinicians. Endoscopy has given us the opportunity to discover such changes in vivo and to follow them up, in order to assess their real malignant potential. This is the aim of one of the research projects of the International Study Group on Gastric Cancer (ISGGC), a free association of researchers interested in stomach cancer (1976). The protocol of this research (Table 5) is centered in the circulation of representative slide among the pathologists of the group, chaired by Dr. S.C. Ming, and in the final agreement on a classification of 'dysplastic' lesions.

Dysplasia is a broad concept but in practice, as Dr. Ming says, it "connotes a sinister aura and implies a high probability of malignant outcome". Disorders are at a cellular level, but also a disorganization of cellular arrangement is present. The essential histological nature of these lesions is the decreased potential for cell differentiation and the increased but disordered proliferating capacity. Up to now dysplasia has been classified according to a different grading system, but there is more and more evidence that only the most advanced degrees may be labelled as real precancerous changes, as in the one proposed by ISGGC (Table 6). A pre-liminary and tentative comparison of the different classifications, prepared by Dr. Ming, is also under trial (Table 7). The main point is to avoid the term dysplasia when no definite evidence of possible malignant transformation is present, in order to avoid misleading information to clinicians. This work is now in progress.

A final topic, on which epidemiological data are attracting a growing interest for its possible implication in the mechanism of gastric carcinogenesis in humans, is the possible implication of the nitrosamines. In fact, the possibly carcinogenic N-nitroso compounds synthesised in vivo from precursors widespread in the environment (nitrates, nitrites, secondary and tertiary amines and amides), may be the 'natural carcinogens' responsible for the peculiar trends observed in the

TABLE 5. Collaborative Study on Atypical Lesions in Gastric Mucosa

INTERNATIONAL STUDY GROUP ON GASTRIC CANCER (ISGGC)

AIMS
  Assessment of histopathological criteria for borderline and dysplastic
  lesions of gastric mucosa with special emphasis to their clinical
  significance

PRELIMINARY AGREEMENT ON CLASSIFICATION
  Mild
  Severe
  Borderline

IMPLEMENTATION
  Circulation of representative slides

INSTITUTIONS INVOLVED
  ISGGC Collaborating Centres

TIME
  1978-1980

FINAL CLASSIFICATION
  ISGGC Committee of pathologists

TABLE 6. Gastric Dysplasia Classification Proposed by the International Study Group
on Gastric Cancer.

CHARACTERISTICS	SIMPLE HYPERPLASIA	ATYPICAL HYPERPLASIA	DYSPLASIA	BORDERLINE
Cystic Dilation	++	++	+	+
Branching of Glands	++	++	+	+
Mucus	+++	+	+/-	-
N/C Ratio	↑	↑	↑	↑
Shape of Nucleus	Normal	Normal	Rod Shape	Rod Shape
Location of Nucleus	Basal	Basal	Central or Superficial	Central or Superficial
Pseudostratification	+/-	+	+++	+++
Mitoses	+/-	+	++	+++

TABLE 7.   Classification of Gastric Dysplasia.

NAGAYO GROUP	1 (Normal)	2 (Slight Atypia)	3 (Borderline Lesion)	4 (Probable Cancer)	5 (Definite Cancer)
MING		1 (Regenerative Changes)	2 (Proliferative Changes)	3 (Dysplasia)	4 (Borderline)
WHO GROUP		(Regenerative Changes)	Mild ←————— Dysplasia —→ Severe		
ISGGC SUGGESTED		Simple Hyperplasia	Atypical ←——— Dysplasia —→ Borderline Hyperplasia	Lesion	

incidence of gastric cancer. These compounds could also be postulated as causative
agents for C.A.G. and I.M. (Correa and co-workers, 1975), as previously discussed,
and these latter lesions may be in their turn responsible for a further increase
in the formation in vivo of carcinogenic nitroso-compounds. A project on nitrosamines and gastric cancer, proposed by Dr. N. Munoz, is among the aims of the ISGGC
and is based on the assessment of individual exposure to in vivo formed nitrosamines in patients with and without precancerous lesions. The dose of total and
volatile nitrosamines in samples of gastric juice, blood, and urines in selected
population groups in countries at different risk for gastric cancer, together with
the histological assessment of gastric mucosa, is part of the protocol. Preliminary
data gathered by the ongoing pilot study performed by the Regina Elena Institute in
cooperation with the International Agency for research on Cancer, show that total
volatile nitrosamines in gastric juice have their highest value at pH 4.5 in C.A.G.
patients and that the values are significantly higher in comparison with normal
controls (Fig. 4).

NITROSAMINES IN GASTRIC JUICES

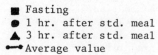

Fasting
1 hr. after std. meal
3 hr. after std. meal
Average value

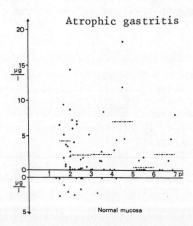

Fig. 4. Nitrosamines in gastric juice.

Furthermore, the nean values of both total volatile nitrosamines and nitrosomethyl-
amine (NDMA) are higher in C.A.G. patients than controls. Although the range is
too wide to provide significance to the data, it is of interest that the highest
values are observed in gastritis patients and not in controls (Fig. 5.).

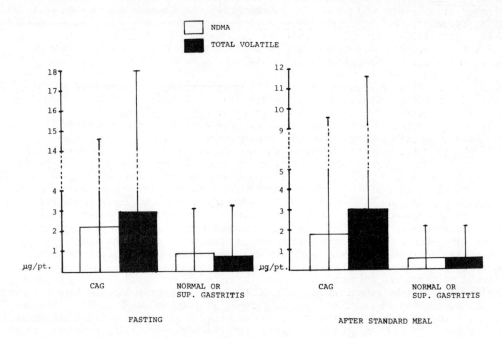

Fig. 5. Level of nitrosamines in gastric juice of 47 subjects submitted to
         endoscopy.

Another point of interest is that a specific nitroso-compound, nitroso-diethylamine,
seems to be formed only in the stomach of chronic gastritis patients. Further
work is in progress. Methods for the measurement of nitrosamines and nitrosamides
are still in a developmental stage, but this line of research seems one of the more
promising in order to elucidate what we may define as the earliest step leading
to 'gastric precancer states'.

REFERENCES

Correa, P., C. Cuello, and E. Duque (1970). Carcinoma and intestinal metaplasia
of the stomach in Colombian migrants. J. Nat. Cancer Inst. 44, 297-306.
Correa, P., N. Sasano, G. Stemmermann, and W. Haenszel (1973). Pathology of gastric
carcinoma in Japanese populations; comparisons between Myagi prefecture, Japan and
Hawaii. J. Nat. Cancer. Inst., 51, 1449-1459.
Correa, P., W. Haenszel, C. Cuello, S. Tannenbaum, M. Archer (1975). A model for
gastric cancer epidemiology. Lancet ii, 58-60.
Crespi, M., V. Casale, A. Grassi, and C. Maggio (1978). Results and prospectives of
a screening for gastric cancer and precancerous lesions of the stomach. Acta
Endoscopica, 8, 73-85.
Dahm, K., and Werner B. (1976). Susceptibility of the resected stomach to experi-
mental carcinogenesis. Z. Krebsforsch, 85, 219-229
Domellof, L.S., Eriksson and K.G. Janunger (1976). Late precancerous changes and
carcinoma of the gastric stump after Billroth I resection. Am. J. Surg., 132, 26-31.

Elster, K., and A. Thomasko (1978). Klinische Wertung der histologischen Typen des Magenfrühkarzinous. Eine Analyse von 300 Fällen. Lever Magen Darm, 8, 319-327.

Haenszel, W., and M. Segi (1967). Stomach cancer among the Japanese. In UICC Monograph Series, vol 10. Springer Verlag, Berlin, pp. 55-63.

Hirayama, T. (1978). Outline of stomach cancer screening in Japan. In A.B. Miller (Ed.), Screening in Cancer, UICC Technical Report Series, Vo. 40, Geneva, pp. 264-278.

Hirota, T. (1980). Personal communication.

Hoover R., T.J. Mason, F.W. Kay, and J.F. Fraumeni (1975). Geographic patterns on cancer mortality in the United States. In J.F. Fraumeni (Ed.), Persons at high risk of cancer, Academic Press, New York, pp. 343-360.

Hoste, P., G. Elewant, G. Mortier, and F. Barbier (1978). The role of endoscopy in the diagnosis of esophageal and gastric disease in patients following gastric surgery. A review of 402 patients. Acta Gastroent. Belg., 41, 18-27.

International Study Group on Gastric Cancer (1976). M. Crespi (Ed.), Report of the first meeting, Siofok, Hungary.

Imai, T., T. Kubo, and H. Watanabe (1971). Chronic gastritis in Japanese with reference to high incidence of gastric carcinoma. J. Nat. Cancer Inst., 47, 179-195.

Jass, J.R. and M.I. Filipe (1979). A variant of intestinal metaplasia associated with gastric carcinoma: a histochemical study. Histopathology, 3, 191-199.

Matsukura, N., K. Suzuki, T. Kawachi, M. Aoyagy, T. Sugimura, H. Kitoaka, H. Numajiri, A. Shirota, M. Habashi, and T. Hirota (1980). Distribution of marker enzymes and mucin in intestinal metaplasia in human stomach and relation of complete and incomplete types of intestinal metaplasia to minute gastric carcinomas. J. Nat. Cancer Inst., in press.

Ming, S.C. (1976). II. Malignant potential of gastric polyps. Gastrointest. Radiol., 1, 121-125.

Mittelstaed, A., F. Borchard, and W.R. Kieker (1978). Zur haufigkeit von epithel-dysplasien im resektionsmagen. Akt. Gastrologie, 7, 433-441

Munoz, N. and J. Asvall (1971). Time trends of intestinal and diffuse types of gastric cancer in Norway. Int. J. Cancer, 8, 144-157.

Munoz, M., and I. Matko (1972). Histologic types of gastric cancer and its rela-tionship with intestinal metaplasia. In Recent Results Cancer Res., 39, 99-105.

Nagayo, T. (1977). Precursors of human gastric cancer: their frequencies and histological characteristics. In E. Farber et al., (Eds.) Pathophysiology of Carcinogenesis in Digestive Organs., Univ. of Tokyo Press, Tokyo, pp. 151-161.

Sasajima, K., T. Kawachi, N. Matsukura, T. Sano, and T. Sugimura (1979). Intestinal metaplasia and adenocarcinoma induced in the stomach of rats by N-propyl-N-nitro-N-nitrosoguandine. J. Cancer Res. Clin. Oncol., 94, 201-206.

Sugimura, T. and T. Kawachi (1973). Experimental stomach cancer. Methods in Cancer Res., 7, 245-308.

Tomasuto, J. (1971). Gastric polyps. Histologic types and their relationship to gastric carcinoma. Cancer, 27, 1346-1355.

Wenger, J., L.L. Brandborg, and F.A. Spellmann (1971). The Veterans Administration cooperative study on gastric ulcer, Chapt. 6, Gastroenterology, 61. 598-605.

DISCUSSION

K. Lewin. We always hear about the question of intestinal metaplasia being so important in the development of carcinoma but if one looks at chronic gastritis, intestinal metaplasia and pyloric metaplasia are almost invariable accompaniments of the damage. Has anyone looked into the question of whether it is the intestinal metaplasia or just the chronic gastritis which predisposes to carcinoma? In other words, is it possible that intestinal metaplasia is something we see but is just part of the chronic gastritis and, therefore, is not really the predisposing lesion, it is the chronic gastritis which is?

M. Crespi. This is the old question, which comes first, the chicken or the egg? This is the reason why I am personally quite shocked by the Japanese data, shown to you by Dr. Hirayama of the National Cancer Centre, because of the degree of accordance that there is between the intestinalisation of the gastric mucosa and the very early cases of cancer that none of us ever see. I am referring to the minute cancers from 1 - 5 mm, and the frequency of their occurrence in metaplastic mucosa. If you consider all the other evidence, mainly epidemiologicl, I would say that this is why we have to go on, after 30 or 40 years, asking this kind of question again. We have a biological lesion which could mean that we have more chance of getting cancer. This biological lesion is epidemiologically associated in a very clear cut fashion with a high incidence area of gastric cancer. The small cancers arise in this kind of mucosa. It is possible that this has nothing to do with it, but there is convincing evidence that it has.

K. Lewin. But if you look at cases of pernicious anaemia, there are a good series of them, you will see that intestinal metaplasia occurs in every single case. Does that mean, therefore, that cancer is related to intestinal metaplasia? It may just mean that this is one of the features of injury to the mucosa.

M. Crespi. It is possible, but what I think is that we have all the evidence in front of our eyes so why don't you trust it? That is the point. There are 20% of cases of cancer which are not associated with intestinal metaplasia, but this is not the problem. The problem is to see if the other 80% has some meaning.

Methods and Results (Cost-Effectiveness) of Gastric Cancer Screening

T. Hirayama

Epidemiology Division, National Cancer Center
Research Institute, Tokyo, Japan

ABSTRACT

Methods and results of gastric cancer mass screening are outlined.

The age adjusted death rate for stomach cancer has been on a downward trend during the past 20 years in Japan. During the same
period gastric cancer mass screening has been actively conducted
using mass radiography, over 3 million people being screened
annually.

Lower stomach cancer mortality was observed in the screened group
compared to the unscreened group by follow-up studies using life
table methods.

The extent of decline in gastric cancer death rates is higher in age
groups where the rate of mass screening is higher.

The extent of decline in gastric cancer death rates in each of 46
prefectures was noted to be associated with both the extent of
dietary improvement and the rate of mass screening.

Possibilities of the effect of lead time bias and length bias are
discussed.

Declining tendency of cost-effectiveness of mass screening in recent
years is shown and possible reasons are   considered.

Measures to enhance the efficiency and to minimize the risk of mass
screening are discussed with special reference to the need for
focussing screening to high risk groups.

KEYWORDS

Gastric cancer; mass screening; cost-effectiveness; Japan.

INTRODUCTION

30,770 men and 19,836 women died of gastric cancer in 1979 in Japan.
Although it is still the leading site of cancer in Japan, the age
adjusted death rate for gastric cancer has steadily come down in
recent years, the rate in men being 45.0 in 1950, 42.1 in 1970 and
32.9 in 1978 and in women 28.6 in 1950, 26.7 in 1970 and 20.4 in
1978. This decreasing tendency is most striking at 40-69 years of
age both in men and women, showing over 40% decline during the past
29 years. A similar downward trend was also observed in incidence
rates in the cancer registries in Osaka and Miyagi. It is important
to note that gastric cancer screening has been actively conducted
using mass radiography during these periods. The purpose of this
paper is to outline methods and results of such mass screening
activities.

RATE OF SCREENING BY AGE GROUPS

Over 3 million people are screened annually by mass gastrography in
Japan and the age specific rates of screened persons per 1,000
population in 1975 were highest at 40-69 years of age in both men
and women. There is a tendency that the extent of decline in
gastric cancer death rate is higher in the age groups where the rate
of mass screening is higher.(Fig. 1)

Fig. 1

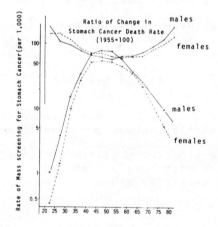

Ratio of Change in Stomach Cancer Death Rate
in 1955 and in 1975 and Rate of Mass screening
for Stomach Cancer in 1975 by Sex and Age Groups

Although the recent decline in gastric cancer in Japan is interpreted as a reflection of dietary improvement of the Japanese people, some of the decrease might be attributed to the effect of a nationwide early detection programme in recent years, since the age groups in which gastric cancer mortality markedly decreased correspond to the age groups for which current mass screening programme was mainly practiced.

METHOD OF MASS SCREENING

Early detection programmes for gastric cancer have been carried out widely since 1960. The number examined by mass radiography for gastric cancer and the number detected in 1975 are 3,087,031 and 3,022 respectively. In nearly 90% of the mass screenings conducted in each prefecture by mobile X-ray unit, 5-7 films were taken and methods were well standardized.

Reasons requiring 6 exposures are as follows:

During mass examinations, one exposure with barium full in the stomach and the patient upright covers only a small part of the stomach, but with increasing numbers of exposures in different positions one can examine more of the stomach. After careful study six exposures in different position were decided as the standard method by the Japanese Society of Mass Screening.

The detectability of gastric cancer has increased substantially using the double contrast technique. With double contrast, radiating folds of mucosa emanating from the lesion show up clearly as one of the important markers which facilitate its identification. Early stage cancers are being found by such method in much higher percentage than conventional methods of X-ray diagnosis.

RESULTS OF MASS SCREENING

57.4% of the cases of gastric cancer detected by screening in 1973-75 were without lymph node metastases.(Table 1)

Table 1 Depth of Cancerous Invasion in Operated Cases and Presence or Absence of Metastasis(1973-75)

		Metastasis (−)	Metastasis (+)	Total	%
Limited in Mucosa	(m)	673	37	710	21.2
Infiltrated to Submucosa	(sm)	685	119	804	24.0
Up to Proper Muscle	(pm)	271	275	546	16.3
Penetrated to Proper Muscle	(ss)	117	302	419	12.5
Penetrated to Serosa	(s)	174	691	865	25.9
Total		1920	1424	3344	100.0
%		57.4	42.6	100.0	

21.2% of lesions were limited to mucosa(m), 24.0% infltrated to
submucosa(sm), 16% to proper muscle(pm), 12.5% penetrated proper
muscle(ss) and 25.9% were penetrated to serosa(s). Percent without
metastasis were 94.8% in m, 85.2% in sm, 49.6% in pm, 27.9% in ss,
and 20.1% in s.

Thus two distinctly different groups of gastric cancer patients are
detected by mass screening, one without metastases mostly limited in
the mucosa (m) or infiltrated to the submucosa only (sm) and one
with metastasis and mostly penetrating to the serosa. The high
frequency of the former group would explain the fact that five and
ten year survival rates are significantly higher in patients detected
by such mass screening, compared to the survival rate in the
unscreened group.

The ten year survival rates for m, sm, pm, ss and s were 90%, 69%
45% and 25% respectively in a follow up study of 470 cases of
gastric cancer by Dr. Hisamichi.

EVALUATION OF MASS SCREENING

The results of follow-up of screened persons clearly showed a significant reduction in gastric cancer adjusted death rate compared
to unscreened persons: 144.32 out of 33,865 screened person-years
and 176.82 out of 388,175 unscreened person-years respectively
(study in Kanagawa Prefecture 1962-71). Similar results have been
reported from Tottori (99.3 in screened versus 139.8 in unscreened
group) and Osaka (162.4 in screened versus 255.2 in unscreened
group). Attention should, however, be paid to the fact none of
these were randomized trials as they would have been extremely
difficult, if not impossible, to carry out in actual situations.
In a study in Kanagawa prefecture, the social and educational back-
grounds of screened and unscreened persons were compared retro-
spectively and no essential difference was found. Such post-
screening comparability study could, but partially, remedy the
drawbacks inherent in unrandomized studies.

Although attention should be given to the possible effect of so-
called lead time bias, 5, and 10 year survival rates in patients
detected by mass screening are too high to be explained by such lead
time bias only. Rather more serious concern is the possible
influence of so-called length bias or bias detecting predominantly
slow glowing tumors. At this moment it is difficult to exclude the
influence possibly arising from such length bias.

COMBINED EFFECT WITH DIETARY IMPROVEMENT

The trends in age-specific mortality rates for gastric cancer were
studied in 46 prefectures in Japan. These prefectures were
classified into four groups according to the extent of decline in
gastric cancer mortality rate in the 40 to 74 age groups. The
extent of decline in age specific gastric cancer death rates was
higher in the prefectures where the rate of screening by mass
gastrography was high. The extent of decline was highest when both
consumption of milk and eggs and also rate of screening was higher
than the national average. Therefore the recent decline in gastric

cancer mortality in Japan should be interpreted as the reflection of
dietary improvement in Japan, just as in other developed countries,
and also partly influenced by the effect of early detection.

SIDE-BENEFIT OF MASS SCREENING

In addition to gastric cancer, many other diseases are detected by
mass-gastrography. In 1975, 8,326 gastric polyps, 41,725 gastric
ulcers, 24,430 duodenal ulcers and 5,226 gastric-duodenum ulcers
were detected in addition to 3,002 gastric cancers.

Observation of detection rates by sex and age revealed interesting
epidemiological patterns such as female preponderance of gastric
polyps, and a younger age peak in duodenal ulcers. Thus mass-
screening is also useful for early detection of these abnormalities
and valuable for the epidemiological study of such diseases.

DECLINING TENDENCY OF COST-EFFECTIVENESS

As shown in Table 2, rate of detection of gastric cancer cases by
mass-screening is declining in recent years. These are considered
to be due to (1) increased proportion of repeatedly examined persons
in screened population and (2) decrease of gastric cancer incidence
as recorded in cancer registry in recent years. Whatever the reason,
one has to admit that the cost-effectiveness of mass-screening is
gradually on the decrease in Japan.

Table 2   STOMACH CANCER MASS SCREENING IN JAPAN
                NUMBER SCREENED AND NUMBER DETECTED

	NUMBER SCREENED	NUMBER DETECTED	RATE PER 1,000
1966	989,762	1,444	1.45
1967	1,334,933	1,839	1.38
1968	1,565,845	2,139	1.37
1969	1,825,861	2,319	1.27
1970	2,165,287	2,360	1.09
1971	2,400,550	2,521	1.05
1972	2,627,156	2,519	0.96
1973	2,707,926	2,721	1.00
1974	2,833,656	2,847	1.00
1975	2,779,399	2,804	1.01
1976	2,965,582	2,821	0.95
1977	3,165,805	2,910	0.92
1978	3,197,594	3,035	0.95

HOW TO IMPROVE COST-EFFECTIVENESS OF MASS SCREENING

Cost-effectiveness   of mass screening programmes in gastric cancer control should be improved by carefully studying these results and also available local resources, funds, and facilities. A focal attack approach is also necessary. One focus would be population groups never examined before. For instance, the screening programme should be focused on sales workers as the existing lower rate of decline of gastric cancer mortality in sales workers was interpreted, at least partly, as a reflection of their exceedingly lower rate of screening especially at 40-54 years of age.

Another focus should be the so-called high risk groups. In order to make the current screening programme more effective, it is of utmost importance to delineate gastric cancer high risk groups as precisely as possible and concentrate screening to such groups. Intensive epidemiological studies on high risk groups are therefore of urgent necessity especially in Japan.

APPROACHES TO MINIMIZE RISK OF MASS SCREENING

To solve realistically existing burning problems of possible radiation effects due to repeated mass radiography, efforts are in progress to improve X-ray apparatus to drastically reduce exposure dose, to enhance film sensitivity, to lengthen examination intervals and, as mentioned above, to concentrate mass screening to groups with the highest risk of gastric cancer and the lowest risk of leukemia and other possible radiation effects. A careful monitoring of leukemia incidence and other radiation related conditions in the screened group is currently in progress. At this time no excess incidence of leukemia has been observed in the screened group compared to the general population in the Osaka Cancer Registry. Out of 33,221 persons screened by mass gastrography in Osaka, 7 cases of leukemia occurred during 6.1 years of follow-up while 7.9 cases were expected. However, in view of the rapid increase in leukemia death rates after age 40 in Japan since 1965, further careful follow-up of the effect of nationwide mass radiography appears to be necessary.

REFERENCES

Hirayama, T. (1975). Cancer Res., 35, 3460-3463.
Hirayama, T. (1963). Bul, Inst. Public Health, 12, 85.
Hirayama, T. (1968). Gann Monogr., 3, 15-27.
Hirayama, T. (1971). Gann Monogr., 11, 3-19.
Hirayama, T. (1975). Proc. XI Int. Cancer Congress., American
    Elsevier.
Kitabatake, T., M. Yoneyama, M. Sakka, and S. Koga (1973). Igaku no
    Ayumi, 84, 445-448.
Hirayama, T. (1977). Origins of Human Cancer. Cold Spring Habor
    Laboratory, New York.

DISCUSSION

M. Keighley. If you once screen the population, when do you re-screen them and how frequently do you do it?

T. Hirayama. Annual examination is recommended. Recently, for various reasons including a possible radiation effect and depending on the efficiency of the examinations, less frequent investigations have been recommended. Because we are examining only 3 million people in a year there are so many people who are never screened. Therefore, administrativly speaking, wider intervals allowing more people to be examined are recommended. Quite recently the Minister of Health and Welfare proposed a budget to examine everybody at the age of 50. I do not know whether this budget has been accepted or not, but this has been proposed officially. This relfects the fact that most of the people involved in gastric mass screening now have a tendency to prolong the interval. I understand that the majority of people agree that intervals of 2 - 3 years would be considered suitable except for some groups which need more careful follow-up, after the initial examination.

V. Brookes. I did not quite understand the figure on the board, Dr. Hirayama, $15.7. Is this for each examination or per patient that you found with gastric cancer?

T. Hirayama. It is for a 6 exposure X-ray examination. Formally it was $3 but because of inflation it went up. This particular figure is obtained when we examine 100,000 people aged 40 and over. I think we found 60 cases of gastric cancer and out of these, 40 were considered to have a very good prognosis. This is the figure given by the Minister of Health. Forty per 100,000 examined. So the cost effectiveness, where you want to calculate this, depends on what value you put on the life of these forty patients.

G. Giles. So these are 40 early gastric cancers and the cost of these 40 is 100,000 x $15.

T. Hirayama. Yes. Of course, in addition, one will need a careful examination and one must allow for the cost of treatment.

F. Smith. For the patients you detected what was the average number of screening times that they had gone through? That might give you an indication of the lag-time and of whether you are dealing with an indolent malignant process.

T. Hirayama. The majority of gastric cancers are detected by initial examination and some are detected by subsequent examination. There is a 2 - 3 times higher detection rate in the initial examination compared to subsequent examinations.

G. Giles. How do you explain that?

T. Hirayama. Well, in the initial examination we detect the prevalent cases.

G. Giles. Are many of these patients symptomatic, which is why they come for screening?

T. Hirayama. They are asymptomatic.

G. Giles. You are picking up a reservoir in the population at first screening?

T. Hirayama. Yes, that is correct.

V. Brookes. One might expect the number to increase every year with a captive population because the age of gastric cancer at first diagnosis is going up. ie. if you find 40 out of 100, 000 in the first year, you would expect to find 40 or

40+ in the second year, and so on.

G. Giles. Dr. Hirayama did say that it is the prevalence in the community that you are screening. It is not the same cohort each time as I understand it. It is the prevalence occuring within the initial screen that is the forty per year. Thereafter the yield for repeated screens would go down, so that the pick-up rate and the cost effectiveness declines with the 2nd, 3rd, 4th and so on, screening.

T. Hirayama. That is right.

F. Smith. Do you follow the patients who are negative on screening? Have any of this group developed gastric cancer? Have there been some patients who have in fact been screened, and then developed gastric cancer? Do you know the number?

T. Hirayama. Yes, many cases. In research projects there is 100% follow-up but even in mass screening the former 'negative' persons are re-examined and actually some new cases are found. These are the incidence cases and, of course, some are misdiagnosed cases, but that kind of rate has also been carefully calculated.

M. Crespi. What is the false negative figure?

T. Hirayama. The false negative rate is sharply on the decline and that is one reason why many experts in this programme accept the idea of prolonging the intervals. Initially the false negaive rate was rather high, but now it is very low.

G. Giles. Do we understand then from what you have said, and from what you have implied, that you now feel that the best cost-effective programme you can have is one screen of everyone aged 50?

T. Hirayama. Yes, and then if it is possible to re-examine them 3-5 years later.

G. Giles. Do you screen before the age of 50?

T. Hirayama. Well, although there is a need to be examined below 50 the cost-effectiveness is not as good.

G. Giles. The best yield is when you screen everybody at the age of 50?

T. Hirayama. This is not my calculation, that is what the Government have decided.

E. Deutch. You showed one graph with males and females starting with gastric ulcer at age 40. If you adopt this later edict about only doing the screening at 50, you will lose this group. If there is an exposure which goes over 20 years, I do not think we should drop the 40 age group, especially for anyone who has a gastric ulcer.

T. Hirayama. I agree.

Application of Serum and Gastric Juice Tumour Markers to Early Diagnosis and Screening of Gastric Cancer

I. Häkkinen

Department of Pathology, University of Turku, Turku, Finland

ABSTRACT

So far no cancer-specific marker has been found for gastric cancer. Consequently, diagnosis using biochemical methods has not been possible. A review of three onco-foetal antigens, AFP, the CEA-group and FSA, gives hope for a screening tool provided that gastric juice is used as the sample source. Until now, only FSA has been studied in practice.

KEYWORDS

Tumour markers; oncofoetal antigens; gastric cancer; cancer screening.

INTRODUCTION

So far, no tumour-specific antigen has been detected in cancerous human gastric cells (when this definition is used in its narrowest sense). Consequently, no immunological or other biochemical test is available which would justify the submission of a patient for a gastric cancer operation. Histological criteria are still the most decisive factors for this.

Nevertheless, tumour-associated antigens have been shown to be associated with gastric cancer. These are α-foetoprotein (AFP), the carcinoembryonic antigen (CEA) group, and foetal sialo glycoprotein antigen (FSA). These three antigens belong to the oncofoetal antigen group. Because of the early spread of gastric cancer its early diagnosis is even more important than e.g. colonic cancer. Therefore, unlike colonic cancer, little benefit is derived from the postoperative monitoring of gastric cancer patients using antigen determinations for the purpose of further investigative operations. An immunological test which gives positive results only in advanced cancer cases is of no use for gastric cancer.

It is surprising how slowly the fact has been accepted that serum determinations are rarely positive in early cancer cases despite the large number of clinical series carried out for both AFP and CEA (Freeman and co-workers, 1979; Fujimoto, Kitsukawa,and Itoh, 1979; Ravry and co-workers, 1974; Satake and co-workers, 1980). A very sensitive test is no solution. To obtain an elevated level of these antigens in the circulation, breakdown of the mucosal microanatomy is necessary,and this results only from tumour invasion. How can it otherwise be explained that there are CEA-like antigen substances in the colonic mucosa (Khoo and co-workers, 1973; Martin and Martin, 1972) and lavages (Egan and co-workers, 1977; Go and co-workers, 1975) but only a minimum basal concentration in the serum even though the colonic mucosa as a producing organ certainly matches the local tumour cell population. Colonic polyps are reported to produce CEA (Isaacson and Le Vann, 1976;Winawer, 1975), but the serum levels are not necessarily elevated (Costanza and co-workers, 1974).

The concept of malignant cell transformation is that it is a stepwise procedure (Culliton, 1972), and the cell can remain in an intermediate stage. Appearance of foetal antigens is one of the early expressions of this development. Examples are colon polyps with elevated CEA (Isaacson and Le Vann, 1976), reappearance of blood group antigen (Cooper, Cox, and Patchefsky, 1980), and FSA in the cancerous gastric mucosa outside the malignant growth (Häkkinen, Järvi,and Grönroos, 1968). The gastric mucosa undergoes morphological changes,and atrophic gastritis is considered in the broad sense as a precancerous state.To what extent oncofoetal antigens are expressed in the gastric mucosa and especially in the gastric juice is a central and interesting question. Studies on this problem are just beginning with regard to AFP and CEA. Limitations to studies on FSA arise from the qualitative nature of this assay. However, this marker has already shown that it can select a risk group which includes a significant number of silent gastric cancers (Häkkinen and co-workers, 1980). Our present knowledge of these three markers in regard to the stomach as well as their usefulness as a screening test for early detection of gastric cancer will be discussed below.

AFP

The study by Gitlin, Pericelli, and Gitlin (1972) indicates that α-foetoprotein is also synthetized in the foetal gastrointestinal epithelium. In some cases gastric cancer cells also produce AFP as is shown by immunohistological techniques (Lee and co-workers, 1979; Okita and co-workers, 1977). Most probably, however, this is an exception and the elevated levels of AFP in the serum of gastric cancer patients which are reported to be found quite frequently (Masseyeff, 1979;Masseyeff and co-workers, 1977) are usually stimulated by liver metastasis.

The occurrence of AFP in gastric juice has not been studied. Due to the ontogenic basis in the gastrointestinal tract for the appearance of AFP (Lee and co-workers, 1979) it is possible that AFP is expressed in the transformation of gastric mucosal cells more frequently than is evident from studies on the gastric cancer cells. This means that we cannot yet exclude AFP as a useful marker for screening when gastric juice is the source material.

CEA

Results of several groups of investigators show that serum determination of CEA does not help much in the diagnosis or screening of gastric cancer (Freeman and co-workers, 1979; Fujimoto, Kitsukawa, and Itoh, 1979; Hine and co-workers, 1978; Plow and Edgington, 1979; Satake and co-workers, 1980).

Healthy gastric mucosa secretes a CEA-like glycoprotein (Go and co-workers, 1975; Vuento and co-workers, 1976) which is not necessarily distinct from the cancerous colonic CEA. The gastric milieu with its digestive properties could be responsible for the minor differences between them. Reproducibility of gastric juice samples and the problem of quantitation of the CEA assay have been discussed in a recent study on gastric juice CEA (Bunn and co-workers, 1979). It is claimed that the determination of either K^+ or total proteins is necessary to give a quantitative

CEA assay. Even so, some error will be caused by variations in protein secretion among other things. It is also necessary to avoid the destruction of CEA by preventing its intragastric digestion by pepsin. When a large-scale screening of CEA is designed it will be necessary to simplify the procedure of collecting samples so that it is quickly performed and tolerated well. Preferably, gastric juice from a stomach fasted overnight could be harvested by washing with a buffer solution, as it is described below.

Immunohistological studies (Mori and co-workers, 1979: Rapp and Wurster, 1979) on the appearance of CEA in gastric cancer cells indicate that both CEA positive and CEA negative gastric cancer cells exist. Of course immunohistological specimens do not exclude the possibility that cancer cells in different parts of the same tumour belong to a different category. Non-malignant but morphologically altered gastric mucosal cells can also be CEA productive,e.g. in metaplasia (Mori and co-workers, 1979; Rapp and Wurster, 1979). Elevated levels of CEA in gastric juice can there- fore derive either from non-malignant or malignant gastric cell populations or from both of them. In cases where an early mucosal cancer of a few mm size is concerned, the majority of elevated amounts of CEA most probably derive from non- malignant cells.

Results of CEA analyses performed on gastric juice are in accordance with the above concept (Bunn and co-workers, 1979: Fujimoto, Kitsukawa, and Itoh, 1979: Kawaharada, Yachi, and Wada, 1979: Satake and co-workers, 1980). According to these studies nearly all gastric cancers and advanced atrophic gastrites are CEA positive. We must,however, regard these results with caution. They are pilot studies. Controls for these materials are few and accidental. Atrophic gastritis or even early cancer cannot be excluded by a few biopsies. The age distribution of the groups, which may be of importance, is also not stated. However, these pilot results justify a thorough study of the problem.

FSA

The first immunological evidence which showed the existence of FSA, a glycoprotein antigen of cancerous gastric juice, came at the time when the first articles on CEA appeared (Häkkinen, 1966, 1967). Since FSA is far less known than the two other oncofoetal antigens, AFP and CEA, a brief survey of its characteristics is justified.

FSA was originally partially purified from cancerous gastric juice. Immunohisto- logical studies revealed that it appears as a normal component of the foetal alimentary canal mucosa (Häkkinen, Saxén, and Korhonen, 1968). It was also observed that except for its regular presence in the gastric cancer cells the antigen could occasionally be found in non-malignant mucosal cells of the cancerous gastric mucosa, thus changing the original concept of its cancer specificity (Häkkinen, Järvi, and Grönroos, 1968).

The first clinical study pointed to the possibility that FSA is a regular component of cancerous gastric juice (96 % of FSA positives out of 78 clinical cancer cases) but it was also found in 12 % of benign conditions of the stomach (material from our Surgical Clinic). Healthy young people (circa 20 years) serving as controls have all been FSA negative (Häkkinen and Viikari, 1969).

A quantitative method lacking (Häkkinen, 1974a), the qualitative immunodiffusion technique remained as the only possibility for demonstration the presence of the antigen in gastric juice. Empirically, a scale was tested where all clinical gastric cancer cases were FSA positive. For this purpose hundreds of proven gastric cancer cases were tested for FSA.

The final procedure is carried out on gastric juice samples which have been
collected from a non-stimulated stomach fasted overnight. The subject swallows
100 ml of PBS[1](0.1 M, pH 6.5) immediately after which an oral tube is introduced
and the gastric washing allowed to run into a collection bottle (yield approximately
100 ml). Addition of phenol red to 100 samples of gastric juice showed that the
PBS diluted the gastric juice by a factor of 1.o - 1.5 (equivalent to 40-50 ml of
gastric juice) with surprisingly little variation. X-ray analysis using gastro-
graphin-labelled PBS demonstrated that buffer swallowed by the subject is quicker
and more thoroughly mixed than buffer introduced by a tube.

FSA is an acid glycoprotein and can therefore be precipitated by polycationic
detergent (cetyl pyridinium chloride) together with other acid glycoproteins which
together form a minority of the gastric juice macromolecules. An approximate 200-
fold concentration is possible with one single precipitation. In practice, 35 ml
of the original sample results in a final sample dissolved in 0.2 ml of saline for
the immunodiffusion run (Häkkinen, 1976).

As the preliminary tests proved encouraging, a mass-screening of a healthy
population of "gastric cancer age" (40 to 70 years) was carried out using the FSA
immunodiffusion test on gastric juice samples. The results of this screening gave
3 % of FSA positives for an industrial population (ca. 12,000 tested samples)(Häkkinen, 1974b), and 8.8 % of FSA positives for an unselected rural population (ca.
40,000 samples tested so far)(Häkkinen and co-workers, 1980). A clinical examination
(gastroscopy) was performed on all FSA positive subjects (95.2 % accepted gastroscopy). In the following, the clinical results of the rural population material
are presented. The percentage of participation was 74.8 %.

TABLE 1   Clinical Findings (Gastroscopy) in 3,508 FSA-Positive
Subjects from 39,706 Rural People in Ages 40-70 Years

Gastroscopy finding and histological diagnosis	Number of cases
Gastric cancer	35
Gastric carcinoid	1
Tubular adenoma	10
Atrophic gastritis	346
Superficial gastritis	
(verified by biopsy)	250
(no biopsy)	614
Erosive gastritis/gastric erosion	43
Peptic ulcer	45
Polyp(s)	153

Detection of all these cancer cases was based solely on the FSA screening. Only in
6 cases clinical symptoms could be noted, all other cases were totally silent.
Table 2 represents the gastric cancer cases according to the depth of invasion.
In 28 cases the operation could be considered radical , and 8 cases were inoperable.
Postoperative follow-up (at present over two years in all but five cases) showed
a stump recurrence in one case (now radically operated); except for one case all
other radically operated cases have remained symptom-free and without clinical
evidence of a recurrence. Table 3 illustrates our results of the 3-year follow-
up of the rural population screening. The benefit ratio for each year is
calculated in Table 4.

[1]PBS - Phosphate buffered saline.

TABLE 2 Extent of Cancerous Invasion
Gastric Cancers Detected by FSA Screening

Depth of invasion	Number of cases
Limited to mucosa	9
to submucosa	10
to musc.propria	4
to subserosa	2
Extending to serosa and surroundings	11
Metastasis in lymph nodes	12

TABLE 3 Distribution of New Gastric Cancer Cases in the FSA-
Positive and FSA-Negative Groups Respectively for
Each Year of Follow-Up

	FSA +			FSA −			All participants		
	Number of cancers			Number of cancers			Number of cancers		
Year	per year	total (up to year)	calcul.* (up to year)	per year	total (up to year)	calcul.* (up to year)	per year	total (up to year)	calcul.* (up tp year)
	per 3,493			per 36,187			per 39,680		
1.	27	27	2	10	10	21	37	37	23
2.	3	30	4	15	25	43	18	55	47
3.	4	34	6	13	38	64	17	72	70

* According to the Finnish Cancer Registry.

TABLE 4 Benefit Ratios (ref.Table 3)

Year	FSA + Rate of cancers	FSA − Rate of cancers FSA −	Benefit ratio
1.	0.773 %	0,028 %	27.6 : 1
2.	0.859 %	0.069 %	12.4 : 1
3.	0.973 %	0.105 %	9.3 : 1

The average duration of the macroscopical latent period of gastric cancer is not known precisely. Some facts point to a two-year latency (Fogh, 1974; Hanai and Fujimoto, 1977; Hisamichi and co-workers, 1978; Kawai, 1978). On the other hand, we know of cases with a fast growing pattern. Some first year cancers "missed" by FSA have been verified as technical laboratory errors or as specimens of inferior quality. This happened more frequently during the beginning of the study, due to inexperience. We have to suppose a biological variation of the onset of elevated FSA secretion prior to the beginning of possible malignant growth. Some of the missed cases may have had a short lead time,and they were in fact non-malignant at the moment of sample collection. Most of these cases belong to the histological diffuse type. A second sample of gastric juice has not been available preoperatively from every FSA negative cancer. Four FSA negative cancer cases have been met where immunohistologically the surgical sample showed the presence of FSA. In 14 cases a technical error in laboratory procedure or sample collection could in retrospect be tracked. But there are cases left which can be true FSA negative. The exact frequency has been difficult to track.

Our 3-year follow-up shows that there is a drop in the number of manifested cancer cases in the years following the active screening. This points to the fact that the early symptom-free cancer cases which were detected belong to the time period considered.

The idea of the FSA screening can be summarized as follows: It is assumed that during the period preceding the development of cancer biochemically transformed mucosal cells secrete FSA. Hence its amount in gastric juice does not directly correspond with the number of cancer cells present. Even early cancers might fall into the group of FSA-positives. If the percentage of FSA-positive subjects in a population were not too great, endoscopy could then be used to confirm the presence of asymptomatic cancers.

The exact quantitation of the secreted components in gastric juice is impossible. The experience gained from the FSA screening shows that a qualitative empirically adjusted method is justified if the results are meaningful as in this case. It is expected that a qualitative FSA-immunodiffusion method will be used in future work side by side with a quantitative FSA-RIA method which is likely to be developed in the near future.

The physicochemical properties of FSA have been clarified only recently. Final purification became possible and chemical analysis of its macromolecular structure has been carried out (Häkkinen, 1980). An earlier immunological observation that a compatible blood group antigen, other than the specific FS-antigen, could co-exist in the same glycoprotein (Häkkinen, 1974c) gained further evidence from the structural nature of FSA being very similar to known blood group substances.

TABLE 5   The Chemical Composition of FSA of Gastric Juice

	Percentage
Galactose	13.5
Fucose	7.4
Glucosamine	24.5
Galactosamine	16.9
Sialic acid	5.4
Sulphate	trace
Amino acids	32.3
Aspartic acid	2.1
Threonine	5.6
Serine	3.2
Glutamic acid	2.9
Proline	2.6
Glycine	1.6
Alanine	1.6
Valine	1.6
Isoleucine	1.7
Leucine	2.5
Tyrosine	0.4
Phenylalanine	0.6
Lysine	1.2
Histidine	0.5

Arginine   1.2
Cystine   0.4
Cysteine+cystine   1.9
Tryptophan   0.8
Molecular size (SDS electrophoresis)   160 000 daltons

FSA appeared not to be sulphonated, the acid character coming apparently from the carboxyl groups. The renomination of the antigen was necessary as foetal sialo glycoprotein antigen (FSA). The tendency to aggregate which is one of the characteristics of FSA explains the many unsuccessful attempts made by other investigators to repeat the purification procedure of FSA, when using too sophisticated methods.

Gastric ulcer is connected with a risk of malignancy (Hauser, 1926; Oota, 1968). We studied the frequency of FSA positivity in clinical stomach ulcer material.

TABLE 6   Frequency of FSA Positives Among Patients with
          Gastric Diseases

Gastric disorder	Frequency of FSA secretion
Duodenal ulcer	17 / 85 = 20.0 %
Pyloric ulcer	9 / 35 = 25.7 %
Chronic gastric ulcer	32 / 59 = 54.2 %
Gastric cancer (all cases)	153 / 168= 91.1 %
Malignant ulcer	14 / 14 = 100.o %

The three oncofoetal antigens AFP, CEA and FSA possess a practical screening capacity for gastric cancer but only FSA has been studied so far. The required condition is that the sample is obtained directly from the target organ,i.e. gastric juice. No evidence exists that any of these markers could be used for the direct diagnosis of gastric cancer. However, it may be possible to use the FSA test as one diagnostic criterium for evaluating the possible risk of malignancy of a gastric ulcer.

ACKNOWLEDGEMENT

This work was supported by National Cancer Institute contract N01-CB-64070 and by a research contract with the Finnish Cancer Society and the KELA.

REFERENCES

Bunn,P.A., M.I.Cohen, L.Widerlite, J.L.Nugent, M.J.Matthews,and J.D.Minna (1979) Gastroenterology, 76, 734-741.
Costanza,M.E., S.Das, L.Nathanson,A.Rule,and R.S.Schwartz (1974). Cancer, 33, 583-590.
Cooper,H.S., J.Cox,and A.S.Patchefsky (1980). Am.J.Clin.Pathol.,73, 345-350.
Culliton,B.J. (1972). Science, 177, 44-47.
Egan,M.L., D.G.Pritchard, C.W.Todd,and V.L.W.Go (1977). Cancer Res.,37, 2638-2643.
Fogh,B. (1974). Ugeskrift for Laeger, 44, 2455-2457.
Freeman,J.G., A.L.Latner, G.A.Turner,and C.W.Venables (1979). Lancet, I, 210.
Fujimoto,S., Y.Kitsukawa,and K.Itoh (1980). Ann.Surg.,189, 34-38.
Gitlin,D., A.Pericelli,and G.Gitlin (1972). Cancer Res.,32, 979-982.
Go,V.L.W., H.V.Ammon, K.H.Holtermuller, E.Krag,and S.F.Phillips (1975). Cancer,

        36, 2346-2350.
Häkkinen,I.(1966). Scand.J.Gastroenterol., 1, 28-32.
Häkkinen,I.(1967). Scand.J.Gastroenterol., 2, 39-43.
Häkkinen,I.(1974a). Transplant.Rev., 20, 61-76.
Häkkinen,I.(1974b). Cancer Res., 34, 3069-3072.
Häkkinen,I.(1974c). Int.Arch.Allergy, 47, 380-387.
Häkkinen,I.(1976). Skandia Internalional Symposia on Health Control in Detection
        of Cancer, Almqvist & Wiksell, Stockholm, pp.105-113.
Häkkinen,I.(1980). Clin.exp.Immunol.,41, in press.
Häkkinen,I., O.Järvi,and J.Grönroos.(1968). Int.J.Cancer, 3, 572-581.
Häkkinen,I.,L.Saxén,and L.Korhonen (1968). Int.J.Cancer, 3, 582-591.
Häkkinen,I.,and S.Viikari (1969). Ann.Surg., 169, 277-281.
Häkkinen,I., R.Heinonen, M.V.Inberg, O.H.Järvi, P.Vaajalahti,and S.Viikari (1980).
        Cancer Res., in press.
Hanai,A.,and I.Fujimoto (1977). Epidemiology of Stomach Cancer: Key Questions and
        Answers, WHO Collaborating Center for Evaluation of Methods of Diagnosis and
        Treatment of Stomach Cancer,c/o National Cancer Center,Tokyo,Japan, pp.21-33.
Hauser,G.(1926).Handb.Spez.Path.Anat.Histol. IV/1, Springer,Berlin.
Hine,K.R., S.N.Booth, J.C.Leonard,and P.W.Dykes (1978). Lancet, II,1337-1340.
Hisamichi,S., M.Sugawara, A.Fuchigami, K.Aikawa, Y.Chuma, Y.Takeuchi, K.Takahashi,
        K.Yoshikawa, R.Fujita, T.Iinuma, T.Yamada,and H.Ichikawa (1978). Gan.No.
        Rinsho, 24, 189-194.
Isaacson,P.,and H.P.Le Vann (1976). Cancer, 38, 1348-1356.
Kawaharada,M., A.Yachi,and T.Wada (1979). Carcino-Embryonic Proteins Chemistry,
        Biology, Clinical Applications, Vol.II, Elsevier/North-Holland Biomedical
        Press, Amsterdam.New York.Oxford, pp.105-108.
Kawai,K.(1978). Clin.Gastroent.,7, 605-622.
Khoo,S.K., N.L.Warner, J.T.Lie,and I.R.Mackay (1973). Int.J.Cancer, 11, 681-687.
Lee,P.K., T.Mori, N.Fujimoto, T.Nakamura, M.Masuzawa,and G.Kosaki (1979). Carcino-
        Embryonic Proteins Chemistry, Biology, Clinical Application, Vil.II, Elsevier/
        North-Holland Biomedical Press, Amsterdam.New York.Oxford, pp.373-378.
Martin,F.,and M.S.Martin (1972). Int.J.Cancer, 9, 641-647.
Masseyeff,R.F.(1979). Immunodiagnosis of Cancer,Part I, Marcel Dekker,Inc.,New
        York and Basel,pp.117-130.
Masseyeff,R., J.F.Rey, R.Maiolini, B.Krebs,and J.Delmont (1977). Rend.Gastroenterol.
        9, 91-96.
Mori,T., P.K.Lee, Y.Nakajo, K.Awata,and G.Kosaki (1979). Carcino-Embryonic Proteins
        Chemistry, Biology, Clinical Application, Vol.II, Elsevier/North-Holland Bio-
        medical Press, Amsterdam.New York.Oxford, pp.23-28.
Okita,K., K.Noda, T.Kodama, T.Takenami, Y.Fukumoto, R.Fuji, M.Odawara, Y.Iida,
        M.Hayakawa, K.Shigeta, Y.Okazaki,and T.Takemoto (1977). Gastroenterologia
        Japonica, 12, 400-406.
Oota,K. (1968). GANN Monogr.,3, 141-151.
Plow,E.F.,and T.S.Edgington (1979). Immunodiagnosis of Cancer,Part I, Marcel Dekker,
        Inc.,New York and Basel,pp.181-239,
Rapp,W.,and K.Wurster (1979). Carcino-Embryonic Proteins Chemistry, Biology,
        Clinical Application,Vol.II, Elsevier/North-Holland Biomedical Press, Amster-
        dam.New York.Oxford, pp.29-38.
Ravry,M., K.R.McIntire, C.G.Moertel, T.A.Waldman, A.J.Schutt,and V.L.W.Go (1974).
        J.Natl.Cancer Inst.,52, 1019-1021.,
Satake,K., K.Yamashita, T.Kitamura, Y.Tei,and K.Umeyama (1980). Am.J.Surg.,139,
        714-718.
Winawer,S.J.(1975). Natl.Large Bowel Cancer Project Newsletter,3, 7-9.
Vuento,M., E.Engvall, M.Seppälä,and E.Ruoslahti (1976). Int.J.Cancer, 18, 156-160.

DISCUSSION

G. Giles. This complements what we have heard from Dr. Hirayama. It looks as though the yield is about the same with the combination of your initial screening and follow-up gastroscopy. Could you tell me what happened to the other 30,000 subjects who were FSA negative? Have you been able to prolong follow-up in this group of patients?

I. Häkkinen. I showed you one slide where we had followed them all. We have a very effective local follow-up. All the hospitals operating in this area have follow-up systems and health personnel make enquiries to help us, so I think that we pick up nearly all cases.

G. Giles. Up to now, have there been any false negatives in your area?

I. Häkkinen. Three years after taking the samples, half of the cancers still fall into the FSA positive group, and the other half are FSA negative.

T. Feizi. What proportion of documented cancers are positive by your standards?

I. Häkkinen. For all established cases of gastric cancer we have a large material and 91-95% are positive. We have very few early gastric cancers in the clinics.

G. Giles. But is it the same high yeild of percentage positives?

I. Häkkinen. Yes.

J. Elder. Do you find your positives are related in any communities: brother, sister, uncles and cousins? Are there any families in which you can see a high incidence of FSA positives or is it not related to clans?

I. Häkkinen. It is not related to clans, but there certainly are differences between different communities. I can detect certain cancer communities, compared with others.

T. Feizi. You mentioned that your substance resembles blood group substances from its composition. Does it have blood group activity?

I. Häkkinen. It has, but not regularly. Immunodiffusion data using anti-blood group antisera and anti-FSA antisera on the same plate showed that we could find blood group activity in some of the antigen preparations, but not all.

D. Day. Do you have any data on the pathology of the gastric cancers which were FSA postive?

I. Häkkinen. We have a slight tendency to find more diffuse cancers in the antigen negative group and the possible explanation could be the faster growth of this type of cancer.

G. Giles. I would like to ask a simplistic question as a clinician. Is there any way in which you can increase the yield of markers in gastric juice by in some way producing a mild mucosal injury? Does that increase the likely yield perhaps of CEA. Peppers, for example, will increase mucosal proliferation and is this likely to be connected with marker-levels?

I. Häkkinen. It is certainly connected with stimulation of mucous secretion because they are mucous components.

G. Giles. Do you think that the combination of some form of stimulant would increase the yield and make it a more sensitive test?

I. Häkkinen. It could be. I don't know that.

H. Thompson. Did any of the patients with carcinoid tumour have pernicious
anaemia? I am interested in this since in the recent literature some patients
with pernicious anaemia have been described with carcinoid polyps, and these polyps
pursue a relatively benign course?

I. Häkkinen. We have only one case so far of real gastric carcinoid in this series
and it was totally without tumour, but was diffusely spread over all the stomach.

K. Ibrahim. Have you looked in the gastric juice for lactic dehydrogenase?

I. Häkkinen. No. I have no experience of this.

T. Feizi. Is you antigen found in the intestinal tract as a normal component? In
other words, is this an aberrant appearance of a normally intestinal antigen in
the stomach?

I. Häkkinen. I have only immunohistological studies which were done in the middle
of the 60's where we examined most tissues and organs in the tumour, and we
could find it only in gastric mucosa. It was also present in certain colonic
tissues but we also found totally negative colonic tissue. We concluded that it
was not prevalent in the colon but how often it is there we cannot say, because
immunohistology is not the right method to look for this.

R. Pichlmayr. Is the ratio of well differentiated cancers higher in the group
which were found by screening than that normally found?

I. Häkkinen. It was about the same as in the clinical material.

R. Pichlmayr. So the better results cannot be a consequence of this?

I. Häkkinen. No.

Histopathology of Gastric Cancer

D.W. Day

Department of Pathology, Duncan Building,
Royal Liverpool Hospital, Liverpool, U.K.

INTRODUCTION

When a large series of cases of gastric adenocarcinoma is examined microscopically there is a marked variation in their structure. This diversity is apparent not only between different tumours but not infrequently occurs as well in different areas of an individual tumour. Perhaps this is not surprising when one considers the complex nature of the normal gastric mucosa with its varied cell types as well as its proneness to undergo transformation to an intestinal type of epithelium-intestinal metaplasia. Because of this variability, a complicated nomenclature arose in an attempt to describe the appearances of the tumour and any products of secretion, as well as the nature of the stroma. This inevitably gave rise to confusion and together with the lack of clear correlation between microscopic grading and gross patterns of the tumours led the American pathologist Stout (1953) to state that histological classification was valueless and that a knowledge of the gross appearance of the tumours was more valuable in diagnosis and assessment of prognosis. However, this view is not held by the majority of pathologists and in this chapter the several systems of classification in current use will be outlined. The histological findings in so-called early gastric cancer will also be discussed together with insights into the possible histogenesis and pathogenesis of gastric cancer that they provide.

HISTOLOGICAL CLASSIFICATIONS OF GASTRIC CANCER

Classification of the World Health Organisation

The classification proposed by the World Health Organisation (Oota, 1977) divides adenocarcinoma of the stomach into papillary, tubular, mucinous and signet-ring cell types, the typing of any particular tumour being based on its predominant component. Papillary adenocarcinomas are composed of pointed or blunt finger-like epithelial processes with fibrous cores. Some tubular formation may be present but the papillary pattern predominates, particularly in cystic structures. Typically this tumour grows as a polypoid mass into the lumen of the stomach. Tubular adenocarcinomas consist of branching glands embedded in or surrounded by a fibrous stroma. Large amounts of mucin are present in the mucinous adenocarcinoma which is often visible in the gross specimen. In some tumours dilated glands contain mucin which may be present as well in the interstitium, whereas in other varieties disintegrated epithelial components are seen as ribbons or groups of cells floating in lakes of mucin. Signet-ring cell carcinomas

are composed mainly of isolated tumour cells with large amounts of intracellular mucin and
often associated with considerable fibrosis. All these types of tumour may be graded as well,
moderately, or poorly-differentiated. In this classification undifferentiated carcinomas and
unclassified carcinomas are separate groups.

The Lauren Classification

This classification, which has been widely used in epidemiological studies, was based on a
pathological examination of operative specimens of gastric cancer collected at the University
of Turku, Finland between 1945 and 1964 (Lauren, 1965). It cuts across the classical descrip-
tions and allocates gastric carcinomas into two main groups, intestinal type and diffuse type.
These differ not only in their general and cellular structure, secretion of mucus and mode of
growth but in their clinical correlations.

In general, intestinal type carcinomas have a glandular structure often with papillary or solid
areas and are made up of large clearly defined pleomorphic cells with large, variably shaped
and hyperchromatic nuclei often in mitosis. Well polarised, columnar cells with a well-
developed brush border are usually observed lining glandular lumina (Fig. 1) and secretion if
present tends to be extra cellular or to occur focally in the cytoplasm in a minority of cells.

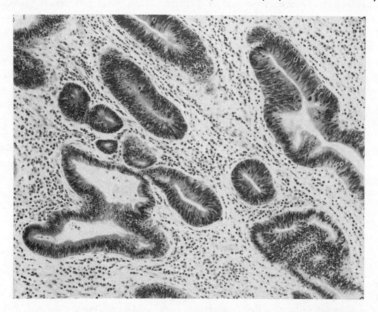

Fig. 1   Intestinal type carcinoma.   H & E, x 132

Diffuse type carcinomas are composed of separated single or small clusters of cells. Occasionally a more solid or aggregated appearance is present but even then the cells are only loosely

attached to each other. A glandular structure is uncommon and when present the lumina are small and poorly defined. Individual cells are small and uniform with indistinct cytoplasm and regular, often pyknotic nuclei in which mitoses are infrequent. In the few tumours with gland ⌐mation the lining cells are unpolarised and when a surface brush border is present it is sparse   ~ Mucin secretion is always present and usually extensive throughout the tumour,   istributed in the cytoplasm of the majority of cells. If extracellular, secreted   ed in the stroma.

            vth in the two types of tumour varies. Thus intestinal carcinomas are mostly   show considerable variation in structure in different parts. Inflammatory cell   ally profuse. Diffuse carcinomas have a more uniform structure, are not so   definea, ..d are characterised by a wider spread in the mucosa. As a rule connective tissue proliferation is more marked and inflammatory cell infiltration less prominent than in intestinal type carcinomas (Fig. 2).

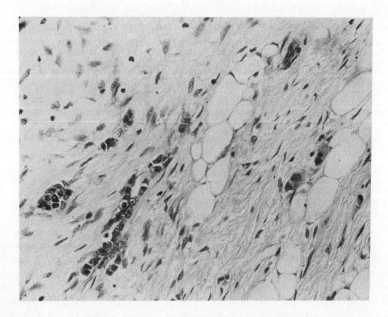

Fig. 2   Diffuse type carcinoma. Small groups of
carcinoma cells are separated by fibrous tissue. H & E, x 132

Solid and mucinous tumours can occur in both groups but are distinguishable on structural grounds.

Grossly in Lauren's series, 60 per cent of the intestinal type tumours were polypoid or fungating, 25 per cent excavated and 15 per cent infiltrating whereas the corresponding figures for diffuse carcinoma were 31, 26 and 43 per cent respectively.

An important difference was the increased frequency and extent of intestinal metaplasia

(Fig. 3) in non-tumorous mucosa in the intestinal group compared with the diffuse type carcinomas.

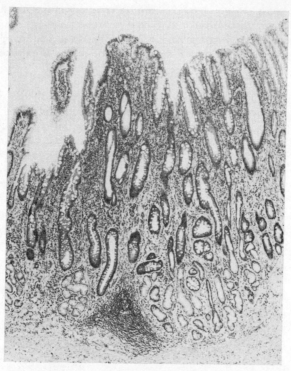

Fig. 3   Intestinal metaplasia.   H & E, x 60

Overall 53 per cent of the tumours were classed as intestinal, 33 per cent diffuse and 14 per cent unclassified because of their atypical or poorly differentiated structure. When the histology was correlated with clinical features it was found that the mean age of patients with intestinal tumours was 55.4 years and there was a 2 to 1 male : female ratio. With diffuse carcinomas the sex ratio was approximately one and the mean age of the patients 47.7 years. The three year survival rate in the 153 patients with 'curative' treatment was 43 per cent in those with intestinal type tumours and 35 per cent in the group with diffuse tumours.

The structural and clinical characteristics of the two types of tumour led Lauren to suggest that their aetiology and pathogenesis might be different.

The Classification of Mulligan and Rember

In their analysis of 297 gastric carcinomas in 290 patients seen at the Colorado General Hospital between 1927 and 1973, Mulligan and Rember (1954) allocated them into three groups: mucous cell carcinoma (45.2 per cent of the total); pylorocardiac gland cell carcinoma (28.3 per cent) and intestinal cell carcinoma (23.4 per cent). In the latter group, five patients had two primary tumours each and one had three separate primary tumours. In nine patients (3.1 per cent) it was not possible to classify the tumour.

The main difference between this classification and that of Lauren is the recognition of the pylorocardiac gland cell carcinoma as a distinct group. These tumours are well demarcated and fungate into the lumen of the stomach or are sometimes widely ulcerated and fibrosed. Microscopically, varying-sized glands are lined by stratified or singly orientated low to tall cylindrical cells. When singly orientated there is often striking vacuolation giving rise to clear cells (Fig. 4) which stain brilliantly with the periodic acid-Schiff reagent. Papillary

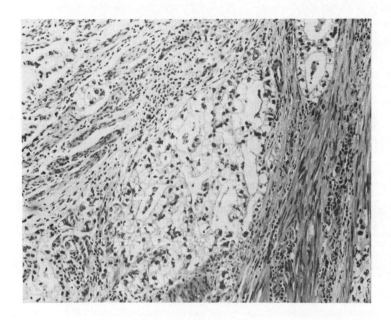

Fig. 4   Pylorocardiac gland cell carcinoma. H & E, x 150

infolding of the glands is sometimes conspicuous or the lining cells may be flattened by inspissated secretion so that an endothelial or mesothelial appearance results. Tumours have a tendency to be sited in the antrum or at the cardia and as their name suggests are presumed to arise from the epithelial cells of the pyloric and cardiac glands deep in the gastric mucosa. The male : female ratio for this type of tumour in Mulligan and Rember's material was 4.13 compared with 2.81 for the whole series.

Classification of Ming

This classification, resulting from a study of 171 gastric carcinomas (Ming, 1977), divides tumours into an expanding type (67 per cent) and an infiltrative type (33 per cent). In the former case tumour cells grow en masse and by expansion, and result in the formation of discrete tumour nodules (Fig. 5), whereas tumour cells of the infiltrative type penetrate individually and widely, eventually resulting in diffuse involvement of the stomach (Fig. 6).

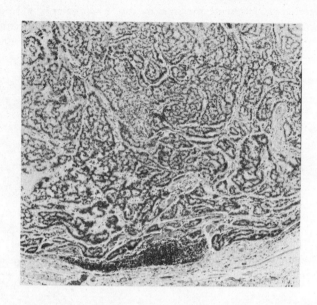

Fig. 5 Expanding type tumour.   H & E, x 60

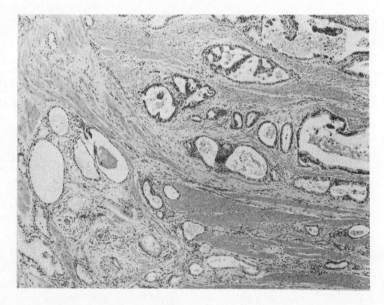

Fig. 6   Infiltrating type tumour.   Glandular structures
invading muscle.   H & E, x 60

The primary emphasis in this classification is not the architectural structure of the tumours but
their biological behaviour as manifest by their growth patterns. Both types of tumour showed
varying degrees of cell maturation but glands were much more common in expanding carcinomas.
Their was some correlation of the two types with their gross appearance. Thus among the expanding type the tumour was fungating in 63 per cent, ulcerated in 20 per cent, polypoid in
10 per cent, superficial in 4 per cent and diffuse in 3 per cent. With the infiltrative type the
carcinoma was diffuse in 68 per cent, ulcerated in 27 per cent and fungated in 5 per cent.
The two types of tumour appeared to have a different histogenesis. Both types were composed
of mucus-producing cells which could vary within the same tumour. Acidic mucin was common,
although many tumour cells secreted neutral glycoprotein, and goblet cells were frequent,
suggesting that both types of tumour originated from metaplastic glands. In the case of expanding tumours there was intestinal metaplasia in the adjacent mucosa of the vast majority which
was extensive in half of the cases, and intraglandular carcinoma and dysplasia of the metaplastic glands was frequent. However, intestinal metaplasia was much less common with infiltrative carcinoma and dysplasia was not seen, with intraglandular carcinoma cells being rare
and when present occurring in non-metaplastic glands. Thus the development of infiltrative
carcinoma did not seem to be related to intestinal metaplasia.

Expanding carcinomas, whatever their degree of differentiation, tended to be surrounded by
small amounts of fibrous tissue often associated with varying numbers of lymphocytes and
plasma cells, whereas the tumour cells of infiltrative carcinoma were mostly embedded in a
densely collagenous and relatively acellular connective tissue. Expanding carcinomas were
twice as common in males as in females. Infiltrative carcinomas were equally distributed
between the sexes. Both types of cancer occurred predominantly in patients older than 50 years
of age but infiltrative carcinoma was more common under the age of 50, particularly in females.

Relative Merits of the Different Classifications

To be of maximum benefit a histological classification of tumours should fulfill three criteria.
Firstly it should be easy to apply by different pathologists and be reproducible. Secondly it
should aid in the assessment of the prognosis of the different types of tumour. Thirdly it should
relate to the histogenesis and if possible the aetiology of the several types of tumour.

The WHO classification fulfils the first criterion if not the latter two, although a considerable
proportion of tumours fall into the undifferentiated and unclassified groups and tumours of
mixed appearance are classified according to the predominant component. However it is of
undoubted value as a standard descriptive classification in routine work and serves as a base
for achieving international uniformity.

The Lauren classification, which is also outlined in the WHO fascicle, has been widely used
in epidemiological investigations and a number of studies have shown that the proportion of
intestinal type tumours is greater in high gastric cancer incidence areas than in low incidence
areas and that when the gastric cancer risk is reduced in a population it is the intestinal type
of tumour that accounts for most of the reduction (Correa, Cuello and Duque, 1970; Munoz
and others, 1968; Munoz and Asvall, 1971). An association of gastric cancer with blood
group A is stronger for the diffuse type tumour than the intestinal type. Opposing results were
found by Kubo (1971, 1973) in studies of the histological types of gastric cancer in the United
States of America, Japan and New Zealand, who found similar proportions of the two types of
cancer in high and low-risk populations. An investigation in Northern Nigeria, where gastric
cancer is uncommon, showed that intestinal type carcinoma predominated in all age groups and

both sexes (Mabogunje, Subbuswamy and Lawrie, 1978). These conflicting results are not
easily explained but they do indicate the need for further checks and standardisation of criteria,
particularly in interpopulation studies.

The classification of Mulligan and Rember is of interest from the point of view of histogenesis,
although it has not been widely used in practice. This is because of difficulty in distinguishing
the pylorocardiac gland cell carcinoma from the intestinal type except when obvious clear cells
are present (Day and Morson, 1978; Teglbjaerg and Vetner, 1977). A single case report on
the ultrastructure of a tumour classified as a pylorocardiac gland cell carcinoma on light microscopy was consistent with an origin from normal, non-metaplastic gastric epithelium, possibly
the pyloro-cardiac glands (Teglbjaerg, 1978). Mulligan (1975) used a modification of Dukes'
classification (1932) for staging and found only 7.6 per cent of mucous cell carcinomas confined to the stomach, compared to 22.2 per cent of pylorocardiac gland cell carcinomas and
41.3 per cent of intestinal cell carcinomas. However in the assessment of prognosis of the
three types staging was not taken into account. The excess male to female sex ratio of the
pyloro-cardiac gland cell carcinoma is of interest in that this has been reported in other studies
of tumours particularly at the cardia but also at the pylorus (Evans and Cleary, 1979; Flamant
and others, 1964; MacDonald, 1972; McPeak and Warren, 1948).

The classification of Ming, although based on biological rather than purely structural patterns,
in practice is similar to Lauren's but has the advantage that it can be applied to those cases
which remain unclassified by the latter system.

In summary the WHO classification should be used for the histological classification of stomach
tumours together with the classification of Lauren and Ming. Whilst pylorocardiac gland cell
carcinoma may be a distinct entity, confirmation of this may depend on histochemical and
ultrastructural techniques.

Histologic Features Related to Prognosis

Study of the pathology of gastric cancer in long-term survivors has shown an association with
particular characteristics of tumours or particular types of tumour. Thus circumscribed growths
with a smooth or scalloped border which advance through the gastric wall en bloc were present
in 25 of 30 patients who survived five years after gastric resection (Steiner and others, 1948).
A 'pushing' margin (Fig. 7) or a combination of a 'pushing' and infiltrating margin was associated with a 52.6 per cent five year survival in a group of 19 patients (12 with tumour in
local lymph nodes) compared with a 12.8 per cent survival in 86 patients where the tumour
margin was entirely infiltrating (Martin and Kay, 1964).

The inflammatory reaction in the stroma of tumours has been investigated in several studies
(Hawley, Westerholm and Morson, 1970; Inberg and others, 1973; Inokuchi and others, 1967;
Larmi and Saxen, 1963; Monafo, Krause and Medina, 1962; Paile, 1977). As a general rule
the prognosis is better in tumours with a pronounced lymphocytic and plasma cell infiltrate.
Thus in a large series of surgically removed tumours 4 per cent had distinctive gross and microscopic features. They were well circumscribed with a homogeneous cut surface and a rather
soft consistency, similar to a malignant lymphoma. Histologically, uniformly distributed
groups of polygonal, small to medium-sized cells with little pleomorphism and only occasional
mitoses were separated by a dense infiltrate of lymphocytes and plasma cells (Fig. 8). The
margin of the tumour was sharply defined. Even with invasion of the serosa the prognosis in
this group of patients was good (Watanabe, Enjoji and Imai, 1976). The same type of tumour

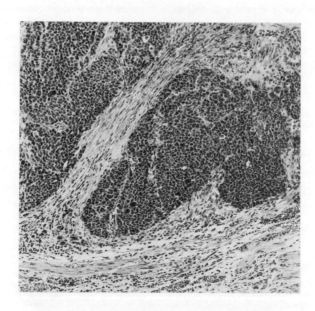

Fig. 7   The edge of this tumour is well demarcated and smooth muscle fibres are being pushed
aside.   H & E, x 114

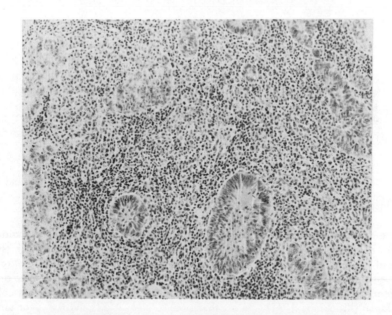

Fig. 8   Groups of tumour cells are separated by a dense
infiltrate of plasma cells and lymphocytes.   H & E, x150

was described by Steiner and others (1948) as a 'blue cell carcinoma' because of its appearance at low magnification, and as 'medullary carcinoma with lymphoid infiltration' by Hamazake, Sawayama and Kuriya (1968) who found only 1.3 per cent of their cases with this histological appearance.

Another type of tumour which although uncommon appears to have a good prognosis is composed of lakes of extracellular mucus in which tumour cells float either singly or in groups often arranged as tubules or ribbons (Fig. 9). Here again the tumour has a rounded or 'pushing' margin (Brander, Needham and Morgan, 1974; Inberg and others, 1973).

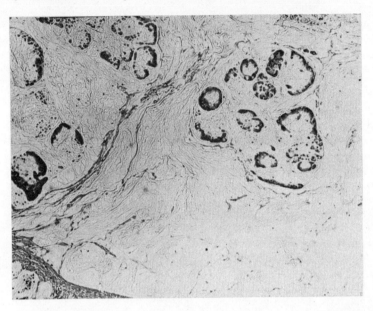

Fig. 9   Tubules and ribbons of carcinoma cells surrounded
by mucin.   H & E, x 186

Staging of Gastric Cancer

As well as the histological appearances and growth patterns of gastric cancer a major factor in the assessment of prognosis is the spread of cancer through the wall of the stomach and the involvement of regional lymph nodes.   This is apparent from the five year survival rate of so-called early gastric cancer, that is cancer limited to the mucosa or to the mucosa and sub-mucosa irrespective of lymph node metastasis, which averaged 95.5 per cent in a collective series from Japan (Kidokoro, 1971).   In another study (Paile, 1977) the five year survival rate was 50 per cent when the tumour was confined to the submucosa but fell to 20 per cent when the muscle coat had been penetrated.   Lymph node invovement in general is associated with a poorer prognosis.   Thus Hawley, Westerholm and Morson (1970) found that the five year survival rate was 40.5 per cent for those without lymph node metastases and 11.8 per cent for

those with node metastases. However the number of lymph nodes involved also influences
the prognosis, patients with few matastases doing better than those with many (Cantrell, 1971;
Hawley, Westerholm and Morson, 1970). In another study involvement of the subpyloric lymph
nodes and metastases in nodes 2.5 centimetres or more from the nearest edge of the primary
tumour were both associated with a considerably worse prognosis (ReMine, Dockerty and
Priestley, 1953).

HISTOPATHOLOGY OF EARLY GASTRIC CANCER

The term early gastric cancer is used to describe tumours in which cancer cells are limited to
the mucosal or mucosal and submucosal layers irrespective of lymph node metastases. The word
'early' was not meant to imply a stage in the genesis of the cancer but was used to mean gastric
cancer which could be cured (Murakami, 1971).

Macroscopic Appearances

On the basis of macroscopic appearances, particularly those seen at endoscopy, these cancers
have been classified by the Japanese into 3 main types, one of which has three subtypes.
Type I - the protruded type. The tumour projects clearly into the lumen and includes all
polypoid, nodular and villous tumours.
Type II - the superficial type, where unevenness of the surface is inconspicuous. This is
further subdivided into three subgroups:
(a) Elevated. This is seen as a flat, plaque-like lesion, well circumscribed and only
slightly raised above the surrounding mucosa.
(b) Flat. No abnormality is macroscopically visible apart from some colour change at
endoscopy. These lesions are usually found incidentally in carefully examined resection
specimens.
(c) Depressed. There is slight depression below the adjacent mucosa. Surface erosion may
be apparent from a thin covering of exudate.
Type III - the excavated type. This is ulceration of variable depth into the gastric wall. It
is rarely seen in pure form and is almost always combined with one or more of the other types.

Microscopic Appearances

Several studies have shown a relationship between the macroscopic appearances of early
gastric cancer and its histological appearances. Thus almost invariably types I and IIa (super-
ficial-elevated) were well differentiated adenocarcinomas (Elster and others, 1975; Nagayo
and others, 1965; Sano, 1971). Among the type IIc (superficial-depressed) cases, well differentiated, poorly differentiated, signet-ring cell, and undifferentiated carcinomas are all seen,
but the degree of differentiation in any one lesion is variable. Type III cancers, often in
combination with another type, had a higher frequency of poorly differentiated and undifferentiated tumour cells. Sano (1971) analysed 300 cases of early gastric cancer, dividing them
into two groups, 211 associated with an ulcer and 89 without ulceration. The latter type
occurred in an older age group (mean age 59.5 years) and were mostly situated in the pylorus.
Multiple tumours were present in 12.4 per cent of the cases. The majority of cancers were well
differentiated. Extension of cancer cells to the submucosa occurred in 68.5 per cent. By contrast the mean age of those cases with an ulcerated tumour was 50.5 years and the preferred site
was on the lesser curve in relation to the gastric angulus. In 5.2 per cent of cases these were

multiple tumours and invasion of tumour into the submucosa occurred in 43.6 per cent. The majority of cases were of signet-ring cell type or undifferentiated type.

The relationship of intestinal metaplasia and early gastric cancer was studied by Nagayo and Komagoe (1961). They examined 42 mucosal carcinomas and divided them into well differentiated adenocarcinoma, poorly differentiated adenocarcinoma and disseminated (signet-ring) carcinoma. There was a close correlation between severe intestinal metaplasia and well differentiated cancers, and the absence of intestinal metaplasia and signet-ring cell carcinomas. In a complementary study using the dye Congo Red at endoscopy, it was found that the gross and histological types of early gastric cancer were closely correlated with the extent of the acid-secreting area (Tatsuta and others, 1979). Thus in general when carcinomas were ulcerated and histologically undifferentiated the acid-secreting area was large, whereas when there was little or no acid-secretion the tumours were polypoid and histologically differentiated.

Nakamura, Sugano and Takagi (1968) examined thirty-three foci of carcinoma in the stomach less than 5 mms. in their largest diameter. In 28 cases the microcarcinoma arose from intestinal-type epithelium, in 4 cases from the ordinary mucosa and one focus was an ulcer-cancer. In another series where 144 foci of superficial carcinomas were studied, the tendency to undergo ulceration or erosion increased with increase in size of the carcinoma. Using strict criteria the incidence of ulcer-cancer was about 1 per cent (Nakamura and others, 1967).

SUMMARY

Accurate histological classification and staging of gastric cancer is essential if valid comparisons of therapeutic results are to be obtained or the data from epidemiological studies assessed. Meticulous examination of gastrectomy specimens by the histopathologist is necessary if meaningful information is to be obtained (Mochizuki, 1971). The study of advanced and early gastric cancers by light microscopy, histochemical methods and the electron microscope is required in order to further clarify the role of both metaplastic intestinal epithelium and ordinary gastric epithelial cells in the genesis of cancer of the stomach.

REFERENCES

Brander, W. L., P. R. G. Needham, and A. D. Morgan (1974). Indolent mucoid carcinoma of stomach. Journal of Clinical Pathology, 27, 536 - 541.

Cantrell, E. G. (1971). The importance of lymph-nodes in the assessment of gastric carcinoma at operation. British Journal of Surgery, 58, 384 - 386.

Correa, P., C. Cuello, and E. Duque (1970). Carcinoma and intestinal metaplasia of the stomach in Colombian migrants. Journal of the National Cancer Institute, 44, 297 - 306.

Day, D. W., and B. C. Morson (1978). Gastric cancer. Recent Advances in Histopathology - 10, ed. Anthony, P. P. and N. Woolf, pp. 159 - 177. Edinburgh, London and New York : Churchill Livingstone.

Dukes, C. E. (1932). The classification of cancer of the rectum. Journal of Pathology and Bacteriology, 35, 323 - 332.

Elster, K., F., Kolaczek, K. Shimamoto, and H. Freitag (1975). Early gastric cancer - experience in Germany. Endoscopy, 7, 5 - 10.

Evans, D. M. D. and B. K. Cleary (1979). The sites of origin of gastric cancers and ulcers in relation to mucosal junctions and the lesser curvature. Investigative and Cell Pathology, 2, 97 - 117.

Flamant, R., O. Lasserre, R. Lazar, J. Leguerinais, P. Denoix and D. Schwartz (1964). Differences in sex ratio according to cancer site and possible relationship with use of tobacco and alcohol. Review of 65,000 cases. Journal of the National Cancer Institute, 32, 1309 - 1316.

Hamazake, M., K. Sawayama, and T. Kuriya (1968). Stomach cancer with lymphoid stroma. Journal of Karyopathology, 12, 115 - 120.

Hawley, P. R., P. Westerholm and B. C. Morson (1970). Pathology and prognosis of carcinoma of the stomach. British Journal of Surgery, 57, 877 - 883.

Inberg, M. V., P. Lauren, J. Vuori, and S. J. Viikari (1973). Prognosis in intestinal-type and diffuse gastric carcinoma with special reference to the effect of the stromal reaction. Acta chirurgica scandinavica, 139, 273 - 278.

Inokuchi, K., S. Inutsuka, M. Furusawa, K. Soejima, and T. Ikeda (1967). Stromal reaction around tumour and metastasis and prognosis after curative gastrectomy for carcinoma of the stomach. Cancer, 20, 1924 - 1929.

Kidokoro, T. (1971). Frequency of resesection, metastasis and five-year survival rate of early gastric carcinoma in a surgical clinic. In Early Gastric Cancer, Gann Monograph on Cancer Research 11, ed. Murakami, T., pp. 45 - 49. University of Tokyo Press.

Kubo, T. (1971). Histologic appearance of gastric carcinoma in high and low mortality countries: comparison between Kyushu, Japan and Minnesota, U.S.A. Cancer, 28, 726 - 734.

Kubo, T. (1973). Gastric carcinoma in New Zealand. Some epidemiologic-pathologic aspects. Cancer, 31, 1498 - 1507.

Larmi, T. K. I. and L. Saxen (1963). 'Host reactions' in gastric cancer; a preliminary study of 119 cases of gastrectomy. Acta chirurgica scandinavica, 125, 144 - 146.

Lauren, P. (1965). The two histological main types of gastric carcinoma: diffuse and so-called intestinal type carcinoma. An attempt at a histo-clinical classification. Acta pathologica et microbiologica scandinavia, 64, 31 - 49.

Mabogunje, O. A., S. G. Subbuswamy and J. H. Lawrie (1978). The two histological types of gastric carcimona in Northern Nigeria. Gut, 19, 425 - 429.

MacDonald, W. C. (1972). Clinical and pathologic features of adenocarcinoma of the gastric cardia. Cancer, 29, 724 - 732.

Martin, C. and S. Kay (1964). The prognosis of gastric carcinoma as related to its morphologic characteristics. Surgery, Gynecology and Obstetrics, 119, 319 - 322.

McPeak, E. and S. Warren (1948). Histologic features of carcinoma of the cardioesophageal junction and cardia. American Journal of Pathology, 24, 971 - 991.

Ming, S. C. (1977). Gastric carcinoma. A pathobiological classification. Cancer, 39, 2475 - 2485.

Mochizuki, T. (1971). Method for histopathological examination of early gastric cancer. In Early Gastric Cancer, Gann Monograph on Cancer Research 11, ed. Murakami, T., pp. 57 - 65. Univesity of Tokyo Press.

Monafo , W. W., G. L. Krause, and J. G. Medina (1962). Carcinoma of the stomach. Morphological characteristics affecting survival. Archives of Surgery, 85, 754 - 763.

Mulligan,. R. M. (1975). Histogenesis and biologic behaviour of gastric carcinoma; study of 138 cases. Gastrointestinal and Hepatic Pathology Decennial, 1966 - 1975, ed. Sommers, S. C., pp. 31 - 101.

Mulligan, R. M. and R. R. Rember (1954). Histogenesis and biologic behaviour of gastric carcinoma. Archives of Pathology, 58, 1 - 25.

Murakami, T. (1971). Pathomorphological diagnosis: definition and gross classification of early gastric cancer. In Early Gastric Cancer, Gann Monograph on Cancer Research 11, ed. Murakami, T., pp. 53 - 55. University of Tokyo Press.

Munoz, N. and J. Asvall (1971). Time trends of intestinal and diffuse types of gastric cancer in Norway. International Journal of Cancer, 8, 144 - 157.

Munoz, N. , P. Correa, P. Cuello and E. Duque (1968). Histologic types of gastric carcinoma in high- and low-risk areas. International Journal of Cancer, 3, 809 - 818

Nagayo, T., M. Ho, H. Yokayama and T. Komagoe (1965). Early phases of human gastric cancer : morphological study. Gann, 56, 101 - 120.

Nagayo, T. and T. Kamagoe (1961). Histological studies of gastric mucosal cancer with special reference to relationship of histological pictures between the mucosal cancer and the cancer-bearing gastric mucosa. Gann, 52, 109 - 119.

Nakamura, K., H. Sugano, K. Takagi and A. Fuchigami (1967). Histopathological study on early carcinoma of the stomach: some considerations on the ulcer-cancer by analysis of 144 foci of the superficial spreading carcinomas. Gann, 58, 377 - 387.

Nakamura, K., H. Sugano, and K. Takagi (1968). Carcinoma of the stomach in incipient phase: its histogenesis and histological appearances. Gann, 59, 251 - 258.

Oota, K. (1977), Histological typing of gastric and oesophageal tumours. WHO, Geneva.

Paile, A. (1977). Morphology and prognosis of carcinoma of the stomach. Annales chirurgiae et gynaecologiae (fenniae) 60, Suppl. 175, 1 - 56.

ReMine, W. H., M. B. Dockerty and J. T. Priestley (1953) Some factors which influence prognosis in surgical treatment of gastric carcinoma. Annals of Surgery, 138, 311 - 317.

Sano, R. (1971). Pathological analysis of 300 cases of early gastric cancer with special reference to cancer associated with ulcers. In Early Gastric Cancer, Gann Monograph on cancer Research II, ed. Murakami, T., pp. 81 - 89. University of Tokyo Press.

Steiner, P. D., S. N. Maimon, W. L. Palmer and J. B. Kirsner (1948). Gastric cancer: morphologic factors in five-year survival after gastrectomy. American Journal of Pathology, 24, 947 - 969.

Stout, A. P. (1953). Tumours of the Stomach. Atlas of Tumour Pathology, Fascide 21, p. 65 Washington US Armed Forces Institute of Pathology.

Tatsuta, M., S. Okuda, H. Taniguchi and H. Tamura, (1979). Gross and histological types of early gastric carcinomas in relation to the acid-secreting area. Cancer, 43, 317 - 321.

Teglbjaerg, P. S. (1978) Highly differentiated gastric adenocarcinoma originating from the normal, non-metaplastic gastric epithilium. An ultrastructural study of a case. Acta pathologica et microbiologica scandinavica, 86, 87 - 89.

Teglbjaerg, P. S. and M. Vetner, (1977). Gastric Carcinoma I. The reproducibility of a histogenetic classification proposed by Mass on, Rember and Mulligan. <u>Act pathologica et microbiologica scandinavica</u>, 85, 519 - 527.

Watanabe, H. M., M. Enjoji and T. Imai (1976). Gastric carcinoma with lymphoid stroma. Its morphological characteristics and prognostic correlations. <u>Cancer, 38,</u> 232 - 243.

Image Analysis in the Cytological Diagnosis of Carcinoma of the Stomach and Oesophagus

H. Thompson*, P. Kurver** and M.E. Boon**

*Department of Histology, General Hospital, Birmingham
**Department of Cytology, Stichting, Samenwerking,
Delftse, Netherlands

ABSTRACT

Brush cytology is extremely valuable in the diagnosis of carcinoma of the stomach
and oesophagus. Morphometry with image analysis equipment provides objective
information on cell size and nuclear/cytoplasmic ratio which has diagnostic significance in difficult cases.

INTRODUCTION

The recent Birmingham study reported by Keighley et al., (1979) emphasises that brush
cytology is of considerable value in the diagnosis of carcinoma of the stomach and
oesophagus. Quantitative statistical studies on gastric cytology have been carried
out by Danno (1975), Shida (1965) and Tajima (1968) and also on cervical cytology and
thyroid cytology by Beyer Boon (1980). It, therefore, seemed logical to subject our
gastric cytology meterial to morphometric analysis to determine whether parameters
could be selected which would be useful in diagnosis.

MATERIAL AND METHODS

Cytological smear preparations were made from gastric brushings in the Department
of Histology, General Hospital, Birmingham, with wet fixation in 74% alcohol. The
smears were stained by the Papanicolauo staining technique and reported by the
cytologist (H.T.) Figs. 1 and 2. Gastric biopsies were also taken from each patient.

A total of 89 smears were submitted to the Department of Cytology, Delft, for
morphometric analysis. The series included the following cases:-

MATERIAL : 89 PATIENTS

A   34 Benign lesions. Negative cytology and tumour negative follow-up.
        40 Positive smears confirmed by Histology.

B   3 cases with positive cytology, negative histology and clinical cancer.

C   3 cases with suspicious cytology (reported as negative) and negative
      follow-up.

D   9 cases with suspicious cytology (reported as negative) and positive
      histology.

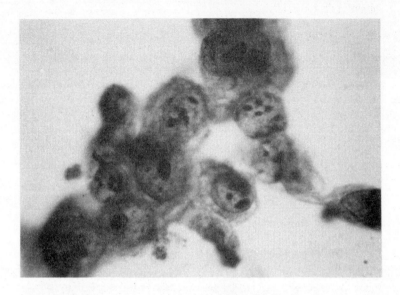

Fig. 1.   Cluster of malignant gastric carcinoma cells showing nuclear
polymorphism and prominent nucleoli.

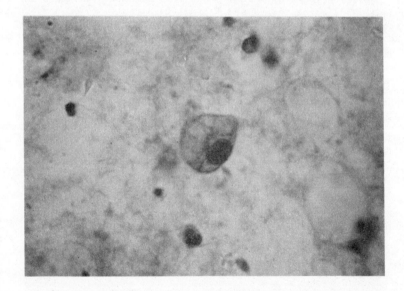

Fig. 2. Malignant gastric mucin secreting cell with eccentric nucleus,
prominent nucleoli and vacuolated cytoplasm.

QUANTITATIVE STUDIES

For the planimetric studies a ASM-Leitz was used, equipped with a camera lucida
system. The digital cursor of the system was seen in the microscopical field under
study, and thus the chosen object could be outlined and its features calculated by
a PET minicomputer attached to the graphic tablet. In each smear, 25 abnormal
cells were chosen: from each cell the contour of the nucleus and the cytoplasm was
delineated on the graphic tablet with the cursor, and from these contours the following five features were calculated by the minicomputer: perimeter nucleus, size
nucleus, perimeter cell, size cell and nuclear/cytoplasmic ratio. From each measured slide, 10 parameters could be calculated, being mean and standard deviation
of the five enumerated features. The measurements were performed by one cytopath-
ologist and one well-instructed cytotechnologist: there were no statistical
differences between the measurements of these two.

STATISTICAL ANALYSIS

Statistical analysis was carried out with a part of the programme STP on a PDP 11
DEC computer (developed by P.H.J.K.). The descriptive statistics were calculated
for the group of benign lesions and for the group of malignant lesions respectively.
Wilcoxon's test was used to establish the difference between the two groups; as a
level of significance, $p\ 0.05$ was adopted.

Consequently, the material of benign lesions and malignant lesions was divided at
random into two groups, a learning population and a testing population. The learning population was used to extract the classification rule, which was consequently
tested on the testing population. Between the learning population and the testing
population were no statistical differences such as patient's age and tumour stage.

RESULTS

The significant differences between the group of benign lesions and malignant
lesions is shown in Table I.

TABLE I.

THE SIGNIFICANT DIFFERENCES BETWEEN THE DIFFERENT GROUPS AND THEIR MEANS

Parameters	Benign	Diff[1]	Malignant
Mean nuclear perimeter	28.01	*	31.58
s.d. nuclear perimeter	3.05	***	5.79
mean nuclear size	53.39		60.15
s.d. nuclear size	10.28	***	21.14
mean cell perimeter	79.32	***	36.59
s.d. cell perimeter	6.33		6.59
mean cell size	156.99	***	73.88
s.d. size	38.03	**	25.28
mean N/C diameter ratio	0.58	***	0.87
s.d. N/C diameter ratio	0.06	***	0.11

1) (*)= p 0.10;   * = p 0.05;   ** = p 0.01;   *** = p 0.001

It is evident that out of the 10 parameters 8 are highly discriminatory, the most
potent parameters being the mean N/C ratio and the standard deviation thereof. It
was computed that there were significant differences between the data of the learning population and the testing population, pointing to an absence of bias. Therefore, it was justifiable to extract a classification rule from the learning
population. It was found that the two parameters mean N/C ratio and standard deviation for the nuclear perimeter were essential for a good discrimination between
the two groups. When the established classification rule was applied on respectively the learning and the testing population, a high probability for a correct
classification was computed, in the learning population ranging from 91-100%,
which was surpassed in the testing population with a range from 99-100%, thus all
cases in both the learning and the testing population were correctly classified
(Table II).

TABLE II

CLASSIFICATION TABLE

LEARNING POPULATION

	Benign[1]	Malignant[1]
1. Benign 19	19	0
2. Malignant 22	0	22

TEST POPULATION

	Benign[1]	Malignant[1]
1. Benign 15	15	0
2. Malignant 18	0	18

1) Computer classification

Figure 3 shows that when a scattergram is made of all cases, with as coordinates
the mean N/C ratio and the standard deviation of the nuclear perimeter, two
clusters are found, one of the benign lesions and one of the malignant lesions.

Two of the three cases with positive cytology and negative histology were classified as malignant, which was in accordance with their follow-up history. The
third was classified as benign: this case proved to be an oesophagus carcinoma,
cytologically of squamous differentiation. Of the suspicious cases, the three
benign cases were classified as benign, and of the malignant cases only one case
was misclassified. The probabilities of the test cases ranged from 0.00 to 0.16
and from 0.24 to 1.00.

DISCUSSION

Keighley et al showed that brush cytology in combination with multiple biopsies
produced a cumulative diagnostic accuracy rate of 97% in the diagnosis of carcinoma of the stomach and oesophagus. Moreover, brush cytology was more sensitive
with an accuracy rate of 87% compared to that of biopsies which was 83%. Brushing
before biopsy produced superior results with a higher diagnostic accuracy rate of
91% compared to that of biopsy which was 82%.

An experienced cytologist is essential for such studies since subjective assessment
of criteria for malignancy is of paramount importance. Since quantitative statistical studies have been employed in cytology, it seemed obvious that our collected
material could be used to determine objective parameters with image analysis
equipment which could be of value in difficult borderline cases. In our clinical

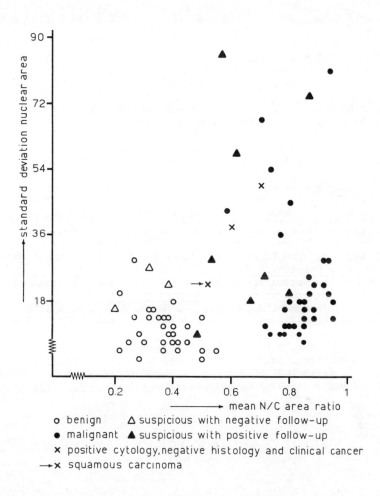

Fig. 3. Image analysis in the cytological dianosis of carcinoma of the stomach
and oesophagus.

series we have recently encountered two cytology positive, biopsy negative patients
who proceeded to gastrectomy with the discovery of early gastric cancer (intra-
mucosal carcinoma) and access to image analysis equipment in such cases would be
invaluable to the cytologist.

Ten morphometric parameters were studied and of these 8 were significantly different in the discrimination of benign and malignant cell populations(Table I). With
these parameters, a classification rule was made with which all benign lesions were
classified as benign and all malignant lesions as malignant (Table II).

The method proved to be valuable in cases with positive cytology and negative biopsy. The only misclassified cases were squamous carcinoma indicating that the parameters for adenocarcinoma cannot be used for squamous carcinoma. The method was also successful in the suspicious cases which had originally been classified as negative. In 2 such cases labelled cytology negative, biopsy positive cases which were subjected to image analysis, the computer identified the cells as malignant indicating that the technique was more sensitive than the experienced cytologist.

It is probable that with the study of larger series of cases, the range of probability will be larger than that described in this material pointing to a continuous scale from atypia to low degree malignancy.

The measurement of smears from one patient with an adequate cell population takes about 15 minutes provided that the equipment is readily available.

These studies show that morphometry provides valuable information for the cytologist and clinician in the diagnosis of carcinoma of the stomach.

REFERENCES

Boon, M. E. and Fox, C. H. (1980). Simultaneous Condyloma Acuminatum and Dysplasia of the Uterine Cervix. In Press. Acta Cytologica Journal.
Boon, M. E., Lonhagen, T. and Willems, J-S. (1980). Planimetric Studies on Fine Needle Aspirates from Follicular adenoma and Follicular carcinoma of the Thyroid. Acta Cytologica Journal, 24, 145.
Danno, M. (1975). Statistical criteria for the cytology of gastric cancer. A proposal of distance index. Acta Cytologica 20, 466.
Keighley, M. R. B., Thompson, H., Moore, J., Hoare, A. M., Allan, R. N. and Dykes, P.W. (1979). Comparison of brush cytology before and after biopsy for the diagnosis of gastric carcinoma. Brit. J. Surg. 66, 246.
Shida, S. (1965). Diagnosis of early gastric cancer. Vol.4. (Gastric Cytology), Bonic Yodo Co. Ltd., Tokyo.
Tajima, M. (1968) Zytomorphologische Darstellong von der verschiedenen zell materialen und ihre untersuchungsmethoden. J. Jap. Soc. Clin. Cytol. 7, 60.

DAY 1. SESSION 2. PANEL DISCUSSION

B. Golematis. I would like to ask Dr. Thompson how he gets the gastric juice, by aspiration, or through the gastroscope?

H. Thompson. These were brushings taken through the endoscope. Mr. Keighley in fact was one of my associates in this study and he will confirm the technique for you.

G. Giles. So this is the standard brushing of suspicious areas?

B. Golematis. This is in accordance with our experience in Greece. Cytology taken by endoscopy is superior.

E. Deutch. Dr. Thompson, could you explain your false positive histology?

H. Thompson. Yes. Of the two cases, one was indeed an error. The biopsies are studied by a large number of people. We have rotating registrars, rotating lecturers going through different departments. The biopsies were looked at independently from myself as cytologist. One of the false positives was from a different hospital with a different pathologist and it was an erronious interpretation that was merely regenerative changes at the edge of a chronic gastric ulcer. The second false positive was initially reported as cancer and then the histologist retracted the diagnosis after discussion with the endoscopist and study of the biopsies, but it was still put down on the list of false positives.

M. Keighley. I would just like to say that although in the trial that Dr. Thompson reported there were no false positive brush cytology results, soon after that study was completed we did have three or four false positives. I think it is worth emphasising to this audience that they were in fact carry overs from the brush used on the previous occasion, and we now feel it is very important to autoclave the brushes in order to avoid this complication.

H. Thompson. I agree entirely with that. I think that there are two possibilities for error in gastric cancer. There is the identity error and secondly there is always the risk of a false diagnosis being made by the pathologist, either on biopsy or cytology.

M. Crespi. We started cytology many years ago and have one of the largest series of brush cytology. I have to say that we never experienced the false positive. Also, simple washing out of brush is satisfactory, without autoclaving it. Secondly, it is very dangerous for data interpretation if you do not have an experienced cytologist. Not only the regenerative changes in chronic ulcer, but also some of the kind of cells you find in chronic gastritis, could be very misleading for the cytologist because we have the nuclei and so on, and everything is there to make the diagnosis of malignancy. So this is another warning signal. I entirely agree that cytology and biopsy combined is around 100%. Our experience in oesophageal cancer is that cytology is much better than biopsy for obtaining morphological confirmation of the diagnosis. We published a series of 30 cases in 1974 in which there was a striking difference in cytology and now we have more than 100 cases of oesophageal cancer and there is the same trend. It means that in the oesophagus, for mechanical reasons of taking the biopsy in a tangential way from the endoscope, the cytology is much superior to histology.

G. Giles. Can we just lay to rest a point, which may have been hinted at, on just sampling gastric juice cytology or gastric lavage? What is the view about the value of gastric lavage and cytology now, is this something which is unlikely to be helpful as a screening procedure, or even as a diagnostic procedure? I think probably it is of no value. Is it?

M. Crespi. I think that it has no value now as a screening procedure because, in fact, screening itself has less value. If you talk about the cost-effectiveness and consider the falling incidence of gastric cancer, I don't think that mass screening has a place today, especially in our country.

G. Giles. But in Finland, do you have cytology done on your samples, Professor Hakkinen?

I. Häkkinen. Not in our clinics.

M. Crespi. There is perhaps only one use for gastric lavage cytology. This is in the follow-up of chronic gastritis patients. As soon as you have got a clear diagnosis of quite advanced chronic gastritis either you submit the individual to yearly, or less than yearly, endoscopic examination. But this is not so easily accepted. Perhaps the best way to pick up an early malignancy is to do lavage cytology. This is the only instance in which I would advise it.

G. Giles. That is an interesting point, and it fits in with the afternoon's discussion. What would you say to that Professor Häkkinen, in terms of following chronic atrophic gastritis? Would you advise that your tumour marker studies be done in such a patient?

I. Häkkinen. No. I think that chronic gastritis cases are very often antigen positive, whether you look at CEA or FSA.

G. Giles. So there is no quantitative immunoassay?

I. Häkkinen. No.

M. Crespi. But the point is to pick up malignancy in cases of chronic gastritis with intestinal metaplasia and it is not too easy to do this?

I. Häkkinen. No, it is not easy.

E. Deutch. Dr. Häkkinen and I have been comparing markers in gastric cancer juice and if, in addition to cytology, a marker is studied it may be possible that a soluble antigen that antecedes the proliferation of cells that Dr. Thompson sees in his cytology would bring us much closer to the aetiological induction of gastric cancer. I have just a solitary gastric cancer in situ in which this happened. A 54 year old man with a peptic ulcer history of four months presented with X-ray evidence that was negative, and on endoscopy showed pre-pyloric ulcer. I took 12 biopsies, one of which was positive. The gastric juice showed a marker, the details of which I won't go into because we do not have adequate data. On resection of that man's stomach, just a simple sub-total resection, all the tissue was negative. So I took his tumour out with one of 12 biopsies. It was a solitary case of gastric cancer in situ. One year later, he had a negative biopsy and the marker was negative.

J. Craven. May I ask Dr. Hirayama and Professor Häkkinen both to address themselves to this particular problem. They both talked of screening for gastric cancer. Now screening means investigation of people who have no symptoms. My very brief experience in Japan led me to conclude that this wasn't screening, it was early diagnosis. The patient presents to a clinic with a complaint, they have dyspepsia perhaps. Now is that correct, or if not, what proportion of the patients in Japan are being diagnosed early and what proportion are being screened, ie. asymptomatic? I would like to ask Professor Häkkinen the same question. What number of his patients were asymptomatic?

T. Hirayama. First of all there is the definition of what is symptomatic. If the people do not consider it is a symptom, then it is not a symptom. This examination is not done in the out-patient clinic, it is done in the field. Many people are taking some form of gastric drugs, but they themselves consider that they are not suffering from gastric disease. The majority of the people who are examined have no symptoms, even after careful enquiry. So I think it is unfair to say the mass screening in Japan is mostly on symptomatic patients. I think it is mostly on healthy people without symptoms.

G. Giles. I think there has been a study in your own centre, Mr. Craven, which has attempted to produce a cohort of so called normal people to compare with your ulcer dyspepsias. Apparently, of several hundred people interviewed in a normal population in York a very significant proportion, 20% or so, had ulcer type symptoms, even though they had never presented to a doctor. So that there will be in a normal population, presumably this is the same in Japan, people with some symptoms. So I think it is a valid point that if they don't complain about it they cannot be regarded as symptomatic.

J. Craven. I am not being critical. I just wanted it to be defined, that's all.

I. Häkkinen. I think the same. Our procedure is as follows. We collect the samples of gastric juice after inviting people by letter. The collectors are nurses. Samples are sent to our laboratory where they are analysed and the result is antigen positive or negative. Up to now we have performed quite a few immuno-diffusion tests and the positives come to me for clinical examination and gastroscopy. So we have no knowledge of their symptoms.

G. Giles. Why did they go for screening? Was it a random sample?

I. Häkkinen. No we sample different communities.

G. Giles. But did you offer this service to them?

I. Häkkinen. Yes.

G. Giles. People who go for a medical test often have some symptoms they are curious to know about.

I. Häkkinen. Yes.

R. Hall. Could I be personal with Dr. Hirayama and ask him if he has been screened and how often is he being screened.

T. Hirayama. This is a good example. I did not have any symptoms, I was forced to be examined. Working in hospitals and companies it is very difficult to refuse the examination, when I am in Japan, of course. So even I have been examined several times.

G. Giles. How often is that?

T. Hirayama. Whenever I am working in Japan and whenever there is the chance to be examined!

G. Giles. I would like to return to the point that Mr. Brookes was making about

the yield from subsequent screenings, which is disappointing in a way. It seemed
to me from what you said, that one examination, about the age of 50, was probably
the best use of screening. You did not feel that there was much to be gained
from screening thereafter.

V. Brookes. In fact I was talking to Dr. Hirayama and that figure of 40 out of
every 100,000 were, as you suggested, the early carcinomas, and the pick up rate
then goes up to 100 per 100,000.

M. Crespi. I am not completely convinced with the case for screening in the pure
sense of screening: the kind of thing done by endoscopy, X-ray and so on. First
of all, they cover only a small part of the population. How many people do you
have aged around 50 or more in Japan? At least 40,000,000? You screen 3 million
per year, so it is a very small number. Secondly, I think that there is always
some self-selection on the basis of symptoms. There is always some bias in the
selection. From the data I saw in Tokyo, at the WHO meeting, in the 24,000 cases
you presented there I saw that many people had symptoms. This means that this
could be the reason why they submitted to examination. A very high percentage
had symptoms, which I do not think is the normal thing. You could not have an
80% symptomatic population in Japan.

T. Hirayama. I think what we are doing is just like fighting fires ie. control.
We believe that primary prevention is much better than secondary prevention, and
we are doing our best. But in addition, an early detection programme is important
as one would do for fire control. You find the fire as soon as possible. We are
not strongly advocating screening but we have to utilize this to fight against this
kind of important disease in the Japanese.

G. Giles. Yes, quite right.

V. Brookes. When one thinks of the number of patients with actual symptoms who are
given some form of treatment by their primary medical contact, the general
practitioners, without investigation it is really important to exclude that section.
To make sure that no preliminary treatment is given without an exact diagnosis
being made.

W. ReMine. Dr. Hirayama, are all of your films read by trained radiologists, or do
you train technicians to do this?

T. Hirayama. We are trying to train as many technicians and as many doctors as
possible. The Minister of Health has a programme to train them. In addition there
are gastric cancer study groups composed mostly of clinicians. They are trying
to train among themselves. This is why I said that each year the technique is
improving.

E. Deutch. Dr. Crespi showed a slide in which gastric ulcer was followed by 1-7%
of cancer. The studies of early gastric cancer using the Japanese Endoscopic
Society criteria in the years 1962 - 1968 showed 2,500 early gastric lesions, of
which 83% were either the depressed IIc lesion or they were the excavated type of
III. The point I am making is that I think there is a larger group that we have
been missing, that have to do with the IIc lesion particularly. We have been
seeing the IIc lesion and thinking that it might be a healed or scarred ulcer. The
yield is pretty good on those, we found 20 lesions in healing scars of this type.
So the IIc and III lesions they describe have an excellent yield by biopsy. It is
in this group particularly that we are interested in the early soluble antigen,
which might get us even closer to that 20 year exposure for the induction of gastric
cancer.

M. Crespi. The point is that in my table I was referring to the proven benign gastric ulcers, which on follow-up were becoming malignant. I was referring to two studies, one was the Cooperative Veterans Administration Study published four or five years ago in Gastroenterology. This was a huge study involving all the Veterans Administration Centres and they reported 6.5% of cancerization of a true benign ulcer. The other is the data from Magy. You can consider it in a different way, that is how many ulcerated cancers you have. You have to distinguish between these two which have completely clear cut differences.

E. Deutch. I think the big mistake that our group makes is that once the gastric ulcer is radiologically healed we call it benign.

M. Crespi. That's alright. The Saito experience showed that the sight of the malignant ulcer is very clear.

E. Deutch. The breakdown of this is the one that we pick out, and then this is being picked up as the early gastric cancer.

M. Crespi. Yes, if you give cimetidine to a nice early ulcerated malignant lesion, you heal it perfectly.

Preoperative Assessment and Palliative Surgery

W.H. ReMine

Department of Surgery, Mayo Clinic and Mayo Foundation,
Rochester, Minnesota, U.S.A.

ABSTRACT

Patients with gastric carcinoma should undergo operation when the diagnosis is
known or tentative and no contraindications are evident. Contraindications include
serious concomitant disease, evidence of distant metastasis and local extension
beyond the point of resectability. Denying a patient the potential benefits of
exploratory laparotomy may eliminate the possibility of cure. After thorough
abdominal exploration, curative resection of gastric cancer involves radical subtotal gastrectomy for lesions restricted to the distal two-thirds of the stomach
and total gastrectomy with splenectomy for lesions in the upper one-third. When
local extension of the cancer is present, adjacent organs should be resected if
the growth can be completely removed. When curative resection is impossible,
palliative resection or gastroenterostomy is often indicated to relieve symptoms.

The experiences of 196 patients who underwent palliative operations for advanced
gastric carcinoma were reviewed to evaluate the effect of treatment. Gastroenterostomy for obstruction alleviated vomiting in most patients, but palliation was
appreciable in only one-third. The associated mortality rate was acceptable, and
the average postoperative hospitalization was 13 days. The results after partial
gastrectomy for patients with obstruction were only slightly better than those
after gastroenterostomy. Approximately one-third of the patients lived comfortably
for more than a year. The poor progress of six patients who underwent total
gastrectomy supports the opinion that this is an unsatisfactory palliative
operation. Esophagogastrectomy for patients with dysphagia yielded results similar
to those after palliative resection of distal lesions. Although the results after
insertion of prostheses for inoperable malignant strictures of the esophagogastric
junction were disappointing, the procedure had definite advantages when compared
with the limitations of jejunostomy and the transient relief afforded by transesophageal dilation. A feeding jejunostomy seldom is indicated in the management
of advanced gastric carcinoma.

KEY WORDS

Operability; curability; "palliation"; palliative "comfort"; quality of life; risk;
definite tissue diagnosis.

GENERAL CONDITION OF PATIENT

In evaluating the patient who is suspected of having cancer of the stomach to
determine whether operative intervention is necessary and feasible, attention
should be directed first to his general physical condition. Of interest are his
age, loss of weight or strength, state of hydration, and general nutritive status.
Any serious concomitant disease, such as cardiovascular, pulmonary, renal, neuro-
logic, or endocrine abnormalities, should be detected, inasmuch as the presence of
such conditions influences the decision for or against operation. Information
obtained from laboratory studies, including values for hemoglobin, serum protein,
and electrolyte balance, should be noted. Such findings, in addition to providing
information about the operative risk, may indicate the need for preoperative preparation or for special prophylactic precautions during the postoperative period.
Because gastric cancer is so serious a disease, relatively few findings in the
patient's general physical status definitely contraindicate an operation. With
proper preparation for operation and utilization of all the special precautions
available, operation usually can be performed with minimal risk.

UNCERTAIN PREOPERATIVE DIAGNOSIS OF GASTRIC CANCER

In most patients with an ulcerating lesion in the stomach, the differential
diagnosis between benignancy and malignancy can be made with a high degree of
certainty. This differential diagnosis is based on the history and results of
physical examination, laboratory studies of gastric secretion, and x-ray examination of the stomach after ingestion of barium. Gastric cytology and intragastric
radiographic procedures may also be helpful. Although gastroscopy is used
occasionally, in our experience it has not helped appreciably in determining a
definite differential diagnosis in the equivocal case. The relative importance
and reliability of these various diagnostic aids have been discussed in preceding
articles. In a few patients, a positive differentiation between a benign and a
malignant gastric lesion cannot be established by any means of clinical investigation.

If the actual diagnosis is uncertain after clinical investigation, the physician
and surgeon must decide whether to advise immediate operation or to suggest a
period of conservative treatment and observation in the hospital to aid in reach-
ing a more certain diagnosis. This decision should be based on numerous factors
carefully evaluated for the individual patient. Among these factors are the
evidence for or against the presence of a malignant lesion, the estimated risk of
operation regardless of whether the lesion is benign or malignant, the wishes of
the patient after the situation has been explained to him, the possible need for
operation even after a period of hospitalization and a trial of medical management,
and the undesirable consequences of delaying operation if a malignant lesion
actually is present.

The reasons for or against surgical treatment of benign gastric ulcer will not be
discussed herein. My colleagues and I believe that operation should be advised
if, after thorough clinical examination, there seems to be a reasonable possibility that a malignant lesion is present. If the patient's general condition is
such that operation will impose an excessive risk, if the patient is strongly
opposed to surgical treatment, or if other equally compelling reasons contraindi-
cating operation are encountered, further efforts should be made to determine a
definite differential diagnosis.

If operative intervention is postponed, the patient is admitted to the hospital
for intensive medical treatment of a benign ulcer; after 2 weeks, he is reexamined
for evidence of healing of the gastric lesion. If a response to the treatment is

evident at reexamination, nonsurgical treatment may be continued. The patient
must be followed up closely by periodic x-ray examination of the stomach to ensure
that the lesion heals completely and remains healed during the next several years.
In the exceptional patient, x-ray evidence of healing may appear relatively early,
and subsequently a definitely malignant lesion may be found in the same site in
the stomach. Such occurrences, although uncommon, are known. If complete healing
does not occur within a reasonable period (2 to 6 weeks at the most), the lesion
should be considered probably malignant or at least unresponsive to medical management and operation should be advised if the patient's general condition permits.

Difficulty in determining whether the lesion in the stomach is benign or malignant
arises most often when the roentgenologist gives an uncertain diagnosis such as
"gastric ulceration, malignancy not excluded" or "gastric ulcer, possibly malignant." Other examples of diagnoses that may leave the clinician and surgeon in
doubt are "prepyloric narrowing," "pyloric obstruction, cause undetermined,"
gastric polyps, and a lesion considered by the roentgenologist as a benign ulcer
in a patient who has no hydrochloric acid in the gastric aspirate.

DEFINITE PREOPERATIVE DIAGNOSIS OF GASTRIC CANCER

In many cases, the diagnosis of gastric cancer can be established with certainty
by clinical examinations that include barium contrast x-ray study of the stomach,
and the decision is made in favor of exploratory laparotomy unless specific findings contraindicate such an operation. These findings include serious disease
elsewhere in the body, evidence of distant metastasis, and evidence of local
extension that might make any surgical effort futile. This last finding is
exceptional because the type and extent of local invasion can seldom be determined
accurately until the abdomen is opened. Contraindications may be relative or
absolute, depending on their nature and on the judgment of the internist and
surgeon who consult after studying the patient's condition.

Serious cardiac insufficiency, advanced pulmonary disease, and pronounced renal
failure are examples of systemic complications that may contraindicate surgical
exploration when weighed against the possible benefit of the operation to the
patient. Because this decision is of great importance, a negative one should be
made only after careful consideration of all of the evidence. In most patients,
however, the decision in favor of laparotomy is reached with relative ease after
the diagnosis of gastric neoplasm has been established.

The finding that most frequently makes an abdominal operation inadvisable is
distant metastasis. The left lower part of the cervical region should always be
carefully examined with the patient in the sitting position, because a Virchow
node may be found behind the medial end of the left clavicle. If detected, this
node should be removed before the abdomen is opened. If cancer is found in the
node, the opportunity for cure is lost, and the abdomen should be opened only when
some type of palliative procedure is indicated and possible. Another region in
which a metastatic lesion may be found in patients who have advanced carcinoma of
the stomach is the pelvic cul-de-sac. Involvement here can be detected by digital
examination of the rectum, a procedure that should always be performed as part of
a general physical examination. With some experience, the examining physician can
be reasonably certain of the nature of what he palpates in this region in most
patients. In some cases in which he is unsure, the findings should not be considered as contraindications to operation.

Metastatic lesions may also be noted in the liver. The diagnosis can usually be
confirmed by percutaneous needle biopsy. Biopsy is recommended when nodularity is
noted in the liver of a patient who has cancer of the stomach. If the biopsy

specimen is negative for cancer, operation is usually advised even though the findings on palpation of the abdomen are most suggestive of hepatic involvement. Occasionally, other lesions in the liver may simulate metastatic involvement on physical examination.

Less commonly, carcinoma may metastasize to the umbilicus or inguinal region. Biopsy specimens may be readily secured from these areas. Metastasis to the lungs from gastric carcinoma is uncommon, as is metastasis to the bones, the central nervous system, or the axillae. If any doubt exists about the actual presence of a metastatic lesion, we advise operation for most patients because of the slight uncertainty of a preoperative opinion and because operation may be the only chance for cure. In general, only definite, objective evidence of metastasis should be considered a contraindication to operation. Suspected, unproved, or questionable distant metastatic involvement generally should not result in denying the patient the possible benefits of surgical treatment.

Perhaps the most exciting developments in recent years have been the advent of computed tomography and ultrasonography. These modalities have added vast dimensions to our diagnostic acumen. As they increase in sophistication, the benefits derived by the patient will be multiplied.

The presence of a mass in the abdomen should not be considered a contraindication to operation. Occasionally, a carcinoma of the stomach of sufficient size to be detected as a palpable abdominal mass may prove to be of a relatively low grade of malignancy and may have remained completely or predominantly confined to the stomach. Such a lesion often can be removed, and the prognosis for the patient may be reasonably good. The surgical approach is more likely to yield good results, of course, if the mass is movable. Although multiple abdominal masses are more serious than a single mass, they should not automatically preclude operative intervention.

If, after thorough investigation of the patient, a definite diagnosis of gastric cancer is made and distant extension has been detected or strongly suspected, the need for and the possibility of performing some palliative procedure should be considered. The indications for such procedures most often are obstruction or substantial recurrent bleeding. If the patient has been vomiting frequently, has been unable to eat in a reasonable manner, and has a lesion in the distal part of the stomach, palliative gastric resection or gastroenterostomy may improve the quality of his remaining life. Conversely, if the lesion is in the proximal portion of the stomach and extends to or involves the lower end of the esophagus, the chance of performing a palliative operation that will prove worthwhile is diminished. In the presence of recurrent and distressing hematemesis, which fortunately is seldom associated with gastric carcinoma, palliative resection also may offer some relief to the patient. The question of whether to perform a palliative operation for gastric pain is rarely posed. Because the pain may be caused by extragastric extension of a neoplasm that cannot be completely removed, such a procedure may have limited success.

PREOPERATIVE PREPARATION

As mentioned earlier, careful consideration should be given to a patient's general condition before surgical treatment; this preliminary investigation will ensure that the operation is performed under the most favorable circumstances possible and will minimize postoperative complications. The patient's general nutritive status, concentration of hemoglobin, state of hydration, electrolyte balance, mental attitude, and pulmonary, cardiovascular, and renal status require evaluation. These considerations apply to all patients who are to undergo major surgical procedures and, therefore, will not be discussed further.

One or two preoperative considerations that are more directly related to the patient who has gastric carcinoma should be mentioned. Because the patient almost invariably has recently ingested a considerable amount of barium, total elimination or removal of all barium should be ensured before operation. In fact, if there is any gastric obstruction, the stomach should be lavaged immediately after the x-ray examination to remove any residual barium. All patients with carcinoma of the stomach should have gastric lavage just before operation so that the stomach is empty and as clean as possible at the time of operation. This procedure aids in preventing contamination by the gastric contents during the operation.

DECISIONS DURING THE OPERATION

Abdominal Exploration

As soon as the abdominal cavity is opened, the surgeon proceeds with a general exploration of the peritoneal cavity regardless of whether the preoperative diagnosis of carcinoma of the stomach was definite or tentative. We prefer to leave the lesion itself and the structures that immediately surround it for the last step in this process. The pelvis is explored first for any evidence of spread into the cul-de-sac. The lower part of the abdomen is then examined; this examination should include the small bowel, retroperitoneal spaces, aorta, and kidneys. A specimen is taken from any area in which neoplastic extension is suspected and is submitted for study by the frozen-section technique. The large bowel also is palpated. Next, the structures in the right upper abdominal quadrant are examined, including the liver, gallbladder, common bile duct, duodenum, and head of the pancreas. A needle biopsy is performed of any area of the liver that suggests hepatic metastasis. The stomach, remaining portion of the pancreas, the left lobe of the liver, the spleen, and the lower end of the esophagus are examined last. At this time, the extent of the lesion in the stomach and the presence or absence of fixation or extension of the growth to surrounding structures are determined. The sites of regional lymph drainage and the omentum are also examined.

After this investigation and evaluation, the surgeon can formulate the plan of management. It is difficult to be completely dogmatic about surgical indications, even after careful exploration of the entire abdomen and the lesion. Many extenuating circumstances might influence the surgeon's judgment in each case. We believe, however, that certain general principles and practices should be followed.

Definitive Operation

If the lesion seems to be confined to the stomach except for possible extension to some of the regional lymph nodes, a curative operation should be attempted. If the lesion is restricted to the distal two-thirds of the stomach, we perform radical subtotal gastrectomy with removal of the omentum and careful resection of all major areas of lymph drainage from the stomach. Some evidence suggests that splenectomy should also be performed, even when the lesion is located in the distal third of the stomach; we have often included this procedure in our cases. Whenever the neoplastic process extends beyond the stomach and suggests involvement in the region of the hilus of the spleen, however, the spleen is removed.

When the growth involves the upper third of the stomach, total gastrectomy is indicated and the spleen is always removed. No pancreatic tissue is resected unless evidence suggests extension to, or involvement of, the pancreas. To our knowledge, postoperative survival rates have not demonstrated the advisability of routine resection of the tail of the pancreas in all cases in which total gastrectomy is performed.

Local Extension

Surgical judgment must be exercised in those patients in whom the growth has extended beyond the stomach and has involved adjacent structures, such as the transverse mesocolon, pancreas, or liver. We think that the growth should be removed en masse with any local extension when this can be done completely. At times, it is difficult or impossible for the surgeon to decide whether complete removal is possible until the involved structures have been somewhat mobilized. After such mobilization, it may be impossible to alter the proposed plan of management. Whenever possible, the surgeon should foresee the evolvement of the entire surgical plan before he becomes irrevocably committed to a given procedure. Rarely is a growth inoperable because of local extension, but this situation can be encountered. Under these circumstances, extensive involvement and fixation of all adjacent retroperitoneal tissues may be found. If the lesion extends to the colon or pancreas or extension is localized to the left lobe of the liver, removal usually can be accomplished satisfactorily.

Distant Extension

When abdominal exploration reveals distant extension within the abdomen, the opportunity for cure probably has passed. Although some surgeons may remove multiple metastatic lesions from the liver and then proceed with a radical operation for gastric cancer, we believe that this procedure is not worthwhile or advisable. One or two isolated nodules may be removed from the liver, but under these circumstances the benefit to the patient is highly questionable. Although a single or even several malignant implants some distance from the growth should not automatically deter the surgeon from performing a curative operation, when multiple areas of involvement are found, palliation is the most that can be accomplished. Often some procedure less than a radical gastric resection may best serve this purpose. In our opinion, total gastrectomy should not be used as a palliative procedure.

The patient usually will be more comfortable for his remaining days if the gastric growth can be removed even though cure is not achieved. Thus, palliative resection of the stomach is frequently used even though some neoplasm remains within the abdomen. Removal of an obstructing carcinoma at the outlet of the stomach may help to relieve vomiting and other symptoms even in the presence of hepatic metastasis.

In some patients who have gastric cancer that causes obstruction and that has extended distally so that the hope of cure is lost, it may be impossible to resect the growth for palliation safely and satisfactorily because of local extension. Under these circumstances, gastroenterostomy may offer some relief, even though the stoma is placed high and proximally in the stomach. Either posterior or anterior gastroenterostomy may be used, as necessitated by the site of the malignant involvement. Obviously, the gastroenteric stoma should be placed in a portion of the gastric wall in which no gross neoplasm is evident. Unfortunately, gastroenterostomy performed under these circumstances does not always provide adequate relief for the patient.

Other procedures have been suggested for palliation when the patient has an inoperable carcinoma of the stomach (Adson, 1964). A plastic tube has been

inserted into the stomach, passing from above down through the neoplasm, in order
to overcome obstruction (Celestin, 1959; Eiseman, Melzer, and Rachiele, 1959;
Mackler and Mayer, 1954). Experience with this procedure has been limited. The
tube may become displaced or plugged and even when it remains in place may not
serve satisfactorily for the transit of the gastric contents. Jejunostomy has
been used for feeding purposes but is infrequently indicated. Similarly, gastrostomy in the distal part of the stomach has been employed for an inoperable lesion
located more proximally. We have not used this procedure for this purpose except
under most unusual circumstances.

The percentage of patients who present with distant metastasis or with local
lesions that are too advanced for cure is a reminder that the surgeon's role in
many cases of gastric cancer is palliative. The recurrence rate and eventual
mortality, even among patients operated on for cure, however, demonstrate that
surgical intervention changes the natural history of the disease in such patients,
delaying death and altering the behavior of the tumor. Thus, the primary focus of
the surgeon should be on obtaining cure, if there is a reasonable possibility that
cure can be achieved. The morbidity and mortality for radical resection of gastric carcinoma in elderly patients reveal that aggressive treatment for possible
cure should be undertaken only by surgeons who have sufficient experience to
assure themselves and their patients that the procedure can be performed safely.
The experience of the surgeon and the surgeon's hospital should be considered.

In my experience in the past decade, the use of the fiberoptic gastroscope has
revolutionized the management of the patient with upper gastrointestinal bleeding
and has repeatedly clarified the situation regarding a gastric ulcer. No longer
must we wait for healing or nonhealing to take place before deciding to operate,
and no longer must we operate on a gastric ulcer without a tissue diagnosis, as
was formerly the case. Although resection of a presumptive malignant lesion of
the colon without a preoperative tissue diagnosis is still appropriate, in most
hospitals it has become unacceptable to operate on a gastric ulcer without at
least an attempt to view and biopsy the ulcer with the fiberoptic gastroscope. If
the biopsy specimen is reported as benign, the presence of cancer is not ruled
out. If the lesion appears to be malignant on direct examination and photography,
however, or if unequivocable evidence of cancer is found in the biopsy specimen,
an appropriate operation can be planned and the patient and family can be coun-
seled appropriately. A well-designed operation can then be performed without
opening the stomach prematurely.

If a preoperative diagnosis of lymphoma can be established with use of gastroscopy,
the preoperative workup should include biopsy of peripheral lymph nodes and bone
marrow and consultation with a medical oncologist. Many patients still require
surgery and can be cured with gastrectomy, but the management is usually different
from that for carcinoma. Radiation therapy and chemotherapy can play a more
substantial role in palliation if a lymphomatous tumor detected at laparotomy is
of a size and extent that suggest that resectability would be questionable.

The frequency of anaerobic contamination of the stomach in patients with gastric
cancer suggests that preoperative antibiotic management is desirable. Certainly,
nasogastric irrigation of the stomach is important.

Further progress is unlikely to evolve from changes in surgical techniques for
gastric cancer but rather from the use of additional therapeutic modalities,
including radiation therapy, chemotherapy (the 5-fluorouracil, Adriamycin, and
mitomycin-C [FAM] program being the preferred drug combination at this time)
(Comis and Carter, 1974; MacDonald and colleagues, in press; Moertel and
colleagues, 1976), and possibly immunotherapy in the future, if clinical trials
demonstrate benefit from the agents currently being studied. The difficulty in

postoperative evaluation of these patients, the uncertain role of carcinoembryonic antigen in follow-up, and the difficulty in prevention of the disease suggest that many years of research will still be necessary.

Although the 5-year survival rate after resection of the stomach for gastric cancer is not as high as desired, no patient with gastric cancer has ever been cured by any means other than surgical removal of the lesion. Therefore, denying a patient the possible benefits of exploratory laparotomy is a great responsibility.

Efforts to cure gastric cancer may be extremely frustrating for the surgeon. He must consider the limitations and benefits of palliative operations in the presence of incurable disease. The nature of the lesion leaves few choices. For the patient with partial or complete obstruction, the risks of definitive surgical treatment become acceptable.

At times, the surgeon must alter his approach in the presence of an incurable lesion. Decisions in management are difficult because objective data may not be available. Benefits of treatment occasionally are merely subjective. Different palliative procedures cannot be compared because operations are varied for numerous reasons and for lesions of varying extent. Despite these limitations, the value of a palliative procedure may be judged by its effect on pain, symptoms of obstruction, and hemorrhage. Although duration of survival is important, the patient's comfort is the most important consideration.

PALLIATIVE SURGICAL PROCEDURES

We reviewed our records (Adson, 1964) for information about selection of palliative operations. Clinical records of patients undergoing palliative procedures for advanced gastric cancer were collected consecutively until a sampling of basic treatment categories considered worthy of study was obtained. The following groups of cases were studied: gastroenterostomy, 98 cases; partial gastrectomy, 46 cases; total gastrectomy, 6 cases; esophagogastrectomy, 17 cases; placement of prosthesis without resection, 16 cases; and jejunostomy, 13 cases. In each case, note was made of preoperative symptoms, operative findings, the surgeon's reasons for selecting a particular procedure, postoperative morbidity, hospital mortality, duration of survival, and effect of operation on the patient's well-being.

Palliative gastroenterostomy was done for some patients with advanced lesions if symptoms of obstruction were predominant and if there was a sufficient area of uninvolved stomach to allow for adequate drainage. Similar bypassing operations were done when pancreatic or duodenal involvement of inoperable lesions precluded safe management of a duodenal stump or when resection of extensively involved adjacent organs did not seem justified.

Palliative resection was done for a variety of indications. Extensive involvement of lymph nodes, inoperable metastatic lesions of moderate size in the liver, and lesser degrees of peritoneal implantation were not strict contraindications to resection, particularly when symptoms could possibly be alleviated by removal of the primary tumor. Removal of the entire stomach for palliation was usually avoided; however, progression to total gastrectomy was necessary in a few cases when partial gastrectomy had been initiated and previously undetected proximal involvement was disclosed on microscopic examination of surgical specimens. Recently, prostheses have been used in some cases in which gastroenterostomy was not feasible and total gastrectomy was considered a poor choice for palliation.

Palliative Gastroenterostomy

Of the 98 patients in the series treated by palliative gastroenterostomy, 3 died in the hospital postoperatively. The average postoperative hospitalization was 13 days. The chief indication for this procedure was obstruction; 79 of the 98 patients had either complete obstruction or a considerable degree of retention. In the remaining patients, the surgeon considered obstruction to be imminent.

The results with respect to survival were discouraging, as might be expected. Approximately a third of the patients died within 3 months after operation, one-third lived 3 to 6 months, and one-third lived more than 6 months. Only 12% of the patients lived for more than 1 year, the longest survival being 16 months.

Other statistical data showed that longevity after palliative gastroenterostomy was similar to that for patients undergoing exploration only. Some surgeons have therefore concluded that gastroenterostomy is of no value. Each group in this comparison, however, comprises a different type of patient, and even a brief respite from obstructive symptoms may be beneficial.

An effort was made to correlate certain pathologic features of the lesions, such as hepatic metastasis, distant peritoneal implants, and ascites, with duration of survival after gastroenterostomy. One of nine patients with ascites lived for more than 6 months after gastroenterostomy. In contrast, neither hepatic involvement nor peritoneal seeding seemed to be a severely limiting factor. Of the 12 patients living more than 1 year, 5 had hepatic metastasis and 4 had diffuse peritoneal implantation of tumor that had been visible at the time of operation. Most patients who survived for only a short time did not return for reevaluation; in these cases, the information was obtained chiefly from correspondence. Because patients are not restored to normal health, statements about relative improvement are influenced by expectations. Rarely does a patient with advanced gastric cancer become completely comfortable after any form of treatment. The results of palliative gastroenterostomy can best be appreciated if the cases are considered in three categories: (1) those in which efforts at palliation failed, (2) those in which benefit followed operation, and (3) those in which the result of treatment was equivocal.

Ineffective operations were the easiest to analyze. Failure of palliation was judged by two criteria: (1) failure to relieve obstruction, and (2) failure to effect relief because of extension of the lesion that was unaffected by gastroenterostomy. Of the 95 patients, 31 were classified in the failure group; however, 10 of these 31 patients had temporary relief of their symptoms of obstruction. Nevertheless, they were included in the group of failures because all but two died in less than 3 months after operation, and it seems important to recognize the discomfort imposed by operation. Although 9 of the other 21 patients became worse abruptly after operation, this could be attributed to non-function of the gastroenterostomy in only 2. In general, failure of palliative efforts could be attributed to manifestations of disease unaffected by gastroenterostomy, such as hepatic metastasis, involvement of the biliary tract precluding decompression, nausea or marked early satiety without vomiting, bleeding and resultant severe anemia, ascites, cerebral metastasis, or extreme weakness.

Nineteen patients definitely benefited from gastroenterostomy, 12 of whom survived 1 year or longer. All 12 had had preoperative obstruction, and all were relieved of symptoms of obstruction for 8 to 12 months. Most of these patients were hospitalized only in the terminal few weeks of their illness, many gained weight postoperatively, and several reported that they felt well enough to return to work for 6 to 8 months. Seven additional patients lived for 9 to 12 months; they had severe symptoms of obstruction preoperatively and failed in health precipitously rather than gradually so that special care was required only during the last few weeks of life. Most of these patients reported a temporary gain in weight and returned briefly to gainful employment.

There remained 45 patients whose progress after operation was classified as inconclusive. These patients lived 3 to 12 months, and all were relieved of obstruction for at least 2 months. Initially, it seemed reasonable to judge results in this group as poor or fair solely on the basis of duration of survival. Ultimately, however, little correlation was noted between comfort and longevity. Of 12 patients who lived for 6 to 12 months after operation, 6 were reasonably comfortable until their terminal month of life and required special care for only a few weeks. Results of treatment for these patients were classified as fair. The other six experienced jaundice, considerable abdominal pain, or discomforting ascites that began 3 to 5 months after operation but did not prove fatal for several more months.

Of 33 patients who lived 3 to 6 months after operation, all were relieved of symptoms of obstruction for at least 2 months but most soon experienced recurrent symptoms of obstruction or disability from the effects of the cancer. Six patients remained relatively comfortable until the terminal month of their illness and required no special care before that time. Results were classified as fair for these 6 patients and as poor for the other 27. Thus, of 45 patients who had equivocal results, the effect of treatment was considered to be fair in 12 and poor in 33.

Gastric Resection

Opinions about the resectability of gastric cancer are widely divergent. Some surgeons apply the term "palliative" to all cases with evidence of residual carcinoma. Some physicians require microscopic proof of residual tumor, whereas others base their opinion on gross appearance. Adson (1964) studied 82 patients who underwent "palliative" resection for gastric cancer. Thirteen were excluded from the study because the operative report did not include microscopic verification or an acceptable description of the residual lesion. Of the remaining 69 patients, 46 had partial gastrectomy, 6 had total gastrectomy, and 17 had esophagogastrectomy.

Of the 46 patients treated by partial gastrectomy, 3 died in the hospital after operation, an operative mortality rate of 6.5%. The average period of postoperative hospitalization was 16.5 days. The duration of survival of the remaining 43 patients was much better than that of the patients who underwent palliative gastroenterostomy. Eight patients survived for more than 2 years, 7 lived for 1 to 2 years, 10 lived for 6 to 12 months, and 18 lived for less than 6 months.

Correlation of survival with pathologic features showed that hepatic metastasis definitely affected the results. More than half of the patients with hepatic spread lived for less than 6 months. Nevertheless, five patients with involvement of the liver lived for 6 to 12 months, and one lived for more than 12 months; thus, hepatic metastasis should not be considered a contraindication to palliative resection. Six of 13 patients having distant peritoneal implantation of tumor survived for 12 months or longer. The one patient with ascites lived for less than 6 months. Only about one-third of the patients treated by partial gastrectomy had symptoms of obstruction before operation. Because the natural history of the disease is less predictable in patients without obstruction, the degree of palliation that can be attributed to operation is uncertain. Of 15 patients who had symptoms of obstruction before operation, all but 2 were relieved of symptoms initially, but only about half of the 15 lived longer than 6 months, and only 3 lived for more than a year.

Five patients lived for 3 months or less, and an additional five patients had persistent, truly disabling discomfort, even though they lived for slightly longer periods. Palliation was not achieved in these 10 patients.

Included in the group having "good" results were 14 of the 15 patients who survived for 12 months or longer. The one patient excluded lived for 14 months; his condition declined gradually. This patient had no symptoms of obstruction preoperatively, and his progress probably would have been similar had resection not been done. Two of the 14 patients had had obstruction before operation and enjoyed eating for 10 to 13 months after operation.

Little correlation existed between length of survival and comfort, and a reasonable estimate of palliation could be made only for those patients who had preoperative obstruction. Results were fair for six patients who were relieved of symptoms of obstruction for 4 to 7 months and who survived for 5 to 10 months, and the effectiveness of treatment for the other 13 was poor.

Two patients who were originally included in the palliative group were later excluded when they were found to be living 5 and 7 years after operation. One of these patients had enlarged, hard nodes in the retroperitoneal region, which could not be removed. The other patient had one obvious superficial hepatic metastatic lesion, which was removed for microscopic confirmation, and several other less definite nodules deeper within the liver, which were "assumed" to be metastatic tumors.

The six patients who had total gastrectomy survived the operation. Although partial gastrectomy had been planned, unsuspected proximal infiltration of the tumor necessitated extension of the procedure. Residual tumor was proved microscopically in five of these patients; in the other case, the surgeon reported obviously inoperable involvement of lymph nodes with extension into the hilus of the liver. The results with respect to survival were disappointing. Five of the patients lived for 3, 4, 5, 5, and 8 months, respectively. The sixth patient, whose resection was described as palliative on the basis of gross diagnosis alone, was reported as living 2 years after operation. Because the five patients who survived for less than 9 months had no dysphagia or other symptoms of obstruction preoperatively, the results with respect to palliation were disappointing. The one long-term survivor was comfortable 22 months postoperatively. Although this series is small, it supports the belief that total gastrectomy for palliation should generally be avoided.

Palliative Esophagogastrectomy

Seventeen patients with hepatic metastasis, distant peritoneal involvement, and involvement of retroperitoneal lymph nodes underwent palliative esophagogastrectomy. One patient died in the hospital. Both the hospital mortality rate and the average postoperative hospitalization period were similar to those after partial gastrectomy.

Dysphagia, the chief indication for resection in patients with advanced disease, was experienced preoperatively by all but 3 of the 17 patients. Although dysphagia was relieved initially in all, palliative resection was considered to have failed in two patients who died in the second postoperative month. Eight patients lived for 5 to 11 months and were relieved of dysphagia for 3 to 8 months. There is no justification for enthusiasm about the progress of these patients; however,

the benefits cannot be ignored, and these results were classified as fair. Of the
remaining six patients, four survived for 13 to 14 months and had relief of
dysphagia for 8 to 12 months. Hepatic metastasis was noted in one of the other
two at operation, and when this patient was seen 20 months later, pain from
metastasis in the right hip was controlled with radiation therapy. The sixth
patient was living 30 months after operation without clinical evidence of residual
disease, although at operation the surgeon had described inoperable nodal involvement posterior to the celiac axis.

Prostheses

Experience at the Mayo Clinic with intraluminal plastic tube prostheses for
palliation of obstructive lesions has been limited. Although some surgeons have
placed tubes intraluminally for the relief of pyloric obstruction, such devices
have been employed here only for obstruction in the esophagus or at the esophagogastric junction. Bernatz recently reviewed the total experience at the Mayo
Clinic with the use of prostheses for esophageal and gastric cancer (Bernatz, P.E.
[1980]. Personal communication). Only those lesions arising in the stomach and
obstructing the esophagogastric junction will be considered here. A variety of
tubes has been used. The Mackler tube, used exclusively in earlier years, has
been inserted less often than the Celestin tube recently. A Tygon tube, employed
in the manner described by Eiseman and associates (1959), was used in only one
Mayo patient.

Of 16 patients who received prostheses, 2 died within the 30-day hospitalization
period, 6 lived 3 months or less, and 4 lived 3 to 6 months. Three other patients
were still living 3 months after operation at last report, but their progress
suggests that survival for more than 6 months is unlikely. Only one patient lived
for more than 6 months.

The prostheses were of no help for 5 of the 16 patients because of short survival,
only transient relief of obstruction, or predominance of symptoms other than
obstruction. Two of these five patients ate well initially but died suddenly 16
and 21 days postoperatively. Two patients lived for 3 months, but correspondence
with relatives indicated that one obtained no help from the prosthesis and the
other "could not keep food down." The fifth patient had no mechanical difficulty
with eating but experienced disabling nausea.

Results were judged as fair in seven patients who obtained relief of dysphagia for
approximately half of their period of survival. The tube became obstructed in two
of these patients, and one had brief postoperative bleeding.

Although the remaining four patients survived for only short periods, their
results were classified as good. The one surviving longest ate satisfactorily for
6 months and died 7 months after operation. At autopsy, the Mackler tube was
found in the ileum. The patient for whom the Tygon tube was used was "comfortable
but weak" until sudden death 4 months after operation; this tube was patent at
autopsy. Another patient, in whom a Mackler tube had been used, ate satisfactorily until sudden death 3 months after operation, and the fourth patient, whose
obstruction had been relieved with a Celestin prosthesis, was eating comfortably
3 months postoperatively at last report.

The alternatives for treatment of inoperable lesions are unattractive. All
physicians are familiar with the undesirable aspects of protracted nasogastric
intubation, gastrostomy, and jejunostomy. Although bougienage may give dramatic
relief, this is too often transient.

Jejunostomy, Gastrostomy, and Miscellaneous Palliative Procedures

Review of the records of 13 patients who had had enterostomy for palliation in earlier years supports the opinion that this procedure is seldom indicated. Seven of the 13 patients lived for 3 months or less, 5 survived for 4 to 6 months, and 1 survived for 13 months. For most patients, symptoms such as pain and nausea that were not alleviated by decompression or stomal feeding were as distressing as the discomforts attributable to obstruction or starvation, and jejunostomy was not truly palliative. For several patients, jejunostomy was done when dysphagia was only minimal. Inasmuch as dysphagia was only slowly progressive in some and was managed by periodic dilations in others, enterostomy had little relationship to progress. Because pain and nausea are not relieved and may be protracted by jejunostomy, this procedure is contraindicated whenever such symptoms are the major complaints.

Occasionally, jejunostomy or gastrostomy seems appropriate. The patient with slowly progressive disease may avoid prolonged hospitalization and may be cared for at home more easily or comfortably if gastrostomy relieves vomiting and precludes the need for nasogastric intubation. Similar benefits accrue if jejunostomy replaces long-term intravenous therapy. Even in this situation, stomal decompression or feeding is of questionable benefit, and the feasibility of relief by insertion of a prosthesis or the advisability of avoiding active treatment should be considered first. A special indication for stomal feeding may be the maintenance of nutrition when chemotherapy offers a reasonable chance of palliation.

Transesophageal dilations for the relief of dysphagia have been attempted. When done by experienced personnel in selected patients (for example, when dysphagia is a major or the sole cause of discomfort), they have definite, although temporary, palliative value. Although the procedure is not without risk, the hazards are less than with open operation, and avoidance of prolonged hospitalization and postoperative convalescence is an advantage. Pain secondary to retroperitoneal neural involvement is occasionally a predominant symptom of advanced gastric carcinoma. In selected cases, splanchnic block with absolute alcohol may give relief.

PHILOSOPHY OF PALLIATIVE SURGERY

Discussion of palliation for patients having advanced cancer is inadequate without some consideration of moral and philosophic aspects of such care. Conservatism is indicated when there is risk of prolonging distress for the incurable patient. In contrast, subjective judgments about apparently incurable disease should be avoided. Clinical observations do not always provide reliable evidence of incurability. Reports of cervical ribs that may simulate Virchow's node, diverticulitis or pelvic inflammation that may seem to be a rectal shelf, or pessimism about incarcerated omentum in a small umbilical hernia make one hesitate to rely solely on clinical judgment. Some huge tumors that appear to be inoperable may be lymphosarcomas and may be amenable to treatment. Another lesion that may cause pessimism is a large posterior penetrating ulcer. Most of these lesions are benign, and the patient with such a lesion, who is judged on the basis of clinical criteria to have an inoperable cancer, may die of the benign disease. Therefore, decisions about inoperability should be based on histologic evidence; usually a specimen may be obtained safely.

Some patients with advanced disease may have only minor disturbances in function, and operation in these patients should not be undertaken indiscriminately. The disability after radical gastrectomy is a fair exchange for hope of cure but not

for the patient with incurable disease whose preoperative disability is minimal.
The procedure for such patients must be chosen carefully.

Modern multimodality therapy, such as systemic or regional infusion with 5-fluoro-
uracil (Moertel and colleagues, 1976)—from which some patients will benefit—or
the use of radiotherapy for localized but inoperable tumors must be considered.

Accordingly, the surgeon must take a discerning look at the "biology of the
tumor." If it is an apparently slow-growing lesion that is still localized, even
with nodal metastases, it should be resected. Resection should be considered even
when the tumor involves multiple viscera, such as the left lobe of the liver, the
transverse colon, and the retroperitoneal nodes. If reconstruction of the gastrointestinal tract is necessary after total gastrectomy for such a lesion, it should
always be done with an esophagojejunostomy combined with a lower enteroenterostomy
at least 20 cm from the esophagojejunostomy. A jejunal interposition of at least
25 cm between the esophagus and the duodenum has also been effective, although the
direct esophagojejunostomy is simpler and can frequently be accomplished with a
stapling device. In no case should the esophagus be anastomosed to the duodenum
or to the jejunum without a lower bypass procedure.

Patients with disseminated tumors that involve the liver or with peritoneal
implants, ascites, or both have a different biologic form of the tumor, yet some
of them respond dramatically to adjunctive therapy, such as chemotherapy with or
without radiotherapy to the major mass. Therefore, every available means should
be used to relieve the symptomatic lesion, particularly if it is causing obstruction. Patients with localized disease should be considered for treatment with
radiotherapy after hepatic artery infusion. All patients who demonstrate a
response to chemotherapy should be considered for weekly treatments with 5-
fluorouracil in a dose of 15 mg/kg.

Perhaps the most important aspect of chemotherapy involves weekly examinations of
the patient; from these examinations, we have derived a better understanding of
the progress of the disease, its complications, and more effective management.

The surgeon must develop guidelines (Lawrence and McNeer, 1958) for selecting the
operative procedure most likely to produce some benefit during the remaining life
of the patient. The choices range from biopsy alone to palliative (or incomplete)
resection, and mortality, morbidity, and potential benefit must all be considered.
The decision depends on both the results of the various procedures that are
technically feasible and the potential for subsequent nonoperative treatment.
This choice must not be made casually.

In choosing optimal treatment, the surgeon must answer the following questions
(Lawrence and McNeer, 1958):

1. If both palliative resection and bypass operations are feasible in a patient,
is it worthwhile to perform the more extensive procedure (resection)?

2. If resection is not feasible without resorting to total gastrectomy, is a
procedure of this extent truly palliative?

3. If resection is not feasible, is bypass gastroenterostomy, gastrostomy, or
jejunostomy beneficial for the patient with gastric cancer and, if so, under what
circumstances?

My opinion in response to the first question is that resection should probably be
done instead of a bypass operation for palliation if both procedures are technically feasible. In response to the second question, I believe that palliative

total gastrectomy is not favorable because of the associated risks. The third question, regarding the advisability of some form of bypass operation when resection is not feasible, is the most difficult to answer. Generally, bypass procedures with use of external tubes (gastrostomy or jejunostomy) have produced no relief of symptoms and have imposed considerable complications in our experience. Such procedures are justifiable in the rare instance when the patient's general condition is such that a reasonable survival time is expected but prolonged intravenous support in the hospital would be necessitated. In this relatively uncommon circumstance, gastrostomy or jejunostomy may allow the patient to return home for his or her remaining months, but most patients with advanced gastric cancer are not candidates for these ineffective procedures. Unless complete or almost complete distal obstruction is present, we also avoid gastroenterostomy as a palliative procedure in patients unsuitable for palliative resection because the gains are minimal.

In most instances, radiation therapy is ineffective as a palliative treatment for gastric cancer because disease in patients found unsuitable for resection is not localized enough for such regional treatment. Alternatively, radiation therapy has been useful in relieving localized areas of obstruction, particularly in the region of the cardia, and patients with chronically bleeding gastric cancers have also benefited from irradiation. The nature of the pattern of spread of gastric cancer in the patient who is not amenable to operative therapy, however, usually makes systemic chemotherapy seem more appropriate than radiation therapy.

REFERENCES

Adson, M. A. (1964). Palliative operations for gastric cancer. In W. H. ReMine, J. T. Priestley, and J. Berkson (Eds.), Cancer of the Stomach. W. B. Saunders Company, Philadelphia. pp. 141-157.
Celestin, L. R. (1959). Permanent intubation in inoperable cancer of the oesophagus and cardia: a new tube. Ann. roy. Coll. Surg. Engl., 25, 165-170.
Comis, R. L., and S. K. Carter (1974). A review of chemotherapy in gastric cancer. Cancer (Philad.), 34, 1576-1586.
Eiseman, B., R. B. Melzer, and F. J. Rachiele (1959). An indwelling plastic conduit for relief of obstruction in unresectable carcinoma of the stomach. Surg. Gynec. Obstet., 109, 460-466.
Lawrence, W., Jr., and G. McNeer (1958). The effectiveness of surgery for palliation of incurable gastric cancer. Cancer (Philad.), 11, 28-32.
MacDonald, J. S., P. V. Wooley, T. Smythe, et al. (in press). 5-Fluorouracil, Adriamycin, and mitomycin-C (FAM) combination chemotherapy in the treatment of advanced gastric cancer. Cancer (Philad.).
Mackler, S. A., and R. M. Mayer (1954). Palliation of esophageal obstruction due to carcinoma with a permanent intraluminal tube. J. Thorac. Surg., 28, 431-443.
Moertel, C. G., J. A. Mittelman, R. F. Bakemeier, P. Engstrom, and J. Hanley (1976). Sequential and combination chemotherapy of advanced gastric cancer. Cancer (Philad.), 38, 678-682.

DISCUSSION

E. Deutch. In the pre-operative assessment of the early lesion, the endoscopist has an advantage, primarily because anaesthesia seems to account for the vascular changes you see with the early lesion. In ten cases where I have got a positive biopsy, the surgeon has called me up and asked me "where is the lesion?"

W. ReMine. What do you tell him?

E. Deutch. Where we found it. I can't put a staple there. I tell him that most of them are in the antrum and a simple sub-total gastrectomy will do. Here is where we have our greatest salvageability, which is what you are talking about particularly in the long term survivors, so I think we can help out with biopsy and with endoscopic description of the vascular changes around the lesion, because they are lost at surgery.

W. ReMine. Would it be possible for you to go back and cauterize an area where you took your biopsies so that the surgeon can identify it?

E. Deutch. I have thought of cauterizing but I would loose my tissue, and that's the reason why I have not cauterized.

W. ReMine. Would it be possible to do that? It would certainly simplify things for the surgeon if he could find a fresh cauterised area.

E. Deutch. I think what you say must be true because even within two or three days of biopsy, you cannot see where I have biopsied. We might try marking the specimen by cautery. I just stayed away from it because I thought I would lose my diagnostic tissue.

W. ReMine. Well, you would at the moment.

E. Deutch. I could get my biopsies first and then mark with cautery. One other area where I think the endoscopist might be of help, particularly in trying to find those that are going to be failures, would be the Bormann type 3 and Bormann type 4 where we see no motillity at all. Would'nt this correlate closely with your failure group?

W. ReMine. I think that is true and it is a very good point. That is also why I operate on these. As you saw from that last slide and heard from the last comment, we had 17 in the group that lived 10 years or longer that required total gastrectomy to get the lesion out because of this type of lesion, the so called linitis plastica. Now you chances of cure of these patients are very slim. It is worth a try because they have no other opportunity and if the surgeon had not been willing to make a try in those 17 patients they would not have been alive.

H. Ellis. I think that any surgeon would say that you can't be put off by the size or shape or consistency of a tumour. I remember in 1948 we had a patient in Oxford who presented with a great big mass in his abdomen and my chief opened him up and there was an enormous tumour. My chief said it was absolutely hopeless but I said "you can't leave this fellow because he has felt the tumour and he wants it removed." So we circumsized this tremendous mass and it was put in the museum and used as one of the teaching specimens in the finals examinations. When I went back to Oxford as a Senior Resident many years later, the first chap I saw in the out-patient clinic was this fellow; so there you are! By the way, gentlemen, in January of next year we will be celebrating the one hundreth anniversary of Billroth's first gastrectomy, so I think it is very appropriate that we saw those pictures of gastrectomy today.

Chemotherapy and Combined Modality Treatment of Gastric Cancer

P.S. Schein, R. Coffey, Jr., and F.P. Smith

Vincent T. Lombardi Cancer Research Center,
Georgetown University, Washington, D.C. 20007, U.S.A.

INTRODUCTION

While gastric carcinoma has decreased in incidence in the United States, it still remains an important health program. It currently ranks as the sixth most common cause of cancer-related death in America (19).

Internationally this tumor has great importance since it represents the major cause of cancer mortality in Japan, Finland, Chile and the U.S.S.R. (17). In the United States, it is projected that 85% of the newly diagnosed cases of stomach cancer will be dead of their disease within five years. The majority of these patients either present with, or soon develop, metastatic tumor requiring chemotherapeutic management. Despite the overall position of this tumor, relatively few anticancer drugs have undergone an adequate clinical trial.

There are several possible explanations. It is widely held that cancer of the stomach is inherently resistant to both chemotherapy and radiation therapy. This preconception coupled with the difficulties in identifying measurable parameters of disease has served to dampen the enthusiasm of clinical investigators. To define an objective response requires that there be measurable tumor. Most patients in whom the tumor mass can be objectively assessed have, by definition, bulk disease and often present with the accompanying clinical features of poor performance status, cachexia and hepatic dysfunction. The latter factor, in particular, may significantly impair the patient's tolerance or ability to receive, many chemotherapeutic agents. In addition, we have long since learned that patients who are bedridden or jaundiced from hepatic metastases have little prospect of benefitting from any form of treatment; they require symptomatic and sympathetic care, but are not suitable candidates for trials of investigational treatment. Nevertheless, many such patients have been included in past studies. To obtain useful and interpretable data patient selection is an essential requirement, and as in the case of surgery, we are dependent on an early identification of the primary or recurrent malignancy.

While the data base for chemotherapy and radiation therapy is still somewhat limited, there are definite indications that advanced gastric cancer can be effectively palliated with chemotherapy in many cases. For patients with locally unresectable tumors, or where "curative" surgery leaves the patient

with a high probability for relapse, the results of a recently completed trial
offers some optimum for the future.

ADVANCED MEASURABLE TUMOR

Single Agent Chemotherapy

Adenocarcinoma of the stomach is one of several tumors for which very few drugs
have been satisfactorily tested. Given for the major class of alkylating
agents, the mustards, the overall denominator of patients to be found in the
literature does not allow for an adequate assessment of their single agent
activity (3). An obvious and important need for the future use of chemotherapy
involves the systematic evaluation of individual anticancer drugs in patients
with advanced disease. We are unfortunately tied to the emperical clinical
trial until there are better and laboratory based rationale for drug selection.

5-Flourouracil (5-FU) is the most extensively studied antitumor drug (3).
Despite over 20 years of clinical use, there is still considerable controversy
as to the optimal method of administration of this agent. The most frequently
reported schedule is the daily intravenous injection for five consecutive days,
the so-called "loading course", in which the cumulative literature suggests an
overall 21% response (in most trials response is defined as a 50% or greater
decrease in the products of the two largest perpendicular diameters of a
measurable tumor).

Many successful programs have selected a weekly method of administration,
although a controlled trial with the loading course has never been reported for
this disease. The oral administration of 5-FU has been evaluated in three
trials involving patients with colorectal cancer metastatic to liver; in all
studies oral 5-FU has proven inferior to intravenous treatment in regard to
percent response and duration. This has been correlated with variation in
absorption from the gastrointestinal trial, and in general oral 5-FU is no
longer considered an accepted route of drug delivery.

While the literature relating to 5-FU in gastric cancer is comparatively vast,
the majority of the reports have failed to analyze these results in
relationship to the known prognostic factors for response; this should include
age, disease-free interval, performance status, histologic grade of the tumor,
and sites of metastasis (10).

Mitomycin-C, an antibiotic alkylating agent, is the second most extensively
investigated agent in gastric cancer (8). The initial enthusiasm resulting
from favorable reports in Japan waned rapidly after the reports of serious and
persistent depression of bone marrow functions when the drug was administered on
a daily schedule. It eventually became recognized that mitomycin-C shares with
the chloroethyl nitrosourea the unusual property of producing delayed and
cumulative hematologic toxicity. In response, recent trials have employed an
intermittent single dose schedule, with much improved patient tolerance (2).
The overall reported response rate for 98 patients reported in the literature
is 24% (3).

The two chloroethyl nitrosoureas that have been adequately evaluated are
1,3-bis-(2-chloroethyl)-1-nitrosourea (BCNU) and methyl-CCNU. BCNU has been
reported to produce an 17% response rate (7). Methyl-CCNU, an agent that has
been employed in many combination chemotherapy programs, has limited single
agent activity with a response rate less than 10% (13). Chlorozotocin, a new
nitrosourea with relative reduced myelosuppressive toxicity is currently being
evaluated in a clinical trial being conducted by the Cancer and Acute Leukemia
Group B (CALGB).

Doxorubicin (adriamycin) has recently been demonstrated to be an important drug for gastric cncer. In trials conducted by the Gastrointestinal Tumor Study Group (GITSG) and the Eastern Cooperative Oncology Group (ECOG) response rates of 22-24% have been reported for patients with advanced and measurable tumors (5,12). Adriamycin has already been incorporated into several active regimens of combination chemotherapy.

There is one unpublished report of the use of cis-platinum in gastric cancer by Brugarolas and co-workers. Nineteen patients who had previously been treated with combination of 5-FU, adriamycin and methyl-CCNU, 5 have demonstrated an objective response. This interesting result awaits confirmation by the current EORTC Phase II trial, but cis-platinum may represent an important new development in the management of gastric cancer.

It must be emphasized that despite the finding of modest therapeutic activity with individual drugs, single agent chemotherapy for advanced gastric cancer is an established exercise in futility. Such treatment is of little value in improving the survival of patients with this stage of disease involvement.

Combination Chemotherapy

The initial approaches to combination chemotherapy during the past decade have involved the use of 5-FU and the chloroethylnitrosoureas. Kovach et al. reported the results of a randomized trial which compared the regimens of BCNU + 5-FU to each single agent in patients with advanced disease (7). The combination was reported to produce a 41% response rate, compared to 29% for 5-FU alone and 17% for BCNU. There was no overall survival advantage for the combination when compared to 5-FU and BCNU alone, but at 18 months, 25% of the patients treated with the combination were alive compared to 5% with the single agents. There was no confirmation of the reported response rate or possible survival benefit with this combination. With the subsequent introduction of methyl-CCNU into clinical trials attention began to focus on this agent in combination chemotherapy.

The ECOG initiated a randomized control trial which compared the combination of methyl-CCNU 175 mg/m^2 po and 5-FU 300 mg/m^2 I.V. daily X5 to methyl-CCNU as a single agent (13). The reported response rate for the combination was 40% compared to 8% for methyl-CCNU; however, a subsequent trial conducted by the ECOG showed no advantage for this combination compared to 5-FU. In a third trial by the same group response rate had dropped to 24%, where the remission rate with 5-FU + mitomycin-C was 32% (12). In a controlled trial the GITSG has recently confirmed a similarly modest response rate with 5-FU + methyl-CCNU, while demonstrating survival superiority for regimens containing 5-FU and adriamycin (18).

While there are very little data on the single agent activity of the antimetabolite cytosine arabinoside in gastric cancer, the drug has been a component of the most common combination used in Japan. This is based upon the study of Ota et al. who reported a high initial response rate with the regimen of mitomycin-C, 5-FU and cytosine arabinoside (MFC) (15). The overall response rate of 36% (129/356), was associated with a mean duration of survival ranging between 4-5 months. The GITSG evaluated the same three-drug combination, employing an intensive course schedule (5); a 17% response rate was recorded with MFC. In addition, the FAMe combination of 5-FU, adriamycin and methyl-CNU produced a superior response rate (47%) and survival (13 weeks) when compared to MFC (9 weeks) in this randomized controlled trial (5).

In 1974 the Vincent T. Lombardi Cancer Research Center initiated a program to evaluate a combination of 5-fluorouracil, adriamycin and mitomycin-C (FAM)

(9). The regimen incorporated the three drugs that we regarded as the most
active single agents for gastric cancer. In addition, mitomycin-C was given in
an intermittent schedule, in recognition of this agent's delayed and cumulative
bone marrow toxicity. Sixty-two patients with advanced and measurable gastric
cancer were entered into this study between Septmber, 1974 and September,
1978. The median age was 62 years, with a range of 28-83 years. There were 38
males and 24 females. Eleven percent of patients were asymptomatic, 35% were
symptomatic but fully ambulatory and 28% were spending part, but less than 50%,
of waking hours in bed. Twenty-six were confined to bed 50-100% of the day.
All patients had biopsy-proven adenocarcinoma of the stomach and none had
previously been treated with chemotherapy or radiation therapy. The majority
of patients had large abdominal masses (50%) and/or followable hepatic
metastases (36%). Eight percent had osseous metastases and 6% had malignant
lymph node masses.

Patients were evaluated for response using the following system. A partial
response (PR) was defined as a 50% or greater decrease in the products of the
two largest perpendicular diameters of the most clearly measurable lesion,
without increase in the size of other known areas of malignant disease. This
result must have been observed at a minimum of four weeks after initiation of
treatment. If hepatomegaly was followed, there must have been a decrease of at
least 30% in the sum of measurements below the xyphoid process and both costal
margins at the midclavicular line, with improvement or stability of
pretreatment liver function tests. If, at the end of a eight-week cycle,
patients demonstrated disease progression they were defined as non-responders
(NR) and alternate therapy was initiated. Duration of survival was measured
from the start of therapy.

The FAM regimen was administered in eight week cycles. 5-Fluorouracil was
administered at a dose of 600 mg/m^2 intravenously on days 1,8,29 and 36.
Adriamycin was was administered intravenously at a dose of 30 mg/m^2 on days 1
and 29 and mitomycin-C, 10 mg/m^2, was administered on day one only of each
course. Drug dosage was modified for subsequent courses according to the
degree of hematologic toxicity as measured by white blood cell and platelet
counts. Blood counts were obtained weekly during the first cycle of
chemotherapy and in subsequent courses immediately prior to each treatment.
Since the nadir of hematologic toxicity produced by mitomycin-C occurs four to
five weeks after administration, blood counts measured during this time period
were used to adjust the dosage of this agent for the subsequent cycle. In
patients in whom myelosuppression temporarily prevented administration of
chemotherapy, blood counts were monitored weekly and treatment initiated as
soon as the white blood cell count was greater than 2,500/mm^3 and the
platelet count greater than 75,000/mm^3.

Twenty-six of 62 patients (42%) achieve a partial remission. The median
duration of response was 9.0 months (range 2-19.5 months). The median duration
of survival in responding patients was 12.5 months. Six of twenty-six (25%)
responding patients survived for greater than 24 months. Of the 36 patients
who failed to respond, all have died and their median survival was 3.5 months
(range 0.5-8.0 months) from the initiation of therapy. The difference in
survival time between the responding and non-responding patients was
statistically significant (p $<$ .01).

Several potential prognostic factors are important in analyzing response to
chemotherapy in patients with advanced cancer. Although there was a slightly
better initial performance status in responding patients compared to
non-responders, there was no statistically significant correlation between
performance status and response.

Another factor that could influence the response to chemotherapy is the presence of a large unresectable primary tumor mass since patients with unresectable gastric tumors are less likely to respond to chemotherapy. Of our total patient group, 28/62 (45%) had undergone a resection of the primary tumor; this included 13/26 (50%) patients evidencing an objective response to chemotheerapy and 15/36 (42%) of the non-responding group (p=0.10). It has been reported that patients with poorly differentiated gastric tumors are less likely to respond to chemotherapy than those with well differentiated neoplasms. Pathological specimens were available for review by a single pathologist for 50 of the 62 cases (25 of the 26 responders and 25 of 36 non-responders). These specimens were categorized into one of two groups: well and moderately well differentiated or poorly differentiated. Sixty-eight percent of patients with poorly differentiated tumor demonstrated a partial response. In contrast, only 32% (8/25) of patients with better differentiated tumors responded.

The FAM regimen was generally well tolerated as outpatient therapy. Vomiting was uncommon, and when noted usually on the first day of treatment. Adriamycin cardiac toxicity was not expected nor was it encountered. With the adriamycin dose employed, 60 mg/m^2 per cycle, the total dose reached after one year of treatment is only 360 mg/m^2. The principal toxicity was bone marrow depression. Significant leukopenia (WBC < 1,500/mm^3) or thrombocytopenia (platelets < 30,000/mm^3) occurred in 11% and 10% of patients respectively. After 12 months of treatment, patients continued to tolerate 75% of their original doses based upon body surface area; which reflected the relatively low cumulative bone marrow toxicity.

These results have stimulated other investigators to attempt to reproduce our findings. In a non-randomized trial Bitram et al. have reported partial responses in 6/11 (55%) of patients with advanced gastric cancer (1). The overall survival for the eleven patients was 6.5 months, with a projectd median survival of 16.5 months for responders. The Southwest Oncology Group (SWOG) has conducted a randomized trial comparing the FAM regimen with the sequential use of the same three drugs. A 44% response was reported with FAM compared to 27% with sequential therapy (15).The FAM combination is now being evaluated as a surgical adjuvant therapy by the SWOG and the CALGB.

The activity of adriamycin-based regimens is further confirmed by the report by Levi et al. of 52% response with the combination of 5-FU, adriamycin and BCNU (FAB) (8). The median duration of response was 48 weeks, and the median survival of responders was one year.

At the Lombardi Cancer Research Center we are conducting a pilot study of a new program for gastric cancer, taking advantage of the report of single efficacy for cis-platinum. The FAP regimen consists of 5-FU, 600 mg/m^2, IV on day 1&8. Adriamycin 40 mg/m^2 IV on day 1, and cis-platinum 75 mg/m^2 IV on day 1. This treatment cycle is repeated every 30 days. The initial results are encouraging, and it is hoped that the addition of cis-platinum to the former two drugs will increase both the percentage of patients responding as well as the quality of the response.

LOCALLY ADVANCED TUMOR

When a cancer of the stomach has involved the regional lymph nodes or adjacent tissues and organs, and cannot be completely resected en bloc, it is designated

as locally advanced. In operational terms, the residual or unresectable tumor
can be encompassed within a moderate sized upper abdominal radiation therapy
field. In this group treated with surgery alone, the median survival has been
estimated to be approximately five months, with essentially all patients dead
within 2 years. The addition of 3500-4000 rads of external beam irradiation to
the region of the stomach has not changed this survival.

Falkson and Falkson studied the combined use of radiation therapy and 5-FU
(4). They reported that 55% of their patients with locally advanced gastric
cancer showed an objective improvement, whereas none responded to radiation
alone and only 17% improved with 5-FU. Subsequently, the Mayo Clinic reported
their experience with 3500-4000 rads of irradiation, with half of the patients
receiving 5-FU by random selection and the remaining patients receiving saline
placebo in addition to their radiation therapy (11). The median survival for
the combined modality approach was approximately 7 months, compared to 5 months
with radiation alone. More importantly, three of 25 patients treated with 5-FU
and radiation therapy survived 5 years, whereas there was no survival in excess
of 15 months with radiation therapy alone (6).

In 1974 the GITSG initiated a randomized controlled trial of chemotherapy
versus combined modality treatment for locally advanced gastric cancer (18).
The chemotherapy regimen chosen was 5-FU + methyl-CCNU. The radiation therapy
arm of this trial consisted of 5000 rads delivered in two 2500 rad courses,
each 3 weeks in duration, separated by a two-week rest interval. The maximum
field size was 400/sq.cm. 5-FU, at a dose of 500 mg/m^2 I.V., was given on
each of the first 3 days of each course of radiation therapy. Two weeks after
completion of this treatment, the patients were placed on 5-FU + methyl-CCNU
until evidence of disease progression. The group randomized to chemotherapy
alone had a median survival of 70 weeks compared to 36 weeks for combined
modalilty (p $<$ .05). With longer followup, however, the survival curve of the
combined modality group has a plateau at 2-4 years at the 20% level, while
patients treated with chemotherapy alone demonstrate a continued probability to
relapse and die. Among patients who had undergone a palliative resection of
the tumor plus combined irradiation and chemotherapy, approximately 25% are
alive and disease-free 4 years after surgery.

The early deaths in the combined modality arm were due to treatment toxicity
(nutritional and hematologic) and tumor progression in the irradiated region.
Intensive nutritional support, including parenteral hyperalimentation, might
have prevented some of the early deaths in this trial. The overall result, a
20% long-term disease-free survival, represents an important advance in the
treatment of locally advanced gastric cancer. It is possible that with greater
attention to reducing the toxicity of upper abdominal irradiation, and the use
of more active forms of chemotherapy such as the FAM or FAMe regimens, these
survival rates can be further improved upon. It should be emphasized that
surgical resection of the primary tumor, while only palliative in intent,
improves the survival results achieved with all forms of post-operative
therapy, and is recommended when it can be safely performed.

SURGICAL ADJUVANT THERAPY

In gastric cancer penetration of the serosa and/or involvement of the regional
lymph nodes by a gastric cancer increases the probability of relapse to at
least 50%, despite an operation with curative intent. If the current
disheartening survival statistics are to change, something must be added to
surgery to eradicate residual and metastatic microscopic foci of cells. The
early trials of adjuvant chemotherapy conducted in the United States were

flawed in their design (3). There was no pre-randomization stratification,
and in the single agent treatment programs the dosages employed were only of
moderate intensity and the duration of treatment was short. The results were
predictably poor in trials employing thio-TEPA, an alkylating agent whose use
in this disease is without rationale.

At the present time, the major cooperative groups are evaluating drug
combinations in randomized controlled trials. The GITSG, ECOG and Veteran's
Administration Surgical Adjuvant Group are comparing the regimens of 5-FU +
methyl-CCNU after surgery versus surgery alone. The SWOG and the CALGB have
initiated controlled trials of the FAM regimen, and the North Central Cancer
Treatment Group is evaluating the combination of 5-FU + adriamycin. The
results of these ongoing adjuvant programs are awaited with great interest;
they represent the most hopeful prospect for improving the survival statistics
of this disease.

FUTURE PROSPECTS FOR THE MANAGEMENT OF GASTRIC CANCER

During the past 6 years it has become apparent that of the major malignancies
of the gastrointestinal tract, gastric cancer is the most sensitive to
chemotherapy. The current response rates for patients with advanced metastatic
disease represent an improvement over the past use of single agent 5-FU and the
combination of 5-FU + nitrosoureas. It is important to recognize that
effective palliative treatment can be delivered in an outpatient setting
without serious or life-threatening toxicity. Nevertheless the duration of
response and survival for patients with advanced disease is limited; we should
not become fixated with our current treatment as had been the case for 5-FU
over 20 years. These advances do not lessen the need to identify new drugs
that might allow for the development of future regimens with greater efficacy
and reduced toxicity.

The current results for locally advanced tumors are promising, and support the
continued investigation of combined modality approaches for this stage of the
disease. The surgeons must be convinced that resection of the primary tumor,
while only palliative in intent, nevertheless results in improved response and
survival with post-operative therapy. The overall approach to radiation
therapy to the upper abdomen can be improved upon. Toxicity must be controlled
by careful monitoring of blood counts, caloric intake and body weight during
the period of treatment. Intensive nutritional support, including intravenous
hyperalimentation, may be required in some patients to enable them to complete
treatment without becoming severely malnourished.

Several new forms of radiation therapy are now being evaluated. Neutron
irradiation presents the theoretical advantages of high linear energy transfer,
decreased oxygen requirement for cytotoxicty and high relative biological
effect when compared to conventional photons. Catterall(20) has presented initial
data supporting the rationale for neutrons; however, our experience at the
Lombardi Cancer Research Center in the treatment of upper abdominal cancers
suggests that late toxicity will be increased, without an improvement in
survival. Intraoperative electron beam irradiation is also undergoing an
initial trial in the United States. In the foreseeable future, the greatest
prospect for improving the survival of patients with gastric cancer will come
with the addition of effective forms of chemotherapy, such as the FAM regimen,
to external photon irradiation. At the Lombardi Cancer Research Center our
current trial consists of an initial 2-month course of FAM followed by 4500
rads of split course irradiation with 5-FU sensitization. After a one-month
period of recovery, the patients are placed on chemotherapy for a minimum

period of one year, assuming adequate hematologic and gastrointestinal
tolerance. The rationale for the initial use of chemotherapy comes from the
recognition that some gastric cancers will continue to grow in the face of
ongoing radiation therapy, and that the period of time required to achieve
tumor control in such cases is too long. Chemotherapy, if it is to be
effective, will produce either a reduction or stabilization of tumor size
during the initial course of treatment.

The most important aspect of clinical investigation is the evaluation of
adjuvant chemotherapy. It is now time to evaluate these regimens in patients
with a minimal residual tumor burden, an approach for which there is ample
precedent in treatment of Wilm's tumor and breast cancer with involvement of
axillary nodes.

REFERENCES

1 Bitran, J.D., R.K. Desser, M.F. Kozloff, A.A. Billings, and C.M. Shapero (1979)
Treatment of metastatic pancreatic and gastric adenocarcinoma with
fluorouracil, adriamycin, and mitomycin- (FAM). Cancer Treatment
Report, 63:2049-2051.

2 Comis, R.L. (1979). Mitomycin-C in gastric cancer in Carter, S.K. and Crooke,
S.T., ed, Mitomycin-C: Current Status and New Developments. New
York, Academic Press, pp 129-132.

3 Comis, R.L. and S.K. Carter (1974). Integration of chemotherapy into combined
modality treatment of solid tumors. III Gastric Cancer. Cancer
Treatment Reviews, 1:221-238.

4 Falkson, G. and H.C. Falkson (1969). Fluorouracil and radiotherapy in gastrointestinal cancer. Lancet, 2:1252-1253.

5 The Gastrointestinal Tumor Study Group (1979). Phase II-III chemotherapy study
in advanced gastric cancer. Cancer Treatment Reports, 63:1871.

6 Holbrook, M.A. (1974). Gastric cancer treatment principles: radiation therapy. J. Am. Med. Assoc., 228:1289-1290.

7 Kovach, J.S., C.G. Moertel, A.J. Schutt, R.G. Hahn, and R.J. Reitemeier
(1974). A controlled study of combined 1,3-bis-(2-chloroethyl-1-
nitrosourea and 5-fluorouracil therapy for advanced gastric and
pancreatic cancer. Cancer, 33:563.

8 Levi, J.A., D.M. Dalley, and R.S. Aroney (1979). Improved combination chemotherapy in advanced gastric cancer. British Med. J., 2:1471.

9 Macdonald, J.S., P.S. Schein, P.V. Woolley, M. Boiron, C. Gisslbrecht,
R. Brunet, and C. Lagarde (In Press). 5-Fluorouracil, doxorubicin
and mitomycin-C (FAM) combination chemotherapy for advanced
gastric cancer. Ann. Int. Med.

10 Moertel, C.G.(1975). Carcinoma of the stomach; prognostic factors and crite-
ria of response to therapy, in: Staquet, M.J., ed., Cancer
Therapy: Prognostic Factors and Criteria of Response. New York:
Raven Press, pp. 229-236.

11 Moertel, C.G., D.S. Childs, R.J. Reitemeier, M.Y. Colby and M.A. Holbrook
(1969). Combined 5-fluorouracil and supervoltage radiation
therapy of locally unresectable gastrointestinal cancer. Lancet,
2:865-867.

12 Moertel, C.G. and P.T. Lavin(1979). Phase II-III chemotherapy studies in
advanced gastric cancer. Cancer Treatment Reports, 63:1863.

13 Moertel, C.G., J.A. Mittelman, R.F. Bakemeier, P. Engstrom, and J. Hanley
(1976). Sequential and combination chemotherapy of advanced
gastric cancer. Cancer, 38:678.

14 Moertel, C.G., M.J. O'Connell, and P.T. Lavin (1979). Chemotherapy of gas-
carcinoma. Proc. Am. Assoc. Cancer Res., 20:288.

15 Ota, K., S. Kurita, M. Nishimura, M. Ogawa, Y. Kamei, K. Imai, Y. Ariyoshi,
        K. Kataoka, M.O. Murakami, A. Oyama, A. Hoshino, H. Amo, and T.
        Kato (1972). Combination therapy with mitomycin-C, 5-fluorouracil
        and cytosine arabinoside for advanced cancer in man. Cancer,
        Chemotherapy Reports, 56:373.
16 Panettiere, F., and L. Heilbrun (1979). Comparison of two different combina-
        tions of adriamycin, mitomycin-C and 5-FU in the management of
        gastric carcinoma. A SWOG study. Proc. Amer. Soc. Clin. Oncol.,
        20:315.
17 Piper, D.W. (1978). Stomach cancer. UICC Technical Report Service, 34:5-26.
18 Schein, P.S., and J. Novak (1980). For the Gastrointestinal Tumor Study
        Group (1980). Combined modality therapy (XRT-chemo) versus
        chemotherapy alone for locally unresectable gastric cancer. Proc.
        Amer. Soc. Clin. Oncol., 21:419.
19 Seidman, H., E. Silverberg, and A.L. Holleb (1974). Cancer Statistics 1976.
        A comparison of white and black populations. CA, 26:2-29.
20 Catterall, M. et al.Gut,1975, 16, 150-156.

DISCUSSION

H. Ellis. One is fascinated by the trials carried on in distinguished centres such as the ones we have heard about today, but the individual surgeon or physician dealing with advanced cases has always got to weigh up whether a few weeks of extra life gained with chemotherapy is worth all the trouble that it involves. I think the man not involved in cancer chemotherapy trials has got to weigh up very carefully before embarking on chemotherapy in an individual patient. What would you think about that? Supposing you were in practice away from your own Unit and you saw some gentleman of 67 with advanced carcinoma of the stomach who lived many miles away from hospital. What would really be the best thing for him? Morphia or chemotherapy?

F. Smith. It is a very important question. I would grant that not all patients are candidates for combination chemotherapy, as we have seen. However, the trials that I have reported, particularly the collaborative group trials, have by and large been carried out outside the major institutions. They have been carried out by physicians, and we have a large group of these in practice in the community. I think we would not want to suggest that every patient with advanced gastric malignancy should be treated with this combination, with any combination of therapy. Certainly the debilitated, near terminal patient is not a candidate for such treatments. But as I tried to point out, the FAM regimen was designed as an out-patient treatment that could be delivered by a private practitioner, and for the most part was done so. We would suggest the treatment and this would be the type of therapy carried out by the private practitioner. Ther majority of our patients maintained a reasonable life-style. They went out and continued to perform their daily tasks, their work, whatever that might be. So I certainly think that for the group of patients in whom some hope of palliation can be expected, the FAM treatment certainly represented a tolerable one.

C. Newman. Have you any correlations with factors which might identify the type of patient who is responding? I am thinking particularly of histology. The microscopic or macroscopic character of the tumour might be able to define a group with a higher chance of response.

F. Smith. I am sorry I did not show the slides but we looked at all the potential characteristics to see if we could predict those patients who might respond. We looked at the initial performance status and although we found very few cases who were debilitated responding, it did not appear to be a significant difference. We looked at the histological type and grade of tumour and found no difference. We were able to obtain responses in all histological varieties.

R. Pichlmayr. Was the study prospective and randomised?

F. Smith. In the last two series, no, they are what are called pilot Phase II trials. They are now being taken in collaborative groups to randomised trials. Most individuals in the United Stages do not feel that a placebo treatment arm is reasonable for gastric cancer. If you are going to treat them at all, some form of chemotherapy should be tested against another. FAM is currently being tested against lesser regimens with 5FU and adriamycin only. 5FU, methyl CCNU and so on.

Nutritional Support for the Cancer Patient

I.D.A. Johnston

Department of Surgery, University of Newcastle upon Tyne,
Newcastle upon Tyne NE1 4LP, U.K.

ABSTRACT

Cachexia is the commonest cause of death in cancer patients. There are many
explanations but a reduced intake of nutrients is the major factor.

Undernourished cancer patients are no different from other undernourished patients
in biochemical or anthropometric terms. Immunological competence is related to
nutritional deprivation as well as the presence of a tumour.

Body protein synthetic and catabolic rates are elevated in patients with large
tumour masses or metastases.

Intravenous feeding while not affecting the outcome of cancer treatment should be
given to all those patients who cannot eat normally for significant periods of
time.

KEYWORDS

Cancer; nutrition; immunology; protein turnover; treatment response.

INTRODUCTION

Cachexia is the commonest cause of death in cancer patients and loss of lean body
mass also contributes to the respiratory problems due to impaired function of the
diaphragm and other muscles of respiration.   There have been many studies carried out to establish the cause of cancer cachexia (Young, 1977). The advent of
total parenteral nutrition led to the enthusiastic application of nutritional therapy as part of the treatment of malignant disease (Copeland and others, 1975) and
there were numerous early and impressive claims of the effectiveness of nutritional
support in the control of malignant disease (Copeland, Daly, Dudrick, 1977).

The early claims of success were soon followed by reports that nutritional support
had nothing to offer the patient with malignant disease.

The causes of cancer cachexia and the role of nutritional support in the management
of different types of cancer in patients with varying degrees of nutritional in-

adequacy undergoing either single, or combinations of treatment are being reviewed
critically at the present time and some of the current problems are:
1.   The relationship between body protein synthesis and breakdown and the metabolic requirements of the tumour.   Is the tumour a nitrogen or protein trap drawing
nutrients away from vital tissues in the host and acting as a metabolic parasite?

2.   What is the true cause of cancer cachexia, how can nutritional inadequacy be
measured or assessed, and can the different causes of cancer wasting be identified
and corrected so that nutritional support can be planned more effectively?

3.   What is the relationship between undernutrition related to cancer and immunological competence?   Can manipulation of the nutritional state alter the immunological profile of patients with cancer and improve survival rates?

4.   What are the metabolic requirements of aggressive cancer treatment and can
these requirements be met easily by intravenous or oral nutritional support?

5.   The most important question of all is whether or not the provision of nutritional support affects the response to treatment by reducing the morbidity or even
mortality related to therapy and in the long run affecting the long-term survival
of patients with different cancers.

Cancer cachexia is not due to a single cause but is related to anorexia associated
with loss of gastrointestinal motility and malabsorption (Blackburn and others,
1977).   The tumour may be undergoing necrosis and infection may have developed
thus making more demands on the energy requirements of the body.   Anaemia related
to bone marrow infiltration by tumour, malabsorption and associated nutrient
deficiencies are other causes.

BIOCHEMICAL CHANGES IN CANCER PATIENTS

Before studying the relationship between under-nutrition in cancer patients,prot-
ein demands and immunological competence, it is necessary to establish whether the
biochemical profile and nutritional assessment in undernourished cancer patients
is any different from undernourished patients with benign disease.   161 patients
suffering from malignant or benign disease referred to a nutritional care team
with nutritional problems were studied.

Significant differences in ketone body production have been recorded in response to
a combination of injury and starvation (Rich, Wright, 1979).   This led to the
hypothesis that there may be two sub-populations of patients - those who can produce
a hyperketonaemia (blood ketone levels >0.2 m-mol per litre) in response to starvation or injury and those who cannot.   It has been shown that there is an inverse
relationship between the concentration of ketone bodies in the blood and the degree
of protein catabolism as measured by nitrogen excretion in the first 24 hours after
injury (Fig.1),and it has been suggested that the protein sparing associated with
hyperketonaemia may be important for survival.   Cachexia in patients with
malignant disease is common and a study was undertaken to compare the serum ketone
response to 24 hour starvation in 161 patients, all of whom had lost more than 15%
of their ideal body weight (I.B.W.).   89 patients (55%) had non-malignant disease
including a variety of conditions ranging from granulomatous disease of the
intestine, benign gastro-intestinal stricture, anorexia nervosa and patients
recovering from multiple trauma.   72 (45%) had malignant disease predominantly of
gastro-intestinal origin.   The groups were matched for age, sex, weight loss, total
serum proteins, serum albumin, serum transferrin and total lymphocyte count(Table 1).

There was no significant difference between the mean serum ketone levels of the two
groups and both groups had mean levels within the normal range following an over-

	Hyperketonaemic (n = 13)	Normoketonaemic (n = 26)	Controls (n = 10)
Urinary Nitrogen Excretion (G/24 hrs)	4.2 ± 0.5**	6.5 ± 0.6**	5.3 ± 0.5
Urinary Urea Excretion (G/24 hrs)	3.1 ± 0.45***	5.3 ± 0.4***	3.5 ± 0.63

means ± s.e.m.   **$p \leqslant 0.01$ ***$p < 0.001$

Fig. 1. The relationship between the blood ketone response to starvation and nitrogen excretion in post operative patients.

TABLE I   Biochemical changes in undernourished patients with cancer

	Cancer Group	Non Cancer Group	P.
Number	72(45%)	89 (55%)	
Mean age years (range)	64 (23 to 85)	56 (14 to 93)	
Sex	Male 47, female 25	Male 43, female 46	
Median % I.B.W. (range)	67% (50 to 85)	70% (44 to 85)	
Mean total proteins g/L	64.5	64.4	0.96
Mean serum albumin g/L	34.5	33.1	0.25
Mean transferrin g/L	2.39	2.14	0.13
Mean peripheral total lymphocyte count. ($x10^3$)	1.41	1.89	0.17

night fast (Fig.2). The cachexia of malignant disease cannot be explained on the basis of any differences in ketone metabolism, and it is more likely to be part of a multifactorial spectrum of under nutrition.   No difference could be detected in biochemical or anthropometric terms between under nourished patients with cancer or benign conditions.   Should nutritional support be required in the patient with malignant disease it should be given along the well proven lines currently used for any other undernourished patient.

A survey of nutritional intakes achieved by different clinical teams caring for undernourished patients revealed that during the first week in hospital all the

Ketone levels in response to 24 hour fasting in 161 patients

	CANCER (72)		NON-CANCER (89)	
	Mean	SEM	Mean	SEM
Ketones mmol/l	0.147	0.024	0.135	0.023

p = 0.71

Fig. 2. Ketone levels in response to starvation in patients with benign and malignant disease.

patients studied were only managing to consume about 80% of their requirements of energy and nutrients even though the clinicians concerned were aware of the under-nourished state of the patients.

These observations indicate that diminished intake of food related to change of environment, fear, pain and the demands of frequent gastro-intestinal investigations is a potent cause of hospital undernutrition.   The significance of this continuing reduced intake on the outcome of treatment has yet to be identified although there is some evidence that nutritional support reduces post-operative morbidity (Collins, Oxby, Hill, 1978).

WHOLE BODY PROTEIN SYNTHESIS AND BREAKDOWN IN CANCER

The metabolic relationships between the growing neoplasm and the host are not fully understood.   The presence of a tumour often causes changes in nitrogen equilibrium disproportionate to the size of the tumour (Goodland, 1967).   These changes in body protein are difficult to interpret by urinary nitrogen balance studies.   Tumour bearing animals fed protein excrete less nitrogen and are in a positive nitrogen balance due to the accumulation of increased amounts of nitrogen in the tumour (Oram Smith and others, 1977).   An increased rate of protein synthesis and break-down has been recorded in cancer patients prior to surgery.

A study was planned to measure whole body protein synthesis and breakdown (g per kg per day) preoperatively using a constant rate infusion of $1-(1-^{14}C)$ leucine.   Twelve apyrexial patients with varying stages of colorectal carcinoma, 7 of whom had normal appetites and 5 with anorexia, were given Clinifeed 400 (0.8 ml kg/hour) for the duration of the study.   The extent of their disease was assessed by the percentage incorporation of the labelled amino-acid into plasma proteins and subsequent Duke's classification.

Protein synthesis increased with advancement of disease in both groups (r = 0.95,
p = 0.001) as did protein breakdown (r = 0.91, p = 0.004).   Protein synthesis and
breakdown were less elevated in the anorexic group suggesting some degree of starvation adaptation (Carmichael and others, 1980).

These results suggest that an increase in protein synthesis with advancement of
disease may be due to tumour utilisation (Fig.3).   As all patients in this study were

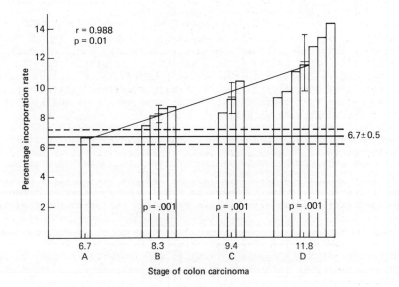

Fig. 3. Relationship between percentage incorporation of ^{14}C leucine
into plasma protein in patients with colon cancer on a
constant intake of nutrients.

in positive balance this suggests that the tumour was "trapping" significant amounts
of protein for tumour growth.   These increases in protein turnover are similar to
those found in the first four days after major injury or surgery, when metabolic
expenditure and protein requirements can be elevated by 10 - 20% above resting
demands.   The extent of the nutritional support for the patient with extensive
cancer should be similar to that required after major surgery.   If the cancer
patient cannot manage the necessary intake from normal hospital diet then supplementary feeding is indicated and on occasions the insertion of a fine bore nasogastric tube can be helpful.

IMMUNOLOGICAL ASPECTS OF CANCER CACHEXIA

Awareness of the prevalence of nutritional depletion among hospital populations and
recognition of the high incidence of postoperative sepsis in malnourished patients
stimulated interest in the effect of malnutrition on the immune system (Douglas,
Schopfer, 1976).   Recent immunological studies of malnutrition have included
investigations of humoral and cell-mediated immunity, phagocytic mechanisms, the
complement system, and various non-specific host defence mechanisms (Chandra, 1975).
These studies confirm that the immune response is depressed in states of malnutrition.

Naturally-occurring substances in plasma capable of suppressing the immune response have been described in several benign and malignant conditions as well as in normal subjects (Cooperband and others, 1976). It has been suggested that lymphocyte depressant factors may also be present in the plasma of patients with acute protein energy malnutrition. Demonstration of the presence of such immuno-inhibitory plasma factors could be of value in understanding the impairment of immunological function in malnourished individuals.

Fifty patients with malignant (n = 25) and non-malignant disease were selected for study. In vitro lymphocyte responses to phytohaemogglutinin (PHA) and purified protein derivative of Mycobacterium tuberculosis (PPD) were measured, and the suppressive activity of each patients' plasma was also measured. For the purposes of the study a nutritional index was calculated on the basis of the patients' weight at the time of hospital admission as a percentage of either their usual pre-illness weight or a standard ideal body weight for individuals of the same height and sex. Patients who were classified as malnourished had suffered illness-related weight loss to the extent that their present weight was less than 85% of either their usual weight or their ideal body weight.

Lymphocyte responses were measured using the Tanned Erythrocyte Electrophoretic Mobility (TEEM) test. Lymphocytes, when stimulated by PHA or PPD to produce a lymphokine which alters the surface electrical charge of tanned sheep erythrocytes; the alteration of surface electrical charge reduces the mobility of the erythrocytes within an electric field and is measured in a cytopherometer. Lymphocyte responses are therefore expressed as a percentage reduction in the mobility of the tanned sheep red blood cells.

Plasma suppressive activity (PSA) was measured in the same test system by adding serial dilutions of the subjects' plasma to the lymphocytes prior to incubation with PPD. Lymphocytes were obtained from each patient (autologous cells) and from a panel of healthy adults (allogeneic cells). The suppressive activity of plasma was calculated as the volume of plasma required to cause 50% inhibition of the lymphocyte response, and so a high plasma suppressive activity is indicated by a small volume of plasma.

The lymphocyte responses of patients with benign and malignant diseases showed positive but weak correlations with nutritional status (Fig.4). The lymphocyte responses were low in severely underweight patients irrespective of the underlying disease. Improvement of nutritional status causes the lymphocyte responses to increase and the difference between the benign and malignant groups becomes apparent. The considerable scatter of results within each group is not altogether unexpected since each group included patients with a variety of diseases differing in pathology, extent and severity. The nutritional index was based on body weight which measures compositive body mass rather than the functional contribution of each tissue compartment.

Plasma suppressive activity was low in well nourished patients with benign disease but was significantly higher in malnourished counterparts. This difference in suppressive activity between the two groups was apparent when both autologous and allogeneic cells were used as test lymphocytes, indicating that the difference was due to an effect of the patients' plasma and not to lower lymphocyte responses in the malnourished group.

In patients with malignant disease plasma suppressive activity was found to be high regardless of the patients' nutritional status or the type of test lymphocyte (Fig.5). Malignancy is frequently associated with high plasma suppressive activity and so any increase or decrease due to the influence of nutritional depletion may not be apparent.

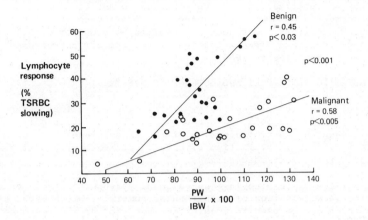

Fig. 4. The relationship between lymphocyte responses to PHA and nutritional status in patients with benign and malignant disease.

PLASMA SUPPRESSIVE ACTIVITY IN PATIENTS WITH MALIGNANT DISEASE

TEST LYMPHOCYTES	AUTOLOGOUS		ALLOGENEIC	
Nutritional status	Well-nourished	Mal-nourished	Well-nourished	Mal-nourished
n	9	16	7	15
Median	1.1 μl	1.14 μl	1.12 μl	0.97 μl
Range	0.48–21.8	0.27–16.5	0.26–16.1	0.28–9.1
	p = NS		p = NS	

(Mann-Whitney U test)

Fig. 5. Plasma suppressive activity in patients with malignant disease.

This study demonstrates that in vitro lymphocyte responses are depressed in malnourished individuals and shows that a positive correlation exists between lymphocyte reactivity and nutritional status.   The finding of raised suppressive activity
in plasma of malnourished patients in the absence of malignant disease is of considerable interest and suggests that the naturally-occurring suppressive activity of
plasma could be an important factor contributing to the reduced immunocompetence so
frequently observed in malnourished subjects.   The source and clinical significance
of these immuno-inhibitory substances have yet to be elucidated.   The detection of
these substances in plasma draws attention to yet another consequence of nutritional
depletion (Francis and others, 1980).

NUTRITIONAL SUPPORT AND OUTCOME OF TREATMENT

Total parenteral nutrition can not only maintain the nutritional status quo but if
provided in an appropriate form can cause a significant increase in lean body cell
mass at a time when the gastro-intestinal tract is completely out of action.   It is
thus possible to eliminate starvation effects in patients with malignant disease
and also cater for any increased demands.

The greatest difficulty in studying the value of parenteral nutrition in cancer
patients is the identification of either anthropometric, biochemical or immunological factors which can be used to predict the need for or the response to nutritional support.

The challenge remains to identify the types of cancer and individual patient where
aggressive nutritional support can improve the results of treatment.

Several studies have demonstrated significant weight gain during cancer treatment
supported by total parenteral nutrition(Holter and Fischer, 1975). The gain in
weight however was not related to the success of the treatment of the malignancy.
There is good evidence that the weight gain is due to the accumulation of water
rather than the deposition of protein and fat.   In one study the improvement in
lean body mass during parenteral nutrition was greater in malnourished patients
with benign rather than the malignant disease(Nixon and others, 1978).

Such reports have not been confirmed and using K_{40} no gain in lean body mass could
be detected in patients with malignant disease given intravenous feeding.   At the
same time no obvious increase in protein turnover or synthesis could be detected
during parenteral nutrition.

The underweight patient with either benign or malignant disease often fails to show
a response to intradermal allergens.   Improvements in body composition produced by
intravenous feeding are associated with improvement in the skin test sensitivity
but a direct cause and effect relationship is difficult to prove and the difficulty
of clinical interpretation of skin testing cannot be over emphasised.

Total parenteral nutrition has been used as part of a programme of palliation in a
number of cancers with no effect on survival or the control of the disease and such
support may even prolong life without improving the quality of life.

In one study total parenteral nutrition appeared to have an adverse effect and
hastened death.

Total parenteral nutrition has not enhanced patients tolerance of treatment or
allowed higher doses of drugs to be used in certain lymphoma patients which have a
high cure and response rate.   One or two studies suggest that the toxicity of cancer
chemotherapeutic agents may be reduced during parenteral nutrition.

Attempts have been made to lower post-operative morbidity and mortality after major cancer surgery by the use of parenteral nutrition.   The results are conflicting with some evidence of a reduced complication rate and a shorter hospital stay in the fed groups.

While nutritional support is not a specific cancer treatment no patient with a reasonable chance of a response to treatment should ever be asked to forego his true nutritional requirements at any time.

The criteria for providing nutritional support in the cancer patient still undergoing active treatment should not differ from those applied in other situations.

The failure to take the measured requirements of nutrients for three or more days before, during or after treatment is an indication for nutritional support. Supplementary oral or tube feeding is safe, simple and effective and intravenous feeding is only required in the presence of alimentary failure.

REFERENCES

Blackburn, G.L., B.S. Nairn, B.R. Bistrian, and W.Y. McDermott (1977).   The effect of cancer on nitrogen,electrolyte and mineral metabolism.   Cancer Res., 37, 2348-2353.

Carmichael, M.J., M.B. Clague, M.J. Kier, and I.D.A. Johnston (1980).   Whole body protein turnover, synthesis and breakdown in patients with colorectal cancer. Brit. J. Surg., 67, 736-740.

Chandra, R.K. (1975).   Serum complement and immunoconglutinin in malnutrition. Arch. Dis. Childh., 50, 225-229.

Collins, J.P., C.B. Oxby, and G.L. Hill (1978).   Intravenous amino acids as protein sparing therapy after major surgery.   Lancet, i, 788-791.

Cooperband, S.R., R. Numberg, K. Schmid, and J.A. Mannick (1976).   Humoral immuno-suppressive factors.   Transplantation proceedings, 2, 225-242.

Copeland, E.M., B.V. Macfadyen, V. Ianzotti, and S.J. Dudrick (1975).   Intravenous hyperalimentation as an adjunct to cancer chemotherapy.   Amer. J. Surg., 129, 167-170.

Copeland, E.M., J.N. Daly, and S.J. Dudrick (1977).   Nutrition as an adjunct to cancer treatment in the adult.   Cancer Res., 37, 2451-2456.

Douglas, S.D., and K. Schopfer (1976).   Host defence mechanisms in protein calorie malnutrition.   Clinical immunology and immunopathology, 5, 1-5.

Francis, D.M.A., B.K. Shenton, G. Proud, P.S. Veitch, and R.M.R. Taylor (1980). Immunosuppressive activity in the plasma of patients with malignant disease. Brit. J. Surg. In Press.

Goodland, G.A.J. (1967).   Protein metabolism and tumour growth.In H.N. Munro and J.B. Allison (Ed.), Mammalian Protein Metabolism, New York Academic Press. pp.415-475.

Holter, A.R., and J.E. Fischer (1977).   The effects of perioperative hyperaliment-ation on complications in patients with carcinoma and weight loss. J. surg. Res., 23, 31-34.

Nixon, D., D. Rudman, S. Heyrusfeld, J. Aynsyley, and M. Kutner (1978).   Responses to nutritional support in cachetic patients.   Amer. Ass. Cancer Res. abst. 689.

Oram Smith, J.C., J.P. Stein, H.W. Wallace, and G.L. Miller (1977).   Intravenous nutrition and tumour host protein metabolism.   J. surg. Res., 22, 499-503.

Rich, A.J., and P.D. Wright (1979).   Ketosis and nitrogen excretion in under-nourished surgical patients.   J.PEN., 3, 350-354.

Young, V.R. ((1977).   Energy metabolism and requirements of the cancer patient. Cancer Res., 37, 2336-2347.

DISCUSSION

W. Gillison. From what you say, cancer is a parasite in a patient. If a patient with cancer has got a reasonable fluid and electrolyte balance, is the time to start your feeding post-operatively or as soon as the tumour is out of the patient?

I. Johnston. On the evidence that we have there is some substance to your suggestion but we tend to assess nutritional requirements on the basis of what the patient has actually been able to take at any one time. I have not been dividing intravenous oral or even the use of hospital diet. So that in a sense we don't really pay attention to whether the tumour is there or not at the moment. The practical answer to your question is yes, one should perhaps not put up that long line until you are sure that you have got weeks of nutritional support ahead of you, and you will certainly do better in the post-operative period, starting a day or so after surgery.

G. Slaney. As a corollary to that question, I think what was in Mr. Gillison's mind was under what circumstances do you spare the surgical attack to correct the nutritional inadequacy? Is it not better to get the tumour out and then start tackling the nutritional problem? Would you comment on that?

I. Johnston. Well that's the other approach. I don't think we have the hard evidence on that at the moment. I wish we had. There is no evidence that the delay of 2 - 3 weeks to convert an anergic patient to perhaps someone who will respond to a foreign stimulus is going to help. There is nothing new about this. Warren Cole in the 50's and 60's used to say that until you got a patient into positive nitrogen balance you should not operate on them, for these sorts of reasons, and we just don't have the evidence to apply this in general terms. If we have a patient who is 60-70% off their ideal weight, who has not been eating for a long time, is dehydrated, then its only reasonable to give them nutrients, as well as fluids, as you build up to surgery. But I don't think one should delay unnecessarily, on the evidence we have at the moment.

G. Slaney. How long will you delay the surgical attack? Five days, 10 days, 3 weeks, or what?

I. Johnston. I shall give you the obvious answer, it depends on the individual patients' requirements. If the plasma proteins and transferins are normal, they are responding to stimulus, they are not anergic and their fluid electrolyte requirements are normal and they are just showing themselves as a 'thinny', they might be a very fit thinny, I would'nt delay. If they have other problems, then I might delay, but not for long.

The Incidence of Early Gastric Cancer since the Advent of Endoscopy

K. Takagi

Department of Surgery, Cancer Institute Hospital, Tokyo, Japan

ABSTRACT

Changes in the incidence of early gastric cancer among the operated cases of gastric cancer at Cancer Institute Hospital, Tokyo during 30 years from 1946 to 1975
were studied. Incidence of early gastric cancer among operated cases of gastric
cancer was 5% in 1950's, 10% in 1960's and over 30% in 1970's. The development of
gastric endoscopy, especially endoscopic biopsy, has played an important role in
the early diagnosis of gastric cancer. Now the microcancer less than 5 mm in diameter is diagnosed by endoscopic biopsy. The increase of early gastric cancer is
due not only to endoscopy, but also the development of X-ray examination and mass
survey. Multiple early cancer and metachronous cancer in the remnant stomach after
gastrectomy for gastric cancer are discussed.

KEYWORDS

Incidence of early gastric cancer; endoscopy of the stomach; microcancer of the
stomach; multiple gastric cancers; metachronous cancer of the remnant stomach.

INTRODUCTION

In Japan, the ratio of gastric cancer to malignant tumors is high, and about 50,000
of 100,000 patients (50%) with malignant tumors die of gastric cancer within a
year. Since the end of the Second World War, there has been a high incidence of
gastric cancer along with a decrease in the incidence of pulmonary tuberculosis.
Since the 1950's quite an effort has been made to combat gastric cancer from the
standpoints of diagnosis and therapy. For the last 30 years, the greatest change
in relation to gastric cancer as experienced in clinical studies has been the diagnosis of gastric cancer in the early stage, which has become very common. The
relationship between the incidence of gastric cancer diagnosed in the early stage
in patients who underwent laparotomy for gastric cancer and the advent of endoscopy
was studied in patients with early gastric cancer who were treated at the Department of Surgery, Cancer Institute Hospital, for 30 years from 1946 to 1975.

In Japan, the relationship between the incidence of early gastric cancer in patients who underwent laparotomy for gastric cancer and the development of gastric
diagnostics, especially endoscopy, is as follows: since the 1950's many cases of

159

gastric cancer have been diagnosed in the early stage owing to the rapid development of gastric diagnostics (Shirakabe, 1966; Sakita, 1971) and to large-scale
mass survey of the stomach (Takahashi, 1971; Ichikawa, 1971; Ariga, 1976). Thus,
gastric cancer, which formerly had been an incurable disease, could be discovered
early and could be treated in the same way as uterine cancer and mammary cancer.

Fig. 1.

YEARLY INCIDENCE OF EARLY CANCER AMONG LAPROTMIZED GASTRIC CANCER

(including multiple cancer)

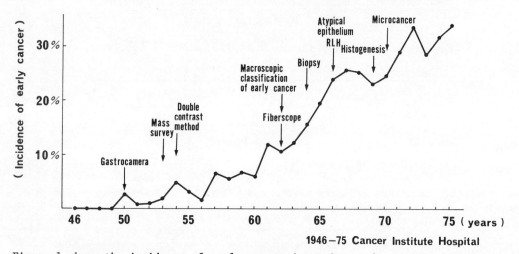

1946—75 Cancer Institute Hospital

Figure 1 shows the incidence of early cancer in patients who were operated on at
our hospital (Takagi, 1980). Changes in the incidence of early gastric cancer
during a 30-year period from 1946 to 1975 were studied. Before 1955 gastric
cancer was diagnosed in the early stage in less than 5% of the patients operated
on for this condition, and it was diagnosed mainly by X-ray examination. After
the gastrocamera (1950), the double contrast method (1954), and mass survey (1953)
of the stomach were introduced, and especially, in 1960 the incidence of early
cancer increased to 10%. The double contrast method (Shirakabe, 1966) came into
use at hospitals specializing in gastroenterology and the gastrocamera was improved and was widely used (Yamaki, 1971). Images of early gastric cancer were
gradually clarified by X-rays and gastrocameras, and case reports were accumulated.
The macroscopical classification of early gastric cancer was reported in close
cooperation with radiologists, endoscopists, surgeons, and pathologists at the
Japan Society for Gastroenterological Endoscopy in 1962 (Tazaka, 1962). Since
then, early gastric cancer came to be studied on a common basis in regard to its
diagnosis in the early stage and its treatment. In 1962, when macroscopic classification of early gastric cancer was performed, Hirschowitz (1958)'s gastroduodenal
fiberscope (from America) was introduced to gastric endoscopy. Immediately after
that, a gastrocamera equipped with a fiberscope (GTF) was produced (Yamaki, 1971),
and the clinical manifestation of early gastric cancer became clearer because more
definite findings could be obtained with a GTF than with a gastrocamera. Gastric
biopsy under direct vision using a fiberscope was introduced in the diagnosis of
early gastric cancer in 1964 (Kurokawa and Takagi, 1964), histological diagnosis
by biopsy was added, and the method of gastric diagnosis was established. After
1964, gastric lesions resembling early gastric cancer were differentiated definitely by gastric biopsy, and new gastric diseases were discovered such as atypical
epithelial lesion (borderline lesion, Takagi, 1967; Sugano, 1971) and reactive
lymphoreticular hyperplasia (Nakamura, 1966). Gastric cancer was diagnosed in the
early stage in 20% of the patients operated on for gastric cancer. In the 1970's

the incidence of early gastric cancer increased to over 30%. Thus, the development of gastric endoscopy, especially endoscopic biopsy of the stomach, has played an important role in the early diagnosis of gastric cancer.

The incidence of early cancer in patients operated on for gastric cancer was studied every ten years for 30 years. As shown in Table 1, from 1946 to 1955 cancer was discovered early in only 28 patients, 2.1% of whom were operated on.

TABLE 1

YEARLY INCIDENCE OF EARLY CANCER AMONG
LAPAROTOMIZED GASTRIC CANCER
(including multiple cancer)

Period	Laparotomy No. of cases	Early cancer No. of cases	%
1946 − 55	1,313	28	2.1
1956 − 65	2,494	241	9.7
1966 − 75	2,413	678	28.1
Total	6,220	947	15.2

From 1956 to 1965 cancer was discovered early in 241 patients. Moreover, from 1966 to 1975 cancer was discovered early in 678 patients, 28.1% of whom were operated on for gastric cancer. In general, laparotomy performed for gastric cancer revealed cancer in the early stage in 1 out of 3 patients. This fact has never been considered. Also, according to Sakita's report (1974) on the "Present State of the Early Discovery of Gastric Cancer" and reports on the total number of patients with early gastric cancer observed at 91 institutes in Japan, cancer was discovered in the early stage in 217 patients (236 cases of cancer) in 1962, and the number rapidly increased, especially in 1966. In 1971 the number increased 5.5 times; that is, 1213 patients (1286 cases of cancer).

Thus, the greatest change regarding gastric cancer in Japan is an increase in the number of cases of gastric cancer discovered in the early stage. Actually, gastric cancer can be diagnosed early thereby improving the results of treatment (Kajitani, 1979).

The Incidence of Early Gastric Cancer According to Macroscopic Classification

At present many cases of gastric cancer are being discovered early. According to macroscopic classification, there is a difference in the incidence of early gastric cancer between the time before invention of the fiberscope—the clinical manifestation of early cancer had still not been clarified (30 years ago)—and the time after techniques for diagnosis were developed (the present time) (Table 2). In the 1950's most of the cases of cancer discovered early have been types III and II_c+III (52%); 8% of the cases have been type II_c. However, at present, the number of cases of cancer discovered type II_c makes up 48% of the total while the number of cases of type III makes up only 4%. Although the number of cases of cancer discovered types I and II_a has increased, it has decreased compared to the total number of cases of gastric cancer discovered early. From a standpoint of the total number of patients with cancer in the early stage, there have been many cases of type III cancer, that is, cancer with open benign ulcer, from the 1950's to the 1960's. However, after 1966 the number of cases of cancer in the early stage (type II_c)

increased and many cases of cancer without open benign ulcer were discovered.

TABLE 2

YEARLY INCIDENCE OF MACROSCOPIC CLASSIFICATION OF EARLY CANCER
(Solitary cancer)

Period	I	IIa	IIb	IIc	III	IIc + III	Total
1946 – 55	3 (12)	7 (28)		2 (8)	5 (20)	8 (32)	25 (100)
1956 – 65	22 (10)	43 (20)	5 (2)	50 (33)	16 (7)	80 (38)	216 (100)
1966 – 75	41 (7)	85 (15)	24 (4)	261 (48)	23 (4)	115 (21)	549 (100)
Total	66 (8)	135 (17)	29 (4)	313 (40)	44 (6)	203 (26)	790 (100)

( )---**Percentage**

As a result of the recent development of gastric endoscopy, cancer with a diameter
of less than 1 cm is being studied as a minute lesion. At present, microcancer
with a diameter of less than 5 mm can be discovered clinically (Takekoshi, 1977).
Takekoshi (1977) reported 10 cases of microcancer with a diameter of less than 5 mm
by performing biopsy of the stomach. As shown in Table 3, the first case was diagnosed in 1968. After that, three cases were diagnosed in 1969, 1970, and 1972,
respectively. The remaining 6 cases were diagnosed as having microcancer after
1974.

TABLE 3

MICROCARCINOMA DIAGNOSED BY BIOPSY

Case	Type	Size mm	Location	Endoscopic diagnosis	Biopsy	Co-existing lesion
0 – 9340	IIa	2	C	Polyp	Adca. tub	(−)
0 – 10401	IIc	5	A	IIc	Adca. tub.	Ulcer (Two micro Ca.)
0 – 11041	IIc	3	A	Erosion	Adca. tub.	IIc
0 – 12511	IIc	5	M	IIc with scar	Adca. mucocell.	(−)
0 – 13164	IIc	4	A	Erosion, ATP	Adca. tub.	IIa-like ATP
0 – 13290	IIb	4	M	IIc	Adca. tub.	IIc, IIb-like ATP
0 – 13377	IIc	4	C	IIc	Adca scirrh	(−)
0 – 13490	IIc	4	A	IIc	Adca. tub.	(−)
0 – 13860	IIc	5	A	IIc. Scar	Adca tub.	Scar
0 – 14536	IIc	5	A	IIc	Adca. tub.	IIc

1968 – 79, Cancer Institute Hospital

Case report (0-13377) of microcancer (type II_c) with a diameter of 4 mm; 57-year-
old male. X-ray: Double contrast picture (Fig. 2, 3) obtained with the patient
in a supine position. Irregular, stellar spots of barium can be observed in the
posterior wall of the upper body. GTF picture (Fig. 4): Slightly-elevated areas
with irregular depression can be observed. Biopsy was performed, and the diagnosis
was undifferentiated adenocarcinoma. Gross findings (Fig. 5): The arrow shows
the microcancer (type II_c) in the posterior wall of the upper body. Histological
findings (Fig. 6): The arrow shows the area of undifferentiated cancer in the
mucosa. Submucosal invasion had already been observed in a part of the area.

Location of Gastric Cancer in the Early Stage

It formerly had been believed that gastric cancer frequently occurs in the lower

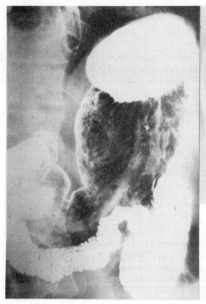

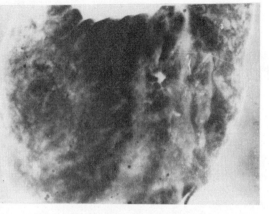

Fig. 3. Double contrast picture (enlargement).

Fig. 2. Double contrast picture in a supine position.

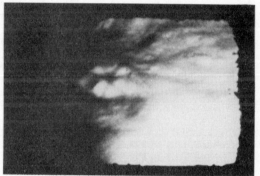

Fig. 4. GTF findings.

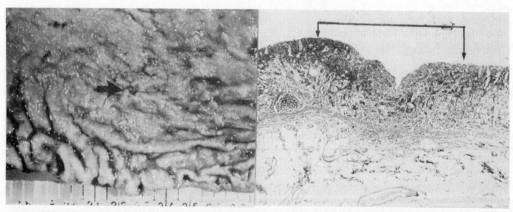

Fig. 5. Gross findings of resected material. Fig. 6. Histological findings.

part of the stomach but rarely occurs in the upper part. However, regarding the
number of cases of gastric cancer discovered in the early stage according to location, as shown in Table 4, the cancer often occurred in the lower part of the
stomach (A) in the 1950's; in the 1960's and the 1970's it often occurred in the
middle part of the stomach (M). However, the number of cases of cancer in the
upper part of the stomach (C) which have been discovered early has not tended to
increase in spite of the development of gastric endoscopy.

TABLE 4

PERIODIC INCIDENCE OF LOCATION

(Early Gastric Cancer)

	A	M	C	Total
1946-55	14 (56)	9 (36)	2 (8)	25 (100)
1956-56	93 (43)	112 (52)	11 (5)	216 (100)
1966-75	192 (35)	309 (56)	48 (9)	549 (100)

( )-percentage   A - Lower Part

M - Middle Part

C - Upper Part

Therefore, a greater effort must be made to discover early cancer in the upper part
of the stomach.

The Number of Cases of Multiple Gastric Cancer Discovered in the Early Stage

Owing to the development of gastric diagnostics, detailed intragastric examination
can be performed. Also, detailed histological examination can be performed and
multiple cancer in the stomach can be found. On the other hand, an increase in the
incidence of early cancer has resulted in an increase in the number of persons who
survive for a long time after operation. It also has resulted in an increase in
the incidence of cancer discovered in other organs.

The incidence of multiple gastric cancer, including cases of multiple intragastric
cancer and cancer in other organs, was 3.1% in the 1950's and 11.4% in the 1970's
(Table 5). Especially, the incidence of multiple early cancer, which was 7.1% in
the 1950's, increased to 18.7% in the 1970's. This remarkable increase should be
noted. When only one lesion is revealed by X-ray examination and endoscopy in the
stomach, other sites, especially the upper part of the stomach, also should be
examined carefully.

Along with the recent increase in the number of cases of early gastric cancer, the
number of persons who survive for a long time after operation is increasing, and
cancer is being discovered in the remnant stomach after gastrectomy has been performed for cancer. There formerly have been reports of patients in whom cancer
occurred in the remnant stomach after gastrectomy had been performed for benign
gastric diseases. However, cases have rarely been reported in which cancer newly

occurs in the remnant stomach after excision of the cancer (Morgenstem, 1960; Takagi, 1977).

TABLE 5

YEARLY INCIDENCE OF MULTIPLE CANCER

Period	Laparotomy cases	Early cancer	Advanced cancer
1946 — 55	3.1% (41/1,313)	7.1% (2/28)	3.0% (39/1,285)
1956 — 65	6.3% (157/2,494)	9.5% (23/241)	5.9% (134/2,253)
1966 — 75	11.4% (275/2,413)	18.7% (127/678)	8.5% (148/1,735)
Total	7.6% (473/6,220)	16.1% (152/947)	6.1% (321/5,273)

Especially, a question remains unsolved regarding cancer in the remnant stomach after gastrectomy has been performed for cancer: Is it a new cancer or a recurrence in the remnant stomach? Excision of a gastric cancer was performed in 13 patients at our hospital. Cancer was observed in the remnant stomach, and detailed histological examination revealed it to be multiple cancer, different from the first cancer. Metachronous multiple cancer occurred in 6 patients (0.25%) in the 1970's, but in 1976 and after 1976 it occurred in 5 patients (1.34%) (Table 6).

TABLE 6   **YEARLY INCIDENCE OF METACHRONOUS MULTIPLE REMNANT STOMACH CANCER AFTER PARTIAL GASTRECTOMY OF GASTRIC CANCER**

Period	Laparotomy No.of cases	Metchronous multiple cancer No.of cases	%
1946 — 55	1,313	0	
1956 — 65	2,494	2	0.08
1966 — 75	2,413	6 (1)	0.25
1976 — 77	373	5 (2)	1.34

( ) Early cancer of remnant stomach

Most of the multiple cancer was advanced, but in 3 patients the cancer in the remnant stomach was in the early stage. In 2 of them it was protuberant cancer in the early stage (types I and II_a), and in the other 1 patient it was depressed cancer in the early stage (type II_c).

Most of the cases of early cancer which are observed in the remnant stomach after gastrectomy are elevated early cancers (Domellöf, 1976; Takagi, 1977), and X-ray examination often reveals abnormal findings. Depressed early cancer (type II_c) has rarely been reported, but it has been discovered by means of endoscopy.

Case report of early cancer (type II_c) in the remnant stomach after gastrectomy has been performed. A 58 year old male underwent gastrectomy (Billroth I) for gastric cancer on May 16, 1972. The cancer, which was 4.3 × 2.8 cm, was located in the anterior wall of the gastric angle. The histological findings revealed that the cancer was scirrhous adenocarcinoma and that it had reached the subserosa without

166 K. Takagi

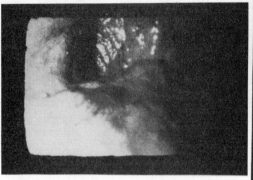

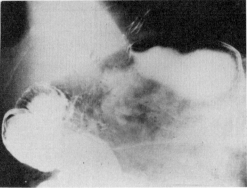

Fig. 8. Double contrast picture
of the remnant stomach.

Fig. 7. GTF findings.

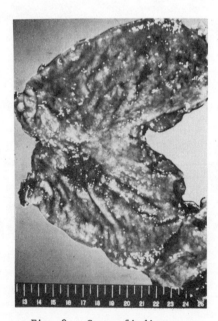

Fig. 9. Gross findings.

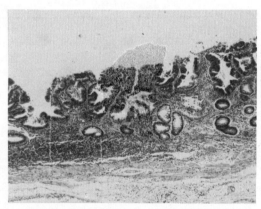

Fig. 10. Histological findings.

metastasis of the lymph node. The patient underwent a follow-up. GTF endoscopic examination made 4 years and 9 months after operation revealed erosion in the posterior wall of the remnant stomach, and the patient was diagnosed as having early cancer (type II_c) (Fig. 7). A biopsy of the stomach revealed that the cancer was well differentiated. Although an X-ray examination was made, it was hard to demonstrate the lesion (Fig. 8). The remnant stomach was excised on January 24, 1977, and observed macroscopically (Fig. 9). A lesion 3.5 × 2.5 cm was present in the posterior wall and the lesion was well-differentiated adenocarcinoma (Fig. 10). Cancer invasion was limited within the mucosa. Three years and five months ago the second operation was performed, and now (June, 1980) the patient is surviving healthfully.

In the examination of the remnant stomach, X-ray examination is not enough, and endoscopic examination should be combined with X-ray examination and a follow-up study should be made.

CONCLUSION

The development of endoscopy is very important for the early discovery of gastric cancer. Also, at our hospital, the number of cases of cancer diagnosed early in patients who underwent gastrectomy for cancer increased owing to the development of endoscopy. However, it was possible to diagnose many cases of cancer due to the development of X-ray examination and mass survey examination of the stomach. In the 1950's and the 1960's X-ray examination and endoscopic examination of the stomach competed with each other owing to their technical development, and the ability to diagnose gastric cancer early was improved.

Due to the development of endoscopy, there is a tendency to overestimate biopsy of the stomach. However, judging from the patients at our hospital who had been diagnosed as having gastric cancer in the early stage during a 20-year period, it is most important to perform biopsy of the stomach on the basis of X-ray diagnosis and morphological examination by means of gastric endoscopy, especially according to definite images produced by the gastrocamera.

Regarding the diagnosis of and the therapy for early cancer, it should be noted that close cooperation among radiologists, endoscopists, surgeons, and pathologists, is very important.

REFERENCES

Ariga, K. and K. Takahashi (1976). Gastric mass survey. In T. Hirayama (Ed.), GANN Monograph on Cancer Research 18. Cancer in Asia. Japan Scientific Societies Press, Tokyo. pp. 99-103.

Domellöf, L., S. Eriksson and K. G. Janunger (1976). Late precancerous changes and carcinoma of the gastric stump after Billroth I resection. Am. J. Surg., 132, 26-31.

Hirschowitz, B. I., L. I. Curtiss, C. W. Peters and H. M. Pollard (1958). Demonstration of a new gastroscope, the "Fiberscope". Gastroenterology, 35, 50-53.

Ichikawa, H. (1971). Detectability of early gastric cancer with indirect fluororadiography. In T. Murakami (Ed.), GANN Monograph on Cancer Research 11. Early gastric cancer. Japan Scientific Societies Press, Tokyo. pp. 27-43.

Kajitani, T. and K. Takagi (1979). Cancer of the stomach at Cancer Institute Hospital, Tokyo. In T. Kajitani, Y. Koyama and Y. Umegaki (Ed.), GANN Monograph on Cancer Research 22. Recent results of cancer treatment in Japan. Japan Scientific Societies Press, Tokyo and University Park Press, Baltimore. pp. 77-87.

Kurokawa, T., A. Fuchigami and K. Takagi (1964). Gastric biopsy under direct vision using gastrofiberscope (Japanese). Clinics of Digestive Diseases, 6, 927-934.

Morgenstern, L. (1960). The late development of gastric cancer after gastrectomy for malignant diseases. Surgery, 47, 557-567.

Nakamura, K., M. Aoki, H. Sugano and K. Takagi (1966). Reactive lymphoreticular hyperplasia of the stomach: Reports of 6 surgical cases (Japanese). Japan. J. Cancer Clin., 12, 691-696.

Sakita, T. and Y. Oguro (1971). Routine gastrocamera examination. In T. Murakami (Ed.), GANN Monograph on Cancer Research 11. Early gastric cancer. Japan Scientific Societies Press, Tokyo. pp. 145-158.

Sakita, T. (1974). Present status on detection of early gastric cancer (Japanese). Gastroenterological Endoscopy, 16, 662-672.

Shirakabe, H., H. Ichikawa, K. Kumakura, M. Nishizawa, K. Higurashi, H. Hayakawa and T. Murakami (1966). Atlas of X-ray diagnosis of early gastric cancer. Igaku-shoin Ltd., Tokyo.

Sugano, H., K. Nakamura and K. Takagi (1971). An atypical epithelium of the stomach. A clinico-pathological entity. In T. Murakami (Ed.), GANN Monograph on Cancer Research 11. Early gastric cancer. Japan Scientific Societies Press, Tokyo. pp. 257-269.

Takagi, K., K. Kumakura, H. Sugano and K. Nakamura (1967). Clinico-pathological study on polypoid lesions of the stomach with special reference to atypical epithelial lesions (Japanese). Jap. J. Cancer Clin., 13, 809-817.

Takagi, K., I. Ohashi, T. Imada and F. Kasumi (1977). Malignant lesions of the remnant stomach (Japanese). Stomach and Intestine, 12, 903-917.

Takagi, K., I. Ohashi, T. Ohta, H. Tokuda, J. Kamiya, R. Nakagoshi, S. Maeda and T. Motohara (1980). Historical transfiguration in gastric cancer (Japanese). Stomach and Intestine, 15, 11-18.

Takahashi, K. (1971). Outline of gastric mass survey by X-ray. In T. Murakami (Ed.), GANN Monograph on Cancer Research 11. Early gastric cancer. Japan Scientific Societies Press, Tokyo. pp. 21-26.

Takekoshi, T., N. Sugiyama and Y. Baba (1977). The diagnostic progress and limitation of gastric carcinoma: Endoscopic study of microcarcinoma of stomach (smaller than 5 mm in diameter) (Japanese). Progress of Digestive Endoscopy, 10, 56-61.

DISCUSSION

M. Keighley. What proportion of your patients with early gastric cancer actually have symptoms and would be referred to the doctor?

K. Takagi. Many people ask about the symptoms of early gastric cancer. There are two types of early cancer. One which is elevated and one which is depressed. The elevated type is not associated with benign ulceration, so there are no symptoms. The depressed type is mainly associated with the benign ulcer and therefore has symptoms. It is very difficult to differentiate between them by clinical symptoms.

H. Ellis. The elevated type, presumably, are picked up by screening?

K. Takagi. Yes, screening is very useful.

H. Ellis. Is this radiological screening, or endoscopic screening?

K. Takagi. Radiological.

W. Longmire. What is the incidence of lymph node involvement in early gastric cancer?

K. Takagi. In Japan, the definition of early gastric carcinoma is invasion of only the mucosa and sub-mucosa, with or without lymphatic involvement. So some cases have lymph node involvement. About 15% overall for early gastric cancer. Where sub mucosal invasion occurs it is more frequent, about 20%. Cancer, limited to the mucosa with intra-mucosal cancer lymph node metastases are found in depressed cancers, types IIc, II or III. In the elevated type of cancer, lymph node metastases are not found.

R. Pichlmayr. Most of the early gastric cancer patients are referred to you by screening?

K. Takagi. Yes, 30 - 40% of the cancers detected by screening are early.

R. Pichlmayr. The proportion may not be representative of a general hospital in your country. Can you give us a percentage for the whole country?

K. Takagi. I don't know exactly but I think the screening pick-up rate for early gastric cancer is about 30 - 40%. Other cases mainly have symptoms and come to out-patient clinics or are discovered by X-ray and endoscopy.

D. Day. What is your explanation for the change in the ratios of the different types of early gastric cancer over the 30 year period? You showed us a table where in the latter part of 1966-75 there was a much higher proportion of the IIc type lesion compared to earlier years.

K. Takagi. The incidence of early gastric cancer may be divided into three decades. In the first decade all the information was obtained with X-rays. Recently the combination of X-rays and endoscopy has made the identification of IIc lesions much easier.

Patterns of Recurrence in Relation
to Therapeutic Strategy

R. Pichlmayr and H.-J. Meyer

Zentrum Chirurgie, Klinik für Abdominal- und
Transplantationschirurgie, Medizinische Hochschule, Hannover,
Hannover, Federal Republic of Germany

ABSTRACT

Surgery is the only available treatment for gastric cancer, but even
in resected cases the survival rate is low and most of the patients
succumbed to a recurrence of this cancer. Recurrence in the gastric
stump may occur in about 10 % to 25 % of all cases, but mainly extensive local recurrence or distant metastases could are obtained at
secondary operations or autopsies. Therefore the resectability rate
is very low and long term survival is achieved only in a few
cases. The main approach to improve the results of primary gastric
cancer and hope to decrease the incidence of recurrence are
now early diagnosis and radical primary operative procedures.

KEYWORDS

Survival rate of gastric cancer; dissemination of gastric cancer;
patterns of recurrence; second operations for recurrent cancer;
treatment of choice for gastric cancer; gastrectomy "de principe".

Introduction

The overall results of treatment in gastric cancer are - as we all
agree - far from satisfactory. The vast majority of the patients
succumb to their disease, except the patients operated in the stage
of early cancer. This unsatisfying situation in advanced gastric cancer - well known and described over several decades - is true nearly
in the same way today despite improvement of surgical technique,
reduction of operative mortality and great efforts in finding adjuvant therapies.
Besides the outstanding importance of an early diagnosis surgery up
till now is the only available treatment with curative or significant
long lasting palliative properties. Thus, although disappointing,
how few patients we are able to cure, we nevertheless have to do our
best in surgery, to save at least the possible curative cases. The
research to find the best kind of surgery is reflected by many discussions about how extensive surgery should be - subtotal gastrectomy,

total gastrectomy, supraradical surgery-, which took place already
forty to fifty years ago and has not come to a final conclusion today. In the assessment of the results of surgery, survival rates and
survival time are of course the leading figures. No great differences
have been found in the overall studies up to now in these parameters,
comparing different surgical methods. But it might well be, that the
survival parameters alone are somewhat insufficient in the judgement
of the proper strategy of surgery. Advantages of a chosen kind of
treatment - for example gastrectomy "de principe" - in some patients
could be equalized or even reversed in the overall results by disadvantages or insignificance of this procedure in other patients. This
undoubtedly happens. A precise knowledge of the patterns of recurrence in relation to the primary stage of tumor and the applied form
of surgery would certainly enable a better individually adapted operative strategy. But it is mentioned that it is very difficult to
find exact data to describe this relationship. Essential prerequisites for this could be precise recording of the categories "tumor",
"surgery","follow up" and "cause of death". (Table 1).

TABLE 1   Prerequisites for Describing the Relation-
           ship between Therapeutic Strategy and
           Patterns of Recurrence

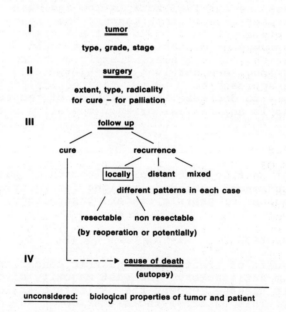

In contrast to this, the evaluation particularly in the conditions
for the local recurrence impeded by the absence of a large prospective study, by the fact that reoperation as well as autopsy are performed only in selected cases respectively by chance and thus does
not strictly allow general conclusions; furthermore the description
of the data is frequently insufficient. Thus, it must be admitted,
that the following statement is more a description than an answer to
the problem and based partly on theoretical considerations instead of
facts.

FACTS AND FREQUENCY OF RECURRENCE

The very low absolute 5-year survival rate in gastric cancer of about
10 % (Gütgemann and Schreiber, 1964) may be the consequence of various factors, as poor general prognosis of the tumor, late stage of
treatment, poor results of treatment and so on; the low survival rate
also in resected cases, even in those resected "for cure", demonstrate,
that recurrence in any form is the probable fate for these patients,
approximately for 70 % of primary resectable cases. Both, local recurrence and distant   spread   are included here. The time of recurrence - in the general sense - can be estimated best by describing
survival curves of "curative" resected patients: most of the patients
dying succumb to their disease within the first three years after
operation. Clinical signs of recurrence proceed death in a range of
three to twelve months with a medium of about four to six months
(Bowden, 1967; Schreiber, Bernhard and Kuss, 1964).
In contrast, recurrence after resections of early gastric cancer is
infrequent, about 2 % to 5 % of all cases; the time period for a potential recurrence is about the same as in advanced cancers.
According to the survival curves, tumor recurrence is the main cause
of death in gastric cancer patients and becomes manifest mostly within the first three years after resection of the primary tumor (Bowden,
1967).

MODES OF DISSEMINATION OF GASTRIC CANCER

Modes and routes of tumor dissemination principally are the base of
radical tumor surgery (Cole and others, 1965; Fly, Dockerty and Waugh,
1956; McNeer, Booher and Bowden, 1950; Wanke and Schwan, 1979). For
gastric cancer spread by the lymphatic system and by contiguity are
the most important routes, followed by hematogenous metastasizing and
tumor cell implantation (Table 2).
The great importance of the lymphatic system for intra- and extragastric tumor spreading has been pointed out very early and confirmed
many times (Coller, Kay and McIntyre, 1941; Eker, 1951; Sunderland,
1967; Zinninger, 1954). According to Coller (Coller, Kay and McIntyre,
1941) three communicating systems play a role in tumor spreading:
The intramural lymphatics with three likewise communicating networks
enables spreading inside the lymphatic vessels or along lymphatic
channels. Particularly in the submucosal and subserosal network tumor
spreading may happen far distant from the primary tumor, which is
hard to ascertain macroscopically or by palpation. It is wellknown,
that anatomical border lines - as the region of the pylorus and of
the cardia - are by no means barriers against tumor spreading. Depending on stage and localisation of the tumor a great variation in the
frequency of crossing these border lines has been described (Wanke
and Schwan, 1979; Zinninger and Collins, 1949).

TABLE 2   Spread of Gastric Cancer

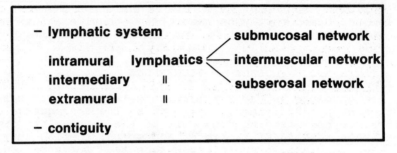

– vascular system
– implantation

Through <u>intermediary</u> lymphatics spreading to the <u>extramural</u> lymphatics
with the four wellknown main zones has taken place in more than 50 %
at the time of operation. Although   spread is common to the tumor
neighboured zones, even distant zones may be affected alone or combined. Particularly the spleno-pancreatic region is of surgical interest; a frequency of involvement of this area up to 23 % independently of the site of the primary tumor has been described (Bengmark,
Domellöf and Olsson, 1971; Fly, Dockerty and Waugh, 1956).
<u>Spread by contiguity</u>, mostly to liver or pancreas, using the lesser
omentum or the bursa omentalis as a bridge, is a sign of deep direct
infiltration; the differentiation from lymphogenic spreading may be
difficult or uncertain.

Metastases in other organs are mostly <u>blood born</u>, particularly in the
liver by portal vein route. Distant metastases are apparent in about
10% to 20% at the time of operation; the frequency of undetected
metastases at this time is unknown and cannot be calculated from the
data available. Peritoneal metastases may come from lymphatic
spreading or from <u>cell implantation</u>. Iatrogenic implantation to the
peritoneal cavity or the gastric remnant is thought to play a minor
role in the mode of origin of recurrence.

Besides spreading beyond the resection lines the multiplicity of the
primary lesions may be the cause of recurrence. The frequency of
multiple primary tumors – investigated mainly in early gastric cancer
– may range between 3% to 10%.

These roughly outlined modes of tumor spread have to be considered
in the surgical strategy as well as in the attempt to distinguish
recurrences between consequences of inadequate treatment and of unavoidable course.

DESCRIBED PATTERNS OF RECURRENCE

a. in reoperated cases: Reoperations in recurrent gastric carcinoma
are relatively seldom performed (Bowden, 1967; Gütgemann and Schreiber,
1964; McNeer, Booher and Bowden, 1950), the resectability of the recurrent tumor is low - thus cure or long lasting palliation is rare -
and findings are frequently inconclusive for clarification of the
origin of the recurrence - because of their mostly widespread or multiple extent (Iwanaga and others, 1978; Koga and others, 1978).
A literature review shows the relatively small number of reoperations
with mainly low resection rates (Table 3).

TABLE 3   Resection Rates in Recurrent Gastric Cancer
          (Literature Review)

author		total cases	sec. resection	
		n	n	%
Schwaiger	(1955)	17	1	5,9
Contzen	(1956)	19	–	–
Hoffmann	(1956)	35	10	29,4
Bauer	(1963)	17	1	5,9
Schreiber	(1964)	44	3	6,8
Bowden	(1967)	57	24	43,8
Koga	(1969)	31	12	38,7
Achatzy	(1973)	44	4	9,1
Bodner	(1977)	15	2	13,3
Kummer	(1977)	59	–	–
Saegesser	(1978)	37	14	37,8
Schlag	(1978)	18	7	38,9
own material	(1980)	61	16	26,2

The patterns of recurrence show great variations (Table 4).

TABLE 4   Patterns of Recurrent Gastric Cancer
          (Literature Review)

author	total	recurrence in gastric or duodenal stump		local (gastric bed)		distant recurrence (liver, peritoneum)	
	n	n	%	n	%	n	%
McNeer and ass. (1951)	88	55	62,5	19	21,6	14	15,9
Berne and Friedman (1951)	26	23	88,5	?	?	3	11,5
Thompson and Robins (1952)	28	5 – 11	18 – 40	13 – 19	46 – 68	?	7
Koga and ass. (1969)	31	20	64,5	7	22,6	4	12,9
Iwanaga and ass. (1978)	154	12	7,8	64	41,6	78	50,6
Koga and ass. (1978)	122	21	17,2	15	12,3	86	70,5
own material (Hannover) (1979)	61	15	24,6	19	31,2	27	44,2

In the reports (Berne and Freedman, 1951; McNeer and others, 1951;
Thompson and Robins, 1952) with high proportions of gastric,
duodenal stump or local recurrence those cases with distal metastases have been excluded before; the low sited reports resemble
more the unselected situation. Of these roughly 30 % local or predominantly local recurrent cases 60 % to 70 % are true gastric stump
recurrences, whereas about 20 % will origin from perigastric lymph
nodes. This means, that about 10 % to 20 % of all cases after partial
resection have recurrence in the gastric stump, which could be
avoidable. But it is not clear to what extent recurrence in the
gastric bed could be diminished by a more radical lymph node dissection.

Amongst 1009 malignant neoplasms we operated on 61 recurrent cases,
irrespective of where the first operation was carried out. The recurrence
was restricted to gastric stump or direct surroundings in one quarter,
was extensively local in 30 % and disseminated in 44 % (Table 5).

TABLE 5   Patterns of Recurrent Gastric Cancer in
          our own Clinical Material

location	n	%	interval ($\bar{x}$, mths.)
gastric remnant only	11		
gastric remnant and bed	4		
	15	24,6	29,3
extensive local recurrence	19	31,2	24,1
peritoneal dissemination	14		
liver metastases only	5		
liver metastases and extensive local recurrence	5		
liver metastases and peritoneal dissemination	3		
	27	44,2	11,5
total	61	100	22,8

In relation to the kind of primary surgery there was a relatively uniform distribution of recurrence after distal, subtotal gastrectomy and of course a high proportion of distant metastases in the total gastrectomy group; in this group all local recurrences were extensive. (Table 6).

TABLE 6   Patterns of Recurrence of Gastric Cancer
in Relation to Primary Operation

pattern of recurrence / op. procedure	gastric stump and bed		extensive local recurrence		distant diss. (liver, peritoneum)		total
	n	%	n	%	n	%	n
distal subtotal gastrectomy	14	35,9	11	28,2	14	35,9	39
proximal subtotal gastrectomy	1	11,2	4	44,4	4	44,4	9
total gastrectomy	–	–	4	30,8	9	69,2	13
total n	15		19		27		61

The interval between first and second operation was shorter in primarily high tumor stages and after total gastrectomy mainly as a consequence of advanced stages of the primary tumor in this group. The survival time did show some positive results in the resected group. Two patients after resection of gastric stump recurrence are alive more than five years after reoperation. None of the patients after total gastrectomy could be resected again (Table 7).

TABLE 7   Dependence of Survival Time on the Patterns
of Recurrence of Gastric Cancer

survival time after operation	local recurrence	extensive local recurrence	liver and peritoneal diss.
	n	n	n
	15	19	27
> 3 months	14	12	7
> 12 months	11	–	–
> 2 years	9	–	–
> 3 years	4	–	–
> 5 years	2	–	–

b. <u>in autopsies</u>: The distribution of recurrence in autopsies is an
expression of the late stage of the disease with mostly combined
manifestations, predominantly in liver, lungs and widespread intra-
abdominal (Donn and McNeer, 1967; Horn, 1955; Warren, 1933; Warwick,
1928). These findings give poor information about the patterns
of early manifestation of recurrence, which is of greater interest
for therapeutic questions (Table 8).

TABLE 8   Distribution of Metastases in Gastric
Cancer According to Findings at Autopsy

	Warwick 1928		Warren 1933		Donn 1967		Dupont 1978	
	n	%	n	%	n	%	n	%
total	176	100	67	100	80	100	348	100
liver	67	38,1	23	34,3	33	41,3	189	54,3
peritoneum	35	19,9	19	28,4	26	32,5	83	23,9
lungs	21	11,9	6	8,9	31	38,8	78	22,4
intestines	7	4,0	4	5,9	17	24,3	100	28,7
bone	1	0,6	4	5,9	14	17,5	3	0,9
adrenals	8	4,6	2	2,9	14	17,5	52	14,9
spleen	4	2,3	1	1,5	9	11,3	45	12,9
ovaries	2	1,1	3	4,5	8	10,0	10	2,9

Summarizing the knowledge about patterns of recurrence with caution
the following conclusions can be drawn:

1.) Gastric stump recurrence is about 10 % to 25 % of all recurrences the only primary, or at least the predominant site of recurrence
and thus could be to a great extent avoided.

2.) Theoretically gastric bed recurrence could be diminished at least
to some extent by a more radical lymph node dissection - but this has
to be stated.

3.) The majority of local and perhaps all of the distant metastases
are unavoidable by the primary surgical method.

CONSEQUENCES TO THE THERAPEUTIC STRATEGY AND RESULTS

Different consequences for the therapeutic strategy in the surgical
treatment of gastric cancer are possible; the aim of reduction of
local recurrences may be fulfilled by a very precise individually adapted surgery as well as by the approach of "total gastrectomy de principe". Personally we have chosen the latter (Pichlmayr and Meyer, 1979;

Pichlmayr, Meyer and van Alste, 1980).
Previous studies de principe gastrectomy were stopped mostly because
of the high post-operative mortality incidence. The lowering of the
mortality rate was a pre-requisite for a wide indication to total
gastrectomy. This could be achieved in their own clinical material.
(Table 9.)

TABLE 9 Postoperative Mortality after Total Gastrectomy for Advanced and Early Gastric Cancer

period	no. of operations	postop. mortality	
	n	n	%
1968 – 1979	299	33	11,0
1968 – 1971	32	5	15,6
1972 – 1975	80	13	16,3
1976 – 1979	187	15	8,0
1974 – 1979	237	22	9,3

The postoperative mortality after this operation in a total of 299
cases has been reduced to 8 % in the last three years. A leakage of
the esophageal-enteral anastomosis was obtained in 32 (10.7 %) patients,
and 15 (46.9%) patients died subsequently. The overall mortality
rate of this complication was 5.0 %.
Using the technique of a long (35 to 40 cm measuring) jejunal interposition according to Longmire, Gütgemann-Schreiber with an end-to-
side esophago-jejunostomy (proposed by Seo), reflux is no longer a
major problem and consecutively the general state of patients, the
nutritional conditions and the quality of life is acceptable or even
excellent over years - recurrence excluded. Radiologically there may
be some reflux, but there are seldom clinical or endoscopic signs of
reflux-esophagitis. The absence of reflux can be shown best by a
sequence scintigraph with m-^{99}Tc (Reichelt, Langenberg and Löhlein,
1977). Thus in achieving an acceptable mortality rate and good functional results total gastrectomy became more and more the treatment of
choice for gastric cancer in our institution (Table 10).

R. Pichlmayr and H.-J. Meyer

TABLE 10   Treatment of Gastric Cancer (own procedure)

advanced and early gastric cancer	gastrectomy "de principe" extensive lymph node dissection splenectomy, resection of the greater and lesser omenta
exceptions: prepyloric localisation	distal subtotal gastrectomy extensive lymph node dissection without splenectomy resection of the distal omenta
high operative risk	individual indications

We can roughly divide between the period before 1974 when subtotal gastrectomy was the routine procedure and total gastrectomies have been only performed by necessity and the period after 1974, where total gastrectomy became the treatment of "de principe", not excluding subtotal gastrectomies in individual cases.
As this is not a prospective trial, only limited conclusions are allowed by comparing these groups respectively periods. Under this aspect the following results have to be mentioned:

1.) The results of total gastrectomy performed in the period of gastrectomy "de principe" are of course superior to those of the gastrectomy "de nécessité", because of the higher proportion of advanced stages in the latter (29 % versus 13 %). A relatively favourable 5-year survival rate of 41 % in the "curative" gastrectomized patients in the group "de principe" may be a positive aspect.

2.) Comparing the results of subtotal and total gastrectomies - which is allowed only in the same remarks mentioned above - subtotal resections are superior in the overall period (Fig. 1.) as well as in the period "de principe", when performance of subtotal gastrectomy has been continued in prepyloric lesions. But this is understandable, because the term "de principe" includes the cases of "de nécessité".

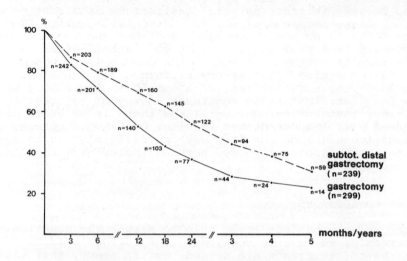

Fig. 1.   5-year survival rate after subtotal, distal
          and total gastrectomy for advanced and
          early gastric cancer.

3.) Comparing the results of both procedures in cancers of the distal
part of the stomach - where the alternative question of the best kind
of surgery is most important - there is no difference to be found
(Table 11). But as in the group of subtotal gastrectomy the percentage
of earlier, well differentiated tumors is higher, these results tend
to be a sign of the advantage of total gastrectomy.

TABLE 11   5-Year Survival Rate for Advanced and
           Early Gastric Cancer (Lesions Located
           in the Distal Part of the Stomach)

	well diff. adv. or early cancer	5 – year survival rate	
		incl. op–mortality	excl. op–mortality
		% ± 2 SE	% ± 2 SE
subtotal, distal gastrectomy n = 141	57%	38,5 ± 8,4	42,4 ± 7,4
total gastrectomy period: "de principe" n = 86	38%	42,1 ± 14,4	44,2 ± 15,0

4.) In comparing the overall results of both periods - the period of
"individual adapted" surgery before 1974 (subtotal gastrectomy as the
method of choice and gastrectomy "de nécessité") with that of the
gastrectomy "de principe" since 1974 - there are some tendencies to
a better outcome in the last period (25 % versus 33 %). This may be
remarked because in training total gastrectomy as a routine procedure
individual cases become - or may be - resectable, which "normally"
would be declared as not resectable, and thus the rate of resectability
has increased from 68 % up to 73 % in the latter period, which should
make the results worse.
In this latter period, gastrectomy performed for "cure" could show a
favourable 5-year survival rate of about 50 %. Personally we use these
results for justification to continue the way of gastrectomy "de principe" in our institution. But until now there is no exact proof, if
this indeed will lead to better results. One should not set the expectations too high; on the long way one certainly has to come to a
stage and tumor adapted surgery, perhaps including a high incidence
of gastrectomies.

CONCLUSIONS

With some reluctance, not to be able to answer the question of the
term correctly, we have to conclude, that further studies in the field
of patterns of recurrence are needed. But it seems, that this is difficult. Considering the unclear situation in the treatment of gastric
cancer we initiated a multicentric study between the university hospitals in Germany. The intention is, to allow in a prospective, non
randomized study, the performance of the operation - in regard to
total or subtotal resection - as used in the individual situation, but
to guarantee a standarized uniform documentation and follow up.
Although it may be difficult even within this study, to find out the
patterns of recurrence in each patient - as reoperation respectively
autopsy cannot be obligatory - it is hoped at least very strongly,
to become able

first to make more precise conclusions as regard to survival time and
the rate, time and kind of recurrence in relation to the performed
operation and to the grade and stage of the tumor and

secondly to have a solid basis to investigate further questions, as
the use of adjuvant therapy, in a standarized manner.

REFERENCES

Achatzky, R., K. Schönwalder and H. Bünte (1973). Chirurgie des
  Magenstumpfkarzinoms. Klinikarzt, 6, 7-12.
Bauer, K. H. (1963). Das Krebsproblem, 2. Auflage. Springer, Berlin-
  Göttingen-Heidelberg.
Bengmark, S., L. Domellöf and A.M. Olsson (1971). The role of splen-
  ectomy in stomach cancer operations. Digestion, 4, 314-320.
Berne, C.J. and M.A. Freedman (1951). Local recurrence following
  subtotal gastrectomy for carcinoma. Am. J. Surg., 82, 5-7.
Bodner, E., K. Schwamberger and S. Weimann (1977). Wiederholung-
  seingriffe nach Magenoperation wegen Karzinoms. Akt. gastrologie,
  6, 129-132.

Bowden, L. (1967). Surgery of locally recurrent gastric cancer. In
  G. McNeer and G.T. Pack (Eds.) Neoplasms of the Stomach.
  J.B. Lippincott, Philadelphia. pp. 332-340.
Cole, W.H., S.S. Roberts, R.S. Webb, F.W. Strehl and G.D. Oates (1965).
  Dissemination of cancer with special emphasis on vascular spread
  and implantation. Ann. Surg., 161, 753-770.
Coller, F.A., E.B. Kay and R.S. McIntyre (1941). Regional lymphatic
  metastases of carcinoma of the stomach. Arch. Surg., 43, 748-761.
Contzen, H. (1956). Ergebnisse der Carcinomrezidivoperationen.
  Langenbecks Arch. klin. Chir., 284, 531-536.
Donn, F. and G. McNeer (1967). Metastasis of gastric cancer to other
  organs. In G. McNeer and G.T. Pack (Eds.), Neoplasms of the Stomach.
  J.B. Lippincott, Philadelphia. pp. 426-440.
Eker, R. (1951). Carcinomas of the stomach. Acta Chir. Scand., 101,
  112-126.
Fly, O.A., M.B. Dockerty and J.M. Waugh (1956). Metastases to the
  regional nodes of the splenic hilus from carcinoma of the stomach.
  Surg. Gynecol. Obstet., 102, 279-286.
Gütgemann, A. and H.-W. Schreiber (1964). Das Magen-und Kardia-Kar-
  zinom. Vorträge aus der praktischen Chirurgie, 69. Enke, Stuttgart.
Hoffmann, V. (1956). Das Problem des Karzinomrezidivs im Magen-
  Darm-Kanal. MMW, 13, 428-433.
Horn, R.C. (1955). Carcinoma of the stomach. Gastroenterology, 29,
  515-525.
Iwanaga, T., H. Koyama, H. Furukawa, H. Taniguchi, A. Wada and
  R. Tateishi (1978). Mechanisms of late recurrence after radical
  surgery for gastric carcinoma. Am. J. Surg., 135, 637-640.
Koga, S., H. Kishimoto, K. Tanaka and H. Kawaguchi (1978). Clinical
  and pathological evaluation of patients with recurrence of gastric
  cancer more than five years post-operatively. Am. J. Surg., 136,
  317-321.
Koga, S. K. Maeda, H. Andachi and T. Iwasaki (1969). Über die
  Re-operation beim Magenkrebsrezidiv. Chirurg, 40, 325-329.
Kummer, D., G. Bertsch, G. Breucha, B. Domres, G.E. Müller and F.
  Sommer (1977). Die Bedeutung der Krebsnachsorge beim Magen-, Dick-
  und Mastdarmkarzinom-Operierten. Med. Welt, 28, 1920-1925.
McNeer, G., R.J. Booher and L. Bowden (1950). The resectability of
  recurrent gastric carcinoma. Cancer. 3, 43-55.
McNeer, G., H. Vandenberg, F.Y. Donn and L. Bowden (1951). A critical
  evaluation of subtotal gastrectomy for the cure of cancer of the
  stomach. Ann. Surg., 134, 2-7.
Pichlmayr, R. and H.-J. Meyer (1979). Value of the gastrectomy "de
  principe". In Ch. Herfarth and P. Schlag (Eds.), Gastric Cancer.
  Springer, Berlin. pp. 196-204.
Pichlmayr, R., H.-J. Meyer and H.E. van Alste (1980). Die Gastrekto-
  mie als Standardoperation beim Magenkarzinom. In H.G. Beger,
  W. Bergemann and H. Oshima (Eds.), Das Magenkarzinom. Thieme, Stutt-
  gart. pp. 238-243.
Reichelt, H.G., G. Langenberg and D. Lölein (1977). Hepatobiliäre
  Sequenzszintigraphie in prä- und postoperativer Oberbauchdiagnostik.
  Chirurg,48. 583-587.
Saegesser, F. and P.V. Ryncki (1978). Malignant tumours of the
  stomach previously operated on for a benign or malignant affection.
  Chir. Gastroent., 12, 111-141.
Schlag, P. (1978). Nachsorge nach Operation eines Magenkarzinoms.
  Z. Allg. Med., 54, 129-132.
Schreiber, H.W., A. Bernhard and B. Kuss (1964). Über das Karzinom
  im Magenstumpf. Zbl. Chir., 16, 577-583.

Schwaiger, M. and K.H. Müller (1955).   Indikation und Ergebnisse der
    operativen Behandlung der Rezidive bösartiger Geschwülste.
    Langenbecks Arch. u. Dtsch. Z. Chir., 280, 536-551.
Sunderland, D.A. (1967).   The lymphatic spread of gastric cancer.
    In G. McNeer and G.T. Pack (Eds.), Neoplasms of the Stomach.
    J. B. Lippincott, Philadelphia. pp. 408-415.
Thompson, F.B. and R.E. Robins (1952).   Local recurrence following
    subtotal resection for gastric carcinoma.   Surg. Gynecol Obstet.,
    95, 341-344.
Wanke, M. and H. Schwan (1979).   Pathology of gastric cancer.
    World J. Surg., 3, 675-684.
Warren, S.   (1933).   Studies on tumor metastasis. N. Engl. J. Med.,
    17, 825-827.
Warwick, M. (1928).   Analysis of one hundred and seventy-six cases of
    carcinoma of the stomach submitted to autopsy.   Ann. Surg., 88,
    216-226.
Zinninger, M.M. and W.T. Collins (1949).   Extension of carcinoma of the
    Stomach into the duodenum and esophagus.   Ann. Surg., 130,
    557-566.
Zinninger, M.M. (1954).   Extension of gastric cancer in the intra-
    mural lymphatics and its relation to gastrectomy.   Am J.Surg., 20,
    920-927.

DISCUSSION

R. Parker. The tail of the pancreas was not removed in the total gastrectomy?

R. Pichlmayr. Not routinely, only if one thinks there could be infiltration do we have an indication to resect the tail of the pancreas. I think that post-operative morbidity would increase significantly with this approach.

J. Craven. You claimed that one of your reasons for the adoption of total gastrectomy was that the splenic nodes are a site of importance but the spleen and the distal pancreas can be resected in a sub-total radical distal gastrectomy without any more difficulty. This does not seem to me to be a good reason for adopting a total gastrectomy.

R. Pichlmayr. Yes, I think we have too few cases to know whether the number of positive lymph nodes in the splenic hilum is a justification for such an operation. One could do a sub-total resection and splenectomy but in this situation one is not radical enough in the lesser curve. In doing a sub-total gastrectomy we do a precise lymphadenectomy taking the gastric artery at its origin from the coeliac axis. In combining a lymphadenectomy with a sub-total gastrectomy I would be concerned about the blood supply of the gastric remnant.

C. Newman. Do you have any anxieties about the validity of this very major undertaking to answer the question of total versus sub-total when you are not randomising cases which could enter either group?

R. Pichlmayr. That is a cruicial point and we have discussed it at length. I think only a randomised study can answer the question precisely. However, it is practically impossible to find clinics that are willing and able to randomise. I think we would end up with incorrect randomisation. If a hospital prefers sub-total resections they will be unable to randomise correctly. It is a big problem and we thought we would overcome it by having a very large number of patients. All Unviersity Hospitals in Germany are now willing to co-operate, and if we have very precise documentation of the pathological data we may have an answer in a few years.

D. Hancock. What is your survival rate for an antral carcinoma with positive splenic node involvement?

R. Pichlmayr. I will call upon Dr. Meyer to help me with this question.

H. Meyer. Looking at retrospective cases the survival rate is 25-28% in patients with positive lymph nodes.

R. Pichlmayr. With positive lymph nodes in the splenic hilum?

D. Hancock. Yes.

R. Pichlmayr. I don't think we have enough data for this. It is a very small group.

D. Hancock. Hawley and Morson in 1970 reported that this group did not do at all well.

R. Pichlmayr. The results of total gastrectomy are good in cases with lesions in the pyloric antrum.

W. Gillison. Accepting your point that you have yet to prove a better survival rate for total gastrectomy for distal gastric lesions, what about the local recurrence rate at the top end of the stomach? Are you like Mckeown of

Darlington who did total gastrectomies for every carcinoma of the cardia, or do you do a resection which preserves the antrum, and have you any data on whether these people are more likely to have gastric recurrence?

R. Pichlmayr. No, I do not perform a proximal partial gastrectomy. I do not know if the recurrence rate would be higher but I think it is quite clear that the rate of insufficiency of the anastomosis is much higher with an oesophago-anterostomy than with interposition or Roux-en-Y oesophago-jejunostomy after gastrectomy.

W. Gillison. So you do a total for technical reasons, but not for cancer reasons?

R. Pichlmayr. Yes.

DAY 2. SESSION 1. PANEL DISCUSSION

V. Brookes. We have talked about extension of the operation proximally. At what level do you divide the duodenum distally, Dr. Pichlmayr, because you talked early on about duodenal and gastric stump recurrence but you did not mention duodenal resection, which I think a lot of people do. At what level do you divide the duodenum distally?

R. Pichlmayr. 2 - 2.5 cms in every case. I prefer the Longmire technique for reconstruction because I find this easier than closing a short duodenal stump.

H. Ellis. It always strikes me as very odd to scrape off, as we sometimes have to do, a carcinoma of the pyloric end of the stomach where our closure, we know, is very close to the tumour edge and then to sacrifice about 12 ins of normal stomach proximally. So what would you do where you have a great big pyloric tumour and you are just a few mm clear of the duodenal side? Are you then happy about having to sacrifice a lot of normal stomach in what you really suspect is a palliative resection?

R. Pichlmayr. I am not happy, but I would do it at the moment becuase I do not know how many lymph nodes might be in the splenic area and how radical I can be with a sub-total gastrectomy. Perhaps in individual cases, I would do a sub-total resection or combine it with pancreatic or duodenal pancreatectomy. We have done this in individual cases and I think one is living now 5 years from surgery. I know it is terrible to take out the whole of the stomach, if one thinks that it is not necessary, but we have no clear guidelines for and against and so this is our approach at the moment.

H. Ellis. Well, I am glad I am in an English University Hospital, not a German one, because I would not be able to join in your trial. Dr. ReMine, what would you do at the Mayo Clinic?

W. ReMine. We would do a radical sub-total. Fly, a number of years ago, showed that 30% of lesions in the lower half of the stomach had positive nodes in the hilus of the spleen and we have forgotten that.

R. Pichlmayr. Is it possible to do a splenectomy, radical lymphadenectomy and take the gastric artery at its origin?

W. ReMine. Yes, you leave the ascending branch of the left gastric artery. A number of years ago it was shown by two men from this country, Berkely and Bentley, I believe, that if you have one good vessel going to your gastric remnant you don't have to worry about you blood supply because you have arteriovenous shunts that open up and they showed it very beautifully with glass microspheres. So for a lesion in the lower half of the stomach we would do a radical sub-total which includes the first portion of the duodenum. You get the sub pyloric nodes and you get the nodes in the hilus of the spleen.

S. Glick. What operation do people primarily do for the early gastric cancer which has developed in a stomach which has got atrophic gastritis, which seems to be the kind of early gastric cancer that we see? Secondly, Dr. ReMine did mention the use of laparoscopy in the workup of the patient with a carcinoma of the stomach. I think it is probably a useful technique, it saves a useless laparotomy, because when you have done a laparotomy in the inoperable case they often go down-hill very quickly.

W. ReMine. I think it is a good thing to do until the doctor comes.

S. Glick. You mean the surgeon?

W. ReMine. Right. We still do a reasonably radical procedure with the early
gastric cancer. In the studies that I reported in 1962, we were able to show that
even with small lesions, if they are high grade lesions and you don't know this
sometimes until you get them out, you may have nodes immediately adjacent or they
may go through the peripheral sinusoides of the nodes, to nodes a little further
along. We treat them all as though they are very dangerous lesions and not just
because they are small. Sometimes the smaller lesions are very high grade and you
have got to be very cautious with those. The bulkier the lesion, the lower the
grade.

H. Ellis. Professor Johnston, what happens in Newcastle?

I. Johnston. We would be moderately radical, not super radical.

W. Longmire. What does Dr. Takagi do with the early superficial lesion?

K. Takagi. For a 2 - 3 cm early cancer located in the upper part of the stomach,
we do a proximal gastrectomy. For a spreading cancer that extends into a body we
do a total gastrectomy. In cases with no metastases along the lesser or greater
curves, we do not remove the spleen and pancreas.

R. Pichlmayr. The problem is that our endoscopists cannot be sure before surgery
if it is an early or an advanced cancer. We have to treat them in the same way,
except perhaps for elevated lesions.

W. ReMine. Unfortunately, you don't know whether the nodes are involved unless
you take them out.

J. Alexander-Williams. I would like to support Dr. Pichlmayr's hypothesis. I am
persuaded by the logic of his argument providing you can have a low mortality and
morbidity. I would like to know about your post-operative mortality with your
interposed loop. It's commendably low, but you have had some patients who have
died, have any of them died because you used an interposition? Did they die
because of the duodenal anastomosis, and might they have lived if you had done a
Roux-en-Y reconstruction?

R. Pichlmayr. We have had one patient with an insufficiency of the jejuno-duoden-
ostomy - one in 300. So I do not know if I would have had duodenal stump rupture
if I had used a Roux-en-Y. The total mortality rate is 8% as I have shown. I do
not know if the interposition would be more beneficial for the nutritional state
than the Roux-en-Y.

H. Ellis. Well, we have got the inventor of the operation sitting in the front
row. What's the latest news about the Longmire Operation? I know you are going
to speak this\afternoon, but perhaps we could have the lowdown!

W. Longmire. I will just summarise by saying that that operation is used much
more in Europe than it is in the United States, including UCLA and California.

B. Golematis. A question for Dr. Smith. Has anyone tried chemotherapy orally before
the operation for gastric cancer? Do you have any experience of that?

F. Smith. Not oral chemotherapy per se. In those few cases where the patient has
been deemed from the beginning to be unresectable, there have been attempts to
give chemotherapy and then a surgical resection is made. I think there are a lot
of problems with that approach and you might be denying the patient the only real
modality of cure, which is surgery. We have had experience where we have had
patients referred to us, initially inoperable and unresectable in spite of

laparotomy. We have then given them FAM and the patient has done well and we have
sent that individual back to surgery to find out if the tumour can then be
resected. But as a primary treatment, no.

P. Wrigley. There are some studies going on in Malaysia where they are giving
pre-operative chemotherapy and when I was there earlier this year, one or two of
the surgeons were speaking very highly of the results. Unfortunately, I have my
doubts as to the quality of the final answer scientifically, but they are
anecdotally speaking highly successful. They often see a lot of late cases.
Dr. Smith, have there been any long term complications of chemotherapy, and has
there been any occurrence of second malignancies in people on chemotherapy?

F. Smith. In the most advanced cases, as you can see from the survival curves,
they don't yet live long enough to experience problems. I think the group of
patients whom we are going to have to follow rather carefully is the group that have
been treated with combined modality therapy to determine in those patients if they
have problems with the nephrotoxicity or carcinogenicity and leucaemogenesis
that's been described with methly-CCNU. The group of patients that we would like
to propose using for chemotherapy treatment will be in the adjuvant setting. I
think that it is in this group that we will learn about late toxicities. Currently
there are on-going studies of 5FU and methyl-CCNU with a median follow-up time of
about two years and to date there has been no long term toxicity noted. There is
also here in Birmingham a study of 5FU and mitomycin-C and perhaps someone here
can tell us if there has been any long-term toxicity with that? I don't think that
any has developed yet.

H. Ellis. Victor, what's the latest news from the Birmingham trial?

V. Brookes. Well we have had some toxicity.

P. Wrigley. It's a multi-centre British trial. About 8% of the patients have
shown some elevation of blood urea, sometimes with accompanying persistent
thrombocytopaenia, and it appears in a number of cases to have preceded death.

F. Smith. I might retract some of my statements. We have seen that feature and we
are not sure whether its a complication of therapy or not. We have observed 6
patients who developed a haemolytic uraemic type of syndrome with erythroid marrow
and there were three linking features in these patients. We have now seen one
patient with adenocarcinoma of the lung and one patient with adenocarcinoma of the
colon. So it appears not to be specifically gastric carcinoma, but the link is
that they all had adenocarcinomas. They have all been treated with mitomycin-C.
The patients that we had were FAM treated patients and since then we have had one
individual treated at the M.D. Anderson with 5FU and mitomycin-C into an hepatic
artery catheter. Of great interest to us is that for the most part these patients
have had very little residual disease. Five of the 6 that we have observed went
on to die and 3 of these individuals had autopsies. In 2 there was no gross
residual disease left, and in the third one there was minimal residual disease left.
We have since identified immune complexes in these patients and we think that
rather than being treatment related, it might be due to the tumour itself. It has
been known that metastatic disease will cause microangiopathic haemolysis and what
we are postulating, at the present time, is that the reduction in tumour bulk may
lead to an antigen balance where immune complexes can be precipitated and we have
been able to measure these immune complexes. In our 6th patient, by combined
treatment with plasmaphoresis and immuran, we have been able to reverse this syndrome.
so we think that this is more disease related.

V. Brookes. The only problem with that argument is that the ones that we have are
all within the treated group. We have had none in the placebo control group.

F. Smith. I think then that the question has to remain because there is the common link with mitomycin-C.

M. Crespi. A question for Dr. Takagi. You say that there are two different types of early gastric carcinoma, one is symptomatic and the other is not symptomatic. The symptomatic one, you say, is the one associated with the benign gastric ulcer. Correct?

K. Takagi. Yes.

M. Crespi. What do you mean exactly? Do you mean that the benign gastric ulcer becomes malignant?

K. Takagi. No. I think that in 1960 after the discovery of very early gastric cancers, they were often associated with benign ulcers. So at that time many doctors believed that benign ulcers became malignant. Then a retrospective study of gastrocamera examinations showed that a IIc lesion may be ulcerated and then heal. When the indicence of cancer was low, the incidence of benign ulceration was low; when the cancer incidence increased so also did the incidence of benign ulceration. I think that benign ulceration occuring in the early gastric cancer is secondary. In Japan many doctors now think cancer with ulceration is not an ulcer cancer.

M. Crespi. In your experience, is it the IIc type of lesion which gives the symptoms or is it another associated type of lesion.

K. Takagi. It is mainly the IIc lesion with ulceration.

R. Pichlmayr. The question of the symptoms of early gastric cancer is so important for us. Our countries are not able to have screening programmes at present. Within our 70 patients with early gastric cancer all, except 2, have been symptomatic and diagnosed by symptoms. I would like to ask again are all IIc early gastric cancers symptomatic, or are there patients also with excavated or ulcerated forms who are asymptomatic and who become advanced without having had symptoms at any time?

K. Takagi. Early gastric cancers with ulceration have symptoms like a benign ulcer.

Stages of Gastric Cancer and Reconstruction after Surgery

K. Takagi

Department of Surgery, Cancer Institute Hospital, Tokyo, Japan

ABSTRACT

Stage classification based on the General Rules for Gastric Cancer Study in Japan
and the TNM classification by UICC (both are used to represent the degree of
advance of gastric cancer) were studied on gastric cancer cases experienced at the
Surgery Department of the Cancer Institute Hospital in 1970-74. The methods of
reconstruction after the curative operations of gastric cancer, i.e., distal, total
and proximal gastrectomy, were examined in relation to the stage of the gastric
cancer. It was suggested that a method of anastomosis which would make it possible
to perform advanced endoscopy should be considered as a method of reconstruction
after surgery of gastric cancer.

KEYWORDS

Cancer stage; TNM classification; reconstruction after operation of gastric cancer;
ERCP after gastric operation.

INTRODUCTION

The stages of gastric cancer are now classified according to the General Rules for
the Gastric Cancer Study in Japan or to the TNM classification by UICC, but classification is still an area of study. The stage classifications of 1054 gastric
cancers which were operated on in 1970-74 at the Surgery Department, Cancer Institute Hospital, were examined. The method of surgery applied in these cases of
gastric cancer and the method of reconstruction were also examined in relation to
the stage of gastric cancer.

The Stage of Gastric Cancer

To examine the method of surgery or review the results of surgery for gastric
cancer, comparative study on different stages of cancer is necessary. However, the
stage of gastric cancer is determined by various factors: that is, the depth of
invasion, size of lesion, regional lymph node metastasis, remote metastasis (peritoneal metastasis, hepatic metastasis, distant lymph node metastasis, etc.). It is
not easy to determine synthetically how these factors are reflected in prognosis.

On the stage of gastric cancer, the General Rules for the Gastric Cancer Study
(First Edition) was published by the Japanese Research Society for Gastric Cancer
in June, 1962 in Japan. It has been revised many times and is now in its 10th
edition (May, 1979).

In the General Rules for the Gastric Cancer Study (hereafter referred to as General
Rules), the factors affecting the stage of gastric cancer are peritoneal metastasis
(P), hepatic metastasis (H), lymph node metastasis (N) and depth of invasion. For
use in diagnosis at the time of surgery, the macroscopic or histologic stage is
used, but for accurate statistics, the histologic stage should be used. The histologic stages are as shown in Table 1.

TABLE 1

CANCER STAGE BASED ON HISTOLOGIC FINDINGS

Stage	Peritoneal Metastasis	Liver Metastasis	Lymph Node Metastasis	Depth of Invasion*
	Macroscopic or Histologic		Histologic	
I	P_0	H_0	$n\ (-)$	$Ps\ (-)$
II	P_0	H_0	$n_1\ (+)$	ss
III	P_0	H_0	$n_2\ (+)$	se
IV	P_1, P_2, P_3	H_1, H_2, H_3	$n_3\ (+), n_4\ (+)$	si, sei

See the "Histostological Classification of Gastrc Cancer" (Part II of The General
Rules for the Gastric Cancer Study in Surgery and Pathology, Section 6.5).

Here, the most advanced stage among the stages obtained for each item is used as
the histologic stage.

There were 1054 cases of gastric cancer operated on at the Surgery Department,
Cancer Institute Hospital in 1970-74. Curative surgery was performed on 830
patients (78.7%) and non-curative surgery on 224 patients (21.3%). The histologic
stages of the patients who received surgery are shown in Table 2; that is, stages
I and IV comprised 32.8% and 29.9% of the patients, respectively.

TABLE 2 Histologic Stage

Stage	Curative Cases No.	Curative Cases %	Non Curative Cases No.	Non Curative Cases %	Total No.	Total %
I	346	41.7			346	32.8
II	188	22.6			188	17.8
III	205	24.7			205	19.5
IV	91	11.0	224		315	29.9
	830	100	224	100	1054	100

1970-74 Cancer Institute Hospital

Of the patients who received curative surgery, 41.7% had stage I cancer. Stage III
was next most common and stage IV comprised only 11.0%. The 5-year survival rate
of the patients on whom curative surgery was performed is shown in Table 3 in relation to the stage of cancer.

TABLE 3   Cancer Stages and 5-Year Survival Rate
(Curative cases)

	5-Year survival rate	
Stage I	97.4%	(337 / 346)
II	65.4%	(123 / 188)
III	39.5%	(81 / 205)
IV	24.2%	(22 / 91)
Total	67.8%	(563 / 830)

The 5-year survival rate of all the patients was 67.8% while that for stage I was
97.4%, and prognosis worsened with the advance of stage. The recent increase in
stage I cancers which now account for half of the gastric cancers operated on, is
due to the fact that early cancers which belong to stage I have increased. By the
way, the frequency of stage I cancers in the gastric cancers operated on was 7.4%
(94/1272) in 1946-55, 14.7% (344/2347) in 1956-65 and 31.7% (665/2098) in 1966-75.
The early cancers belonging to stage I during these periods were 18.1% (17/94),
50.0% (172/344) and 74.3% (494/665), respectively. This clearly shows the importance of early cancers in improving the results of gastric cancer treatment.

Macroscopic classification is not included in the factors that affect the stage of
gastric cancer, but is important for treatment. From the pattern of the cancer
growth into the surrounding tissue which was observed in sections of the lesions
in formaldehyde-fixed resected stomachs, Kajitani (1950) assigned three types:
localized type, intermediate type and infiltrative type, and he reported on the
significance of such a classification (Kajitani, 1979). The relationship between
the macroscopic type of gastric cancer and the stage with respect to prognosis are
shown in Table 4.

TABLE 4

Macroscopic Classification and Stage : Prognosis

	Stage I	Stage II	Stage III	Stage IV	Total
Superficial type	100%	100%			100%
	(257/257)	(21/21)			(278/278)
Localised type	92.3%	56.5%	49.1%	27.3%	55.7%
	(24/26)	(39/69)	(28/57)	(6/22)	(97/174)
Intermediate type	62.5%	57.1%	31.8%	54.5%	48.4%
	(5/8)	(12/21)	(7/22)	(6/11)	(30/62)
Infiltrative type	92.7%	66.2%	35.7%	17.2%	49.7%
	(51/55)	51/77)	(45/126)	(10/58)	(157/316)
TOTAL	97.4%	65.4%	39.0%	24.2%	67.7%
	(337/346)	(123/188)	(80/205)	(22/91)	(562/830)

In stage I, though 74.3% (257/346) were superficial cancer (synonymous to early cancer), a 90% or higher 5-year survival rate was observed even in advanced cancer of both localized and infiltrative types. In stage III and IV cases, the prognosis of the localized type was better than that of the infiltrative type. Thus, in advanced cancer, extensive radical surgery should be performed aggressively for localized type cases.

In the General Rules, patients with P_{1-3}, H_{1-3} or para-aortic lymph node metastasis are not included as subjects of curative surgery. However, Kajitani and Takagi (1979) have experienced 10 patients with such metastasis who survived more than 5 years after dissection of distant metastasis. They were 2 patients with wedge-resection of solitary small metastasis in left lobe of liver, 2 patients with peritoneal metastasis of Douglas pouch removed and 6/83 patients with para-aortic lymph node metastasis dissected (Ohhashi, 1976). Especially, when no other factor hinders curative surgery, patients with para-aortic lymph node metastasis can be expected to survive for more than 5 years with aggressive dissection.

TNM Classification of UICC

Clinical classification of gastric cancer was proposed by UICC in 1966. The TNM classification was only a clinical classification. However, in Japan, with the progress of gastric diagnosis, it has become possible to clinically diagnose early gastric cancer by radiology and endoscopy, and in 1974 the Classification of Early Gastric Cancer was introduced (second edition). This was also a clinical classi-fication and T_{1-4}, N_x, $M_{0,1}$ were described. In 1978, clinical classification of TNM and post-surgical histopathological classification (p-TNM) were reported and stages were divided into stages I-IV.

We examined the gastric cancers operated on (1970-74) for this TNM classification. The TNM classification (1968, second edition) is as shown in Table 5.

TABLE 5
TNM CLASSIFICATION
(1970-74,Laparotomized cases)

			No. of cases	5-Year Survival No.of cases	%
T_0	N_x	M_0	7	7	100.0
T_1	N_x	M_0	271	265	97.8
T_2	N_x	M_0	34	27	79.4
T_3	N_x	M_0	530	218	41.1
T_4	N_x	M_0	193	42	21.8
T_{1-4}	N_x	M_1	19	0	
Total			**1054**	**559**	**53.0**

$T_1N_xM_0$ comprised 25.7% (271/1054) of all the laparotomies and $T_2N_xM_0$, only 3.2% (34/1054). The 5-year survival rate for T_0 and T_1 was 100% and 97.8%, respective-ly, that for T_2 was 79.4%, but that for T_2 and T_4 was only 41.1% and 21.8%, respec-tively. There were 19 patients with $T_{1-4}N_xM_1$, but none survived for 5 years.

The TNM classification and p-TNM of the stage groupings of gastric cancer (1978, third edition) are as shown in Table 6. Particularly in TNM classification, as laparotomy findings were included in the pre-surgery findings, the earlier the stage of the cancer, the harder it is to determine the lesion inside the stomach. Therefore, in the present study, we used only the findings obtained by radiology and endoscopy for T_{1-3}, and the laparotomy findings for N and M.

TABLE 6   Stage Grouping (provisional)

TNM

Stage I	T_1	N_0	M_0
Stage II	T_2	N_0	M_0
	T_3	N_0	M_0
Stage III	T_1, T_2, T_3	N_1, N_2	M_0
	T_1, T_2, T_3	N_3	M_0
	(Resectable for cure)		
	T_4	Any N	M_0
	(Resectable for cure)		
Stage IV	T_1, T_2, T_3	N_3	M_0
	(Not resectable for cure)		
	T_4	Any N	M_0
	(Not resectable for cure)		
	Any T	Any N	M_1

P-TNM

Stage I	pT_1	pN_0	pM_0
Stage II	pT_2	pN_0	pM_0
	pT_3	pN_0	pM_0
Stage III	pT_1, pT_2, pT_3	pN_1, pN_2	pM_0
	pT_1, pT_2, pT_3	pN_3	
	(Resected for cure)		
	pT_4	Any pN	pM_0
	(Resected for cure)		
Stage IV	pT_1, pT_2, pT_3	pN_3	pM_0
	(Not resected for cure)		
	pT_4	Any pN	pM_0
	(Not resected for cure)		
	Any pT	Any pN	pM_1

The TNM Pre-treatment Clinical Classification of the Gastric Cancers operated on in 1970-74 (Table 7) shows that 25.5% of all the patients operated on had stage I

cancer, and their 5-year survival rate was 100%. Of all the patients, 22.2% had
stage II cancer and their 5-year survival rate was 76.5% (179/234). In $T_2N_0M_0$, it
was 88.9% and almost as good as for stage I, but in $T_3N_xM_0$ it was 73.4%. Stage III
comprised 29.5% of all the patients, and their 5-year survival rate was 35.7%.

TABLE 7

STAGE GROUPING, TNM

	(1970–74 Laparotomized cases)	
	No. of cases	5 – Year Survival rate
Stage I $T_1 N_0 M_0$	269 (25.5 %)	100 % (269 / 269)
Stage II $T_2 N_0 M_0$	50 (4.7 %)	88.0 % (44 / 50)
$T_3 N_0 M_0$	184 (17.5 %)	73.4 % (135 / 184)
Stage III $T_1 T_2 T_3 N_1 N_2 M_0$	213 (20.2 %)	42.2 % (90 / 213)
$T_1 T_2 T_3 N_3$ M_0	34 (3.2 %)	(0 / 34)
Resectable for cure		
T_4 Any N M_0	64 (6.1 %)	32.8 % (21 / 64)
Resectable for cure		
Stage IV $T_1 T_2 T_3 N_3 M_0$	43 (4.1 %)	(0 / 43)
Not resectable for cure		
T_4 Any N M_0	29 (2.8 %)	(0 / 29)
Not resectable for cure		
Any T Any N M_1	168 (15.9 %)	(0 / 168)
Total	1,054 (100 %)	53.0 % (559 / 1054)

There were no patients with T_1, T_2, T_3 N_3M_0 who survived for 5 years, and their
prognosis was very bad. Stage IV comprised 22.8% of all the patients, but none of
them survived for 5 years.

As classified according to the p-TNM post-surgical histopathological classification
(Table 8), stage I comprised 25.8% of all the patients and the 5-year survival rate
was 100% for these patients; stage II comprised 15.8%, and the 5-year survival rate
was 60.1%; stage III, 38.3% and the 5-year survival rate was 40.9%. Of the stage
III cases, the 5-year survival rate of pT_{1-3}, pN_3pM_0 was 2.2% and prognosis was
bad.

Thus, of the stage groupings of the new TNM and p-TNM classifications, stages I,
II and IV were closely in parallel to prognosis, but the prognosis of $T_{1-3}N_3M_0$ and
$pT_{1-3}pN_3pM_0$ of stage III was extremely bad and the prognosis in these cases was the
same as for stage IV cases.

In Japan, it is now possible to accurately diagnose early cancer before surgery
due to the progress in gastric cancer diagnosis. Of the 277 cases diagnosed as T_1
early cancer before surgery, 234 cases (84.5%) were found to be pT_1 early cancer
by histologic diagnosis. On the other hand, of the 280 cases diagnosed as pT_1
early cancer after surgery, 234 cases (83.5%) were found to be early cancer by
pre-surgery diagnosis. However, such early diagnosis of gastric cancer was not
made possible in a day, but is in fact the result of about thirty years of progress

in the technology of diagnosis.

TABLE 8

STAGE GROUPING, p.TNM

(1970-74 Lapalotomized cases)

		No. of Cases	5-Year Survival rate
Stage I	pT1 pN0 pM0	261 (24.8 %)	100 % (261/261)
Stage II	pT2 pN0 pM0	107 (10.2 %)	82.2 % (88/107)
	pT3 pN0 pM0	59 (5.6 %)	76.3 % (45 / 59)
Stage III	pT1 pT2 pT3 pN1 pN2 pM0	322 (30.6 %)	47.8 % (154/322)
	pT1 pT2 pT3 pN³ pM0	45 (4.3 %)	2.2 % (1 / 45)
	Resectable for cure		
	pT4 Any pN pM0	36 (3.4 %)	27.8 % (10 / 36)
	Resectable for cure		
Stage IV	pT1 pT2 pT3 pN3 pM0	44 (4.2 %)	
	Not resectable for cure		
	pT4 Any pN pM0	50 (4.7 %)	
	Not resectable for cure		
	Any pT1 Any pN pM1	130 (12.3 %)	
Total		1,054 (100 %)	53.0 % (559 /1054)

Reconstruction

Curative operations for gastric cancer can roughly be classified into distal gastrectomy, total gastrectomy and proximal gastrectomy. Various combined resections
using these three methods are performed depending on the stage and location of the
gastric cancer. The reconstruction performed at our hospital in 1970-74 were
examined.

Distal gastrectomy and reconstruction. Distal gastrectomy is performed when the
gastric cancer is located in the middle or lower part of the stomach. For reconstruction there are two methods, i.e., Billroth I and II (hereafter referred to as
B-I, B-II). However, the B-I method is more physiological and is the recommended
method. When the area of the resected stomach is large, such as when subtotal
gastrectomy is performed, the B-II method is used. At our hospital after distal
gastrectomy, the B-I method was applied in 94% (544/576) as shown in Table 9.
Judged from the stage classification in the General Rules B-I was often used for
stage I-III but, B-II was often used for stage IV advanced cancer. The prognosis
of patients on whom B-I was used was good, i.e., the 5-year survival rate was
78.9%. However, when B-II was used, the 5-year survival rate was 31.1%, and the
prognosis of the patients with stage IV cancer was bad.

Total gastrectomy and reconstruction. Total gastrectomy at our hospital is performed in the following cases: When the distance from the cancer to the cardia is
less than 5-6 cm, when the cancer is spreading into the pancreas or spleen and
when lymph node metastasis is found in the upper part of the lesser curvature, in
the cardia or along the splenic hilus or splenic artery.

TABLE 9

CANCER STAGES AND RECONSTRUCTION
AFTER DISTAL GASTRECTOMY

1970-74, Curative cases

	Billroth-I		Billroth-II		Total	
	No.	5-Y.s.	No.	5-Y.s.	No.	5-Y.s.
Stage I	300	296	4	4	304	300
Stage II	123	89	5	4	128	92
Stage III	99 (2)	42	11	2	110 (2)	44
Stage IV	22	2	12	0	34	2
Total	544 (2)	429	32	10	576 (2)	438

( )--- Operative mortality cases

5-Y.s.--- 5-Year survival cases

Since 1950, we have been performing combined resection of pancreatosplenectomy with total gastrectomy for advanced cancer in the upper or middle stomach as a typical method of surgery. The frequency of total gastrectomy combined with pancreato-splenectomy to total gastrectomy was 72.3% (149/206) and the total gastrectomy alone was performed when the gastric cancer was stage I or II (fairly early cancer).

There are no general methods of reconstruction after total gastrectomy, as the Billroth I and II methods after distal gastrectomy, and various methods of anastomosis are employed at each hospital, each after consideration of the safety of the anastomosis and post-surgery nutrition. At our hospital, we use mainly three methods of reconstruction: The jejunal interposition method, double tract method and Roux-Y method (Fig. 1).

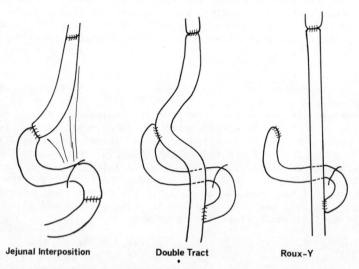

Jejunal Interposition   Double Tract   Roux-Y

Fig. 1. **RECONSTRUCTION PROCEDURES AFTER TOTAL GASTRECTOMY**

The double tract method is a modified Roux-Y method in which side to end anastomosis of the jejunum anastomosed to the esophagus and duodenal stump was added.
The benefit of this method is that food can also pass into the duodenum. The
direct mortality of patients who received total gastrectomy was 1.5% (3/206), that
of patients on which jejunal interposition was used was 4.8% (1/21), and that when
the double tract method was used was 1.4% (2/141).

The method of reconstruction to be used after total gastrectomy is selected after
consideration of the stage of gastric cancer. Jejunal interposition, double tract
and Roux-Y methods were selected at the rate of 10.2%, 68.4% and 18.4%, respectively. The method of reconstruction of the cases of total gastrectomy and the
frequency of each method used for the cancers at each stage are shown in Table 10.

TABLE 10

CANCER STAGES AND RECONSTRUCTIONS AFTER TOTAL GASTRECTOMY

(1970 - 74, Curative cases)

	Jejunal Interposition		Double tract		Roux-Y		Others		Total	
	No.	5-Y.s.	No.	5-Y.s.	No.	5-Y.s.	No.	5-Y.s.	No.	5-Y.s.
Stage I	8	8	29	28			1	1	38	37
Stage II	2(1)	1	34(1)	20	4	1	1	1	41(2)	23
Stage III	8	3	52	25	17	2	2(1)	1	79(1)	31
Stage IV	3	1	26(1)	11	17	3	2	0	48(1)	15
Total	21(1)	13	141(2)	84	38	6	6(1)	3	206(4)	106

( ) --- Operative mortality cases

5-Y.s. --- 5-Year survival cases

The double tract method is most often used, and it is used for all stages of cancer.
The jejunal interposition method is used on early gastric cancer patients who are
expected to live for a long time. The Roux-Y method is used on stage III and IV
advanced cancers, and is often used when serosal involvement is marked.
The 5-year survival rates when jejunal interposition and double tract methods were
used were high; 61.9% and 59.6%, respectively. However, when the Roux-Y method
was used it was low, 15.8%.

Proximal gastrectomy. Proximal gastrectomy is performed for early cancer in the
upper stomach and for fairly early cancer in the cardiac. In spite of the progress
in gastric diagnosis, however, there are few early cancers in the upper stomach,
and we performed proximal gastrectomy on only 35 patients (4.2%).

The methods of proximal gastrectomy are shown in Fig. 2 and the relationship
between the method of reconstruction and the stage of cancer in Table 11. The
jejunal interposition method was used for stage I early cancers and the 5-year
survival rate was high. The double tract, esophago-gastric anastomosis and Roux-Y
methods were used for more advanced cases in this order, and the prognosis of the
patients on whom the Roux-Y method was used was bad. Though careful consideration
is needed when a method of reconstruction after curative surgery of gastric cancer
is to be selected, recently, patients who survive for a long time after resection

of gastric cancer are increasing.

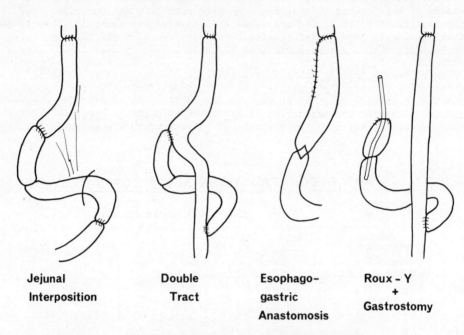

| Jejunal Interposition | Double Tract | Esophago-gastric Anastomosis | Roux - Y + Gastrostomy |

Fig. 2. **RECONSTRUCTION PROCEDURES AFTER PROXIMAL GASTRECTOMY**

TABLE 11

CANCER STAGE AND RECONSTRUCTIONS AFTER PROXIMAL GASTRECTOMY

1970–74 Curative Cases

	Jejunal interposition		Double Tract		Esophago-gastrie Anast.		Roux-Y.		Others		Total	
	No.	5-Y.s.	No.	5-Y.s.	No.	5-Y.s.	No.	5-Y.s.	No.	5-Y.s.	No.	5-Y.s.
Stage I	5	5	3	3	1	1					9	9
Stage II					1 0	2	1	0	2	0	1 3	2
Stage III			1	0			4	0			5	0
Stage IV	1	1	1	0	1	1	3	1	1	0	8	3
Total	6	6	5	3	1 2	4	8	1	3	0	3 5	1 4

5-Y.s. ----- 5-Year. survival cases

It has become possible to check for abnormalities of the biliary and pancreatic organs with the advancement in endoscopy examinations in such long-term survivals. It is very helpful if endoscopic retrograde cholangio-pancreatography (ERCP) can be performed on these patients after surgery.

Examination by ERCP is possible on patients who had Billroth II after distal gas-trectomy (Safrany, 1973) and we experienced cases in which ERCP could be performed

after total gastrectomy. In a case in which double tract reconstruction was performed after total gastrectomy, a duodenal fiberscope was passed from the jejunum
anastomosed to the esophagus through the jejuno-duodenal anastomosis into the
descending portion of the duodenum: ERCP was thus performed and mild chronic pancreatitis was diagnosed (Fig. 3).

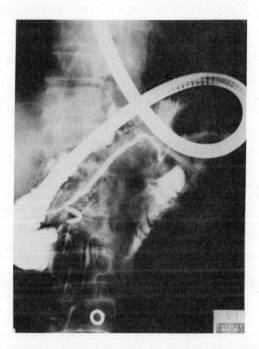

Fig. 3. ERCP of patients subjected to total gastrectomy.

Sixty-eight year old male; double tract anastomosis was
performed after total gastrectomy because of multiple early
cancer 2 years ago. ERCP was performed after complaints of
heaviness in upper abdomen and of increase in serum amylase
level. Mild distention of pancreatic branch and formation
of a small cyst were observed in the pancreatogram, and the
case was diagnosed to be mild chronic pancreatitis.

In another patient on whom the jejunal interposition was used after proximal gastrectomy the direct vision fiberscope was inserted into the duodenum, and endoscopic observations were done (Takagi, 1976).

Thus, methods of anastomosis which make it possible to use advanced endoscopy after
surgery of gastric cancer need to be considered.

REFERENCES

The General Rules for the Gastric Cancer Study in Surgery and Pathology (1979).
    Edited by Japanese Research Society for Gastric Cancer. 10th Edition, Kanahara
    Shuppan, Tokyo.
Kajitani, T. (1950). Clinical classification of gastric cancer and its signifi-
    cance (Japanese). Gann, 41, 76-77.

Kajitani, T. and K. Takagi (1979). Cancer of the stomach at Cancer Institute
    Hospital, Tokyo. In T. Kajitani, Y. Koyama and Y. Umegaki (Ed.), GANN
    Monograph on Cancer Research 22. Recent results of cancer treatment in Japan.
    Japan Scientific Societies Press, Tokyo and University Park Press, Baltimore,
    pp. 77-87.
Ohhashi, I., K. Takagi, T. Konishi, S. Izumoi, A. Fukami and T. Kajitani (1976).
    Five year survival cases with dissection of para-aortic lymph-node metastases
    from gastric cancer (Japanese). Japan. J. Gastroenterol. Surg., 9, 112-116.
Safrany, L. (1973). Endoscopy of the efferent loop and cannulation of the papilla
    of Vater after Billroth II operation. In Demling, L. and M. Classen (Ed.),
    Endoscopy of the small intestine with retrograde pancreato-cholangiography.
    George Thieme, Stuttgart, pp. 101-107.
Takagi, K. (1976). Pan-endoscope (Japanese). Cancer & Chemotherapy, 3, 1281-1284.
UICC: TNM, Classification of malignant tumours. Stomach. Livre de Poche 1974,
    Second edition. Livre de Poche 1978, Third edition. Geneve.

The Place of Radical Surgery in Gastric Cancer

W.P. Longmire, Jr.

Department of Surgery UCLA School of Medicine,
Los Angeles, California, U.S.A.

ABSTRACT

Radical surgery for gastric cancer may involve extensive or total removal of the
stomach itself, extensive dissection of regional lymphatics, or the removal of all
or a part of adjacent organs. The unresolved questions today concern (1) the removal of all or almost all of the stomach for cancer that by gross examination and
frozen section monitoring of the resection margins might be removed by a lesser
operation, and (2) the extensive dissection of regional lymph nodes for tumors that
have little if any serosal extension.

Although both of these procedures deserve further evaluation, at present there is
insufficient evidence of their contribution to increased patient survival to warrant their widespread adoption.

KEYWORDS

Gastric cancer; radical surgery; radical lymph node dissection; elective total
gastrectomy.

INTRODUCTION

In discussing the role of radical surgery for gastric cancer, a number of variables
must be defined. First, there are different operations for the treatment of gastric cancer that might be included in the general category of "radical." With some
modifications, most of these could be classified as one of the following:

1. Radical distal subtotal gastrectomy
2. Subtotal gastrectomy plus radical lymph node dissection
3. Total gastrectomy
4. Extended total gastrectomy plus distal pancreatectomy and radical
   lymph node dissection
5. Radical proximal subtotal gastrectomy

Second, the site of tumor origin in the stomach plays an important role in selecting the operation and deciding whether it is "radical" or not. Is the tumor confined to the antrum where almost 50% of malignant tumors originate, in the

body (18%), fundus (24%) or at the esophagogastric junction (9.5%) (Paulino and Roselli, 1973)?

Third, operations performed for gastric cancer under certain conditions must be extensive or "radical" if a surgical approach is to be used at all (required or de necessité); in other situations, a "radical" surgical approach may be elected (en principe) over a lesser procedure even though the superiority of a more extensive operation has not as yet been clearly demonstrated.

Certain indications for radical operation are:

1. Extensive tumor involvement of gastric wall, including linitis plastica and multiple cancers that can be removed only by total gastrectomy.
2. Cancer of the gastric remnant after subtotal gastrectomy for cancer or for ulcer.
3. Gastric cancer arising in a patient with pernicious anemia.
4. Miscellaneous mucosal changes, e.g., chronic diffuse atrophic gastritis or diffuse hypertrophic gastritis (Ménétrier's disease) with cellular atypia, and diffuse polyposis.

The principal conditions under which elective radical operation might be considered are:

1. Total gastrectomy for early localized tumors, both proximal and distal that could be cleared by a lesser operation.
2. Routine radical lymph node dissection with total or subtotal gastric resection.

HISTORICAL

The first successful radical operation for gastric cancer was a total gastrectomy reported by Schlatter (1897, 1898), a 33-year-old Swiss surgeon. He realized the importance of evaluating digestive functions after removal of the stomach, and therefore hospitalized the patient for observation during the 14-month period of survival. No significant abnormalities in fat and protein digestion were found. The patient regained weight and ate normally. Anemia that developed late in the postoperative period was thought to be due to recurrent cancer.

Numerous isolated accounts of total gastrectomy were published during the first four decades of this century including a report by Moynihan (1911), who first called attention to severe anemia as a serious late postgastrectomy complication, a proposal by Graham (1943) of an invaginating type of esophagojejunal anastomosis inasmuch as he recognized that this suture line was the most treacherous step in the operation, and Roux-en-Y esophagojejunal anastomosis described by Orr (1947) to prevent reflux esophagitis.

Throughout the early 1900's, the operation continued to be associated with a high mortality rate of 35 to 40%, even in the reportable series; postoperative complications were frequent and severe, and survival for longer than a year generally prompted a case report.

The decades of the 40's and 50's, however, brought forth fresh new surgical attacks on cancer of the stomach. The subsequent dramatic decline in its incidence had not yet removed gastric cancer from first place as the cause of death from malignant disease among males in the United States and it was still a surgical disease of primary importance in North America.

Significant developments in the fields of anesthesia, antibacterial therapy, fluid and electrolyte balance and the banking of blood for transfusion greatly improved the safety of the earlier radical operations and encouraged evaluation of even more extensive procedures. Therefore, an unacceptable operative mortality rate no longer prohibited extending the then sacrosanct principle of en bloc resection of the grossly visible primary cancer and its lymphatic drainage area to the surgical management of gastric cancer.

Although various radical operations for gastric cancer were tested during this period, the results were not found to be sufficiently encouraging to warrant their widespread adoption. However, once again the use of radical operations for gastric cancer is being proposed and the questions to be answered would seem to be: what conditions might indicate radical gastric cancer operations and what type of radical procedures would be the most useful at the present time?

CURRENT GENERALLY ACCEPTED PRINCIPLES

Palliative total gastrectomy, in which the surgeon is aware of leaving unresectable tumor, has been found to be unrewarding (Longmire and associates, 1968). Similarly, although linitis plastica is frequently given as an indication for total resection, the results are poor. Of nine patients with linitis plastica treated by total gastrectomy, none survived more than 18 months (Paulino and Roselli, 1973), and the majority succumbed within six months. However, for the large fungating tumor that cannot be widely excised by subtotal gastrectomy, and in which all identifiable tumor tissue can be removed by total gastrectomy, the procedure is generally accepted. In a recent international review of 15 reports, total gastrectomy was performed in approximately 25% of the resections (a low of 6.5% and a high of 48.8%) (Longmire, 1980). Presumably, the size and extent of the tumor were indications for total resection in the majority of these cases.

Similarly, there seems to be no argument against accepting total resection for cancer developing in the gastric remnant after subtotal resection, for gastric cancer arising in a patient with pernicious anemia or in a patient who has other types of diffuse mucosal lesions with malignant or premalignant changes such as hypertrophic gastritis (Menetrier's disease) or severe atrophic gastritis. Diffuse polyposis of the stomach, although extremely rare, would also warrant total gastrectomy.

TODAY'S PROBLEMS

The chief problems to be considered today regarding radical resections are:
(1) What is the role of the supraradical subtotal resection, (2) should elective (en principe) total gastrectomy be performed, (3) should total gastrectomy, elective or required, be extended to include other organs and secondary and tertiary lymph node areas, (4) should total gastrectomy be performed for cancer of the cardia, and (5) should elective extended lymph node dissection be carried out with subtotal gastric resection?

Radical Distal Subtotal Resection

In an effort to completely eradicate the tumor from the gastric wall while avoiding the precarious esophagojejunal anastomosis, a number of surgeons have advocated radical distal subtotal gastrectomy, "leaving a gastric pouch no larger than a man's thumb." After reviewing 246 total gastrectomies performed at the Lahey clinic during the 1940's and 50's, Marshal stated in 1957 that the pre-

ferred operation for cancer of the stomach was a radical subtotal gastrectomy, and
splenectomy with removal of the omentum and lymph nodes. It was his opinion that
total gastrectomy should be performed in approximately one-third of gastric resections for cancer.

In an excellent monograph on gastric cancer Paulino and Roselli (1973) reviewed
their experiences with over 200 resections. For carcinoma of the distal portion
of the stomach (restricted to the pylorus and antrum) they recommend subtotal gastrectomy with resection of 3-5 cm of the duodenum and the entire lesser curvature,
omentectomy and extensive dissection of subpyloric, hepatic and preaortic lymph
nodes. The left gastric artery they divided at its origin after completely dis-
secting the nodes in the preaortic fat--an operation that might be considered a
"high" but not "radical" subtotal gastrectomy. We have likewise recommended a similar "high" but not "radical" subtotal gastrectomy for distal gastric cancer, preserving the spleen and the vasa breva (Longmire, 1977).

Of the cases reported by Paulino and Roselli (1973), 18% had extensive tumors in
the body of the stomach, not invading the fundus. They believed that tumors of
this type could be treated by extensive, nine-tenths subtotal resection, with en
bloc distal pancreatectomy and splenectomy. In addition to the hazards of distal
pancreatectomy, to be discussed later, they noted the danger of depriving the gastric remnant of its blood supply in such an extensive resection. Similar concerns
have been noted by others (Marshal, 1957; Longmire, 1977; Spencer, 1956). To
insure the blood supply of a 5 to 7 cm cuff of gastric wall, the phrenic and periesophageal vessels must be preserved. This has two disadvantages: (1) it is
unwise to dissect out and divide the vagus nerves, a step that allows the descent
of the gastric remnant and greatly facilitates the subsequent anastomosis, and
(2) periesophageal lymph nodes, which might be expected to be involved in over 25%
of extensive cancers of this type, cannot be adequately dissected without danger
of devascularizing the gastric remnant.

In our experience the postoperative sequelae of such extensive resections of the
gastric wall are identical to those of total gastrectomy. We are inclined to dis-
count the technical advantage of leaving such a small cuff of gastric wall, and
thus the only remaining advantage of radical subtotal gastrectomy appears to be the
possible prevention of late postgastrectomy macrocytic anemia. However, the nine
patients of Paulino and Roselli (1973) required treatment for vitamin B12 deficiency and anemia. Tumors inviting this type of extensive radical subtotal resection, we believe, are best treated by total gastrectomy.

Radical Proximal Subtotal Gastrectomy

The "expansive" period of cancer surgery (1940-1950) directed new efforts toward
the treatment of cancer of the gastric cardia and esophagogastric junction. Adams
and Phemister (1938), Garlock (1948), and Sweet (1948) in the United States,
Allison (1949) in England, Lortat-Jacob (1957) in France and Koch (1969) in Sweden,
among others, made early contributions to surgery in this difficult area.

A survey of cancer treatment in various regions of the stomach makes it quickly
apparent that the least favorable results among all series have been achieved in
lesions of the cardia and esophagogastric region. Dupont (1978), for example,
reported that among 1,222 operations for adenocarcinoma of the stomach, there were
25 esophagogastrectomies with a 27.3% operative mortality and a five-year survival
rate as low as 1.97%. Unless the cancer originates in the lower esophagus or quite
near the esophagogastric junction, symptoms are apt to be delayed and metastasis
advanced by direct extension and/or by lymphatic spread when surgery is performed.

In general, resectable tumors at this site may be treated by one of two operations:
(1) resection of the proximal stomach and lower esophagus followed by an esophagogastrostomy and pyloromyotomy, or (2) total gastrectomy and distal esophagectomy
followed by esophagojejunostomy.

The choice of procedure will depend upon (1) the histologic type of the tumor,
(2) the extent of proximal stomach involved, and (3) the apparent direction of direct extension and lymphatic spread of the tumor.

The squamous cell tumor which originates in the mucosa of the lower esophagus may
involve a relatively small area of the proximal stomach but invade the lymphatic
drainage along the lesser curvature and extend into the celiac lymph nodes. These
tumors also tend to spread upward in the intramural and paraesophageal lymphatics,
usually requiring a generous resection of at least one-half of the intrathoracic
esophagus. The limits of the gastric resection will be determined by the area of
tumor involvement but should include at least one-half of the lesser curvature, the
left gastric artery to its origin, the fundus of the stomach and the spleen.

The true gastric cancer of the cardia is an adenocarcinoma arising in the gastric
mucosa. It grows more extensively in the gastric wall, and esophageal involvement,
although usually present, is limited. Unless the extent of the tumor in the esophagus and stomach has been defined by x-ray and endoscopic studies, the surgeon must
be prepared to proceed with a radical subdiaphragmatic operation or a combined
thoracoabdominal procedure. In Koch's report of 46 patients with adenocarcinoma of
the cardia, proximal gastric resection including resection of the distal esophagus
was performed in 17 patients and total gastrectomy with lower esophageal resection
was performed in 29 patients. These procedures were carried out by the abdominal
approach in eight patients; in the other 38, separate abdominal and right-sided
thoracic incisions were used. None of the patients who underwent proximal gastric
resection survived five years, but 10 of the 29 patients on whom a total gastrectomy
was performed lived more than five years. Koch recommended an operation that would
include a total gastrectomy, omentectomy, splenectomy, and resection of the pancreatic tail. The lower one-third of the esophagus was excised through the thoracotomy and the esophagus anastomosed to a Roux-Y jejunal limb at the level of the
hilus of the right lung.

In the series of Lortat-Jacob (1975) no patient lived longer than four years after
a partial gastrectomy for carcinoma of the fundus, whereas 40% survived after
total gastrectomy.

Sixty-two carcinomas of the gastroesophageal junction reported by Stone and others
(1977) were adenocarcinomas and 24 were squamous cell carcinomas. Fifty-two
lesions (60%) were resected by combined midline laparotomy and right thoracotomy.
The spleen and celiac lymph nodes were encompassed with the gastric resection and
a pyloroplasty or pyloromyotomy was performed. Continuity was restored by esophagogastrectomy. Total gastrectomy was utilized in only five patients. Six deaths
occurred, two owing to anastomotic leaks. The mean survival was 2.1 years with a
22% three-year life table survival (10/52). Five of 14 patients with negative
nodes were alive after more than five years at the time of their report. Palliative
resection in 17 patients achieved a mean survival of 10.5 months but no five-year
survivals. The mean survival of the 18 nonoperative patients was three months.

The five-year survival results of McNeer and others (1974) for carcinoma of the
proximal one-third of the stomach were not as good with extended total gastrectomy
(12.7%) as with partial proximal gastrectomy (19%). For carcinoma of the cardia,
Paulino and Roselli (1973) recommended an extensive (nine-tenths) proximal gastrectomy with resection of the lower third of the esophagus through a left thoracoabdominal incision. A jejunal segment was interposed between the esophagus and the

small antral remnant.

Any excision of a cancer of the cardia and esophagogastric junction will require a
radical operation. In most instances a combined thoracoabdominal approach will be
required for adequate resection of the lower esophagus and exposure for the esophagogastric anastomosis. With any type of resection, the margins of the esophagus
and stomach or duodenum should be checked for microscopic tumor by frozen section
at the time of operation. While Koch's results with total gastrectomy are impressive, the decision to remove the entire stomach will depend in part upon the type,
location and spread of the original tumor. In most instances of gastric cancers
of the cardia, total gastrectomy will be advisable.

Elective Total and Extended Total Gastrectomy

After a brief but rather vigorous experience with the routine use of total gastrectomy in the U.S. in the late 1940's and early 1950's, the concept was abandoned.
Paulino and Roselli (1973) relate the turning point to Marshal's repudiation in
1957 of routine total gastrectomy based on 246 cases and the retrospective evaluation of the Johns Hopkins Hospital experience by Rush, Brown and Ravitch in 1960
and the collective review by Rush and Ravitch in 1962. Ten years later Paulino and
Roselli noted that no further serious suggestions had been made favoring the routine use of total gastrectomy for gastric malignancy. Instead, with somewhat less
than spectacular results, attention shifted toward emulating Japanese surgeons in
their effort to diagnose and treat early superficial gastric cancer, and to achieve
results comparable to the 92.5% five-year survival rate they reported in certain
types of gastric cancer.

There also developed a greater awareness that despite our best efforts at early
diagnosis, more than 70% of our patients admitted to hospitals in the Western
countries who were diagnosed as having gastric cancer had recognizable disseminated
disease at or before operation; and that of the remaining group, less than 40%
would survive five years after resection. These persistent results over the years
tended to emphasize that extirpative surgery would be effective in only a very small
percent of cases and that efforts should therefore be directed toward finding a
"compromise" operation to provide an effective tumor excision in a high percentage
of cases without grossly disseminated disease, an operation that could be generally
performed with an acceptable operative mortality rate and one which would have minimal undesirable side effects. Such operations have been described by a number of
surgeons. There has also been general recognition that when total gastrectomy is
necessary, digestive function can be greatly improved by using one of several
methods of reconstruction to prevent alkaline reflux esophagitis (Paulino and
Roselli, 1973; Longmire and associates, 1952, 1977; Hoerr and Hodgman, 1973; Orr,
1947; Lima-Basta, 1959; Hunt, 1952; Lawrence, 1962) (Figs. 1 and 2).

Now, some 20 years after total gastrectomy seemed to have been relegated to a fairly limited role in the surgical armamentarium for the treatment of certain types of
gastric cancer, accounting for about one-fourth of resectable cases, elective or
en principé resection is again being considered.

McNeer and others reported in 1974 that total gastrectomy had consistently been
performed at the New York Memorial Hospital for the past 20 years and that in all
but 19 of the 94 total gastrectomies, the body and tail of the pancreas had been
included in what they identified as an extended total gastrectomy. Fifteen of the
patients had a partial excision of an additional organ. The five-year survival of
patients with tumors in the distal third of the stomach was improved from 29.8% for
subtotal resection to 43.7% by elective total gastrectomy. Although the survival
of patients with carcinoma of the mid one-third of the stomach was not improved by

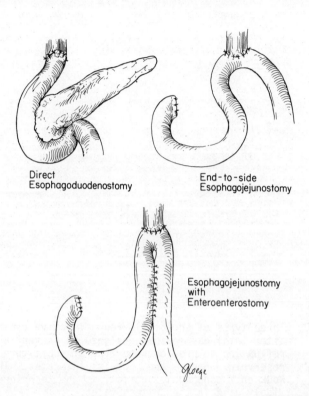

Direct
Esophagoduodenostomy

End-to-side
Esophagojejunostomy

Esophagojejunostomy
with
Enteroenterostomy

Fig. 1.   Three methods of reconstruction following total gas-
          trectomy that are associated with a high incidence
          of reflux alkaline esophagitis and should not be used.
          Anastomotic leakage is a frequent complication of
          esophagoduodenostomy, another contraindication to its
          use.

elective total gastrectomy, they found that patients undergoing total resection
had three times as many lymph nodes involved as those undergoing subtotal resection. Despite this unfavorable finding, the five-year survival for the total
resection group of mid-body cancers was as good or better than that in the subtotal group. These authors recommended elective total gastrectomy for operable
carcinoma arising in the mid one-third or distal third of the stomach. However,
the number of cases in these two groups in their series was limited: 23 in the

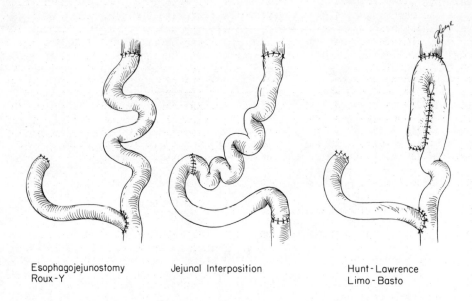

Esophagojejunostomy   Jejunal Interposition   Hunt-Lawrence
Roux-Y   Limo-Basto

Fig. 2.   Three types of acceptable reconstructive procedures
          after total gastrectomy designed to prevent alkaline
          reflux and to provide some type of substitute gastric
          reservoir. Each method has its advocates. The
          Roux-en-Y esophagojejunostomy is the technique most
          widely used in the United States.

mid one-third and 16 in the distal third.

Lortat-Jacob and colleagues in 1975 reported a 50% five-year survival when total
gastrectomy was performed en principé. Fourteen of these cases had carcinoma of
the cardia, 15 were located in the antropyloric area and four were on the lesser
curvature. In the same series of 482 radical operations for gastric cancer there
were 118 total gastrectomies de necessité and 331 partial gastrectomies. In cases
of cancer of the pylorus and antrum, the chances of surviving five years were
given as 20% after partial gastrectomy and 50% after total resection. Their
operative mortality was 16.5% for subtotal resection, 35.6% for totales de necessité, and one of two was alive when an elective total gastrectomy was carried out.

Shiu and co-workers in a recent report from the Memorial Hospital in New York
found five-year survival to be improved for early-stage tumors treated by total
gastrectomy or extended total gastrectomy (distal pancreatectomy and splenectomy).
They pointed out that when all stages of disease were analyzed together there was
no statistically significant difference in five-year survival rates of patients
treated by subtotal resection, total gastrectomy or extended total gastrectomy.
However, when the early stage patients (TI-4 NO MO and TI-4 NI MO) only were

considered, there was a remarkable difference in survival. When treated by distal subtotal gastrectomy these patients had a very low five-year survival rate (2/12, 17%) as compared with those treated by total gastrectomy (6/8) and the much higher survival rate after extended total gastrectomy (15/36, 42%). A retrospective review of the pathology and operative records indicated that the tumor in these cases could have been managed by a high distal subtotal gastrectomy, thereby avoiding the risk attendant upon an esophagojejunal anastomosis. In the entire series the operative mortality for high distal subtotal resection was 13%, for total gastrectomy 23%, and for extended total gastrectomy 22%. However, the overall operative mortality rate for the last five years had dropped to 8% (3/36). These authors also questioned the need for distal pancreatectomy when the pancreas was not directly invaded by cancer, for they indicated that the celiac and superior pancreatic lymph nodes could be dissected off the capsule of the pancreas while preserving the splenic artery without pancreatic resection. We agree that omission of pancreatectomy would avoid the postoperative morbidity associated with the frequent leakage of pancreatic fluid and associated septic complications.

Arhelger and colleagues (1955) were among the first to call attention to the fact that the usual radical subtotal or total gastric resection, although possibly including splenectomy, dissection of the juxtacardiac lymph nodes, and dissection of the splenic artery, celiac axis and aorta, did not include some of the most frequent sites of lymph node metastases. Utilizing the unique opportunity afforded by "second-look" operations, they identified histologically the site of residual cancer in 30 such "second-look" procedures. In 15 cases cancer was found within lymph nodes, fibrous tissue or fat of the hepatic pedicle. Residual cancer was found in the retropancreaticoduodenal areas (superior or posterior retropancreaticoduodenal nodes) in six of the 30 operations.

On the basis of these observations, they performed 24 primary extended lymphatic dissections including the hepatic pedicle and the retropancreaticoduodenal areas. The operation consisted of total or near-total removal of the stomach, excision of the greater and lesser omenta, splenectomy, and dissection of the lymphatic channels and lymph nodes of the hepatic pedicle, the retropancreaticoduodenal area, the suprapancreatic areas along the horizontal hepatic and splenic arteries, the celiac and aortic areas, and the abdomino-paraesophageal and juxtacardiac chains. Metastases to the lymph nodes of the hepatic pedicle were found in 11 of the 24 specimens and in the retropancreaticoduodenal area in four. In a subsequent review by Gilbertson (1969) of this well-directed radical approach, the results were found to be disappointing. The operative mortality for partial gastrectomy for cure rose from 13.3 to 25.6% and for total gastrectomy from 22.5 to 33.3%. During this same time, the five-year survival rate for those operated upon for cure, which had reached a peak of 28% in the period prior to instituting the radical resection, fell to 17%. Five-year survival for patients with positive lymph node gastric cancer declined more sharply--from 18 to 9%. The overall five-year survival rate for all patients seen fell from 12.2% for the earlier group to 8.8% for those seen during the later period. Gilbertson concluded that further improvement in patient survival would not likely occur as a result of more extensive surgical excisions and lymph node dissections in the treatment of patients with cancer of the stomach.

Hawley and associates (1970) reported on 205 patients treated by total or partial gastrectomy for carcinoma of the stomach, 116 of whom (61%) had a partial gastrectomy and 74 (39%) had a total gastrectomy. Lymph node involvement had the greatest influence on prognosis; there was a 40% five-year survival in the absence of node involvement which decreased to 11% with positive nodes. These authors observed no benefit from total rather than subtotal gastrectomy if the cancer and regional lymph nodes could be removed with the simpler procedure.

Early deaths (within three months) were attributed to the operation. There were
51 (27%) early deaths, 58% of which followed total gastrectomy. The overall survival rate was 19.4% at five years and 11.5% at 10 years. They concluded that
total gastrectomy had a high postoperative mortality and should be avoided unless
it was impossible to remove the tumor with a lesser procedure.

In the series of 1,497 cases of adenocarcinoma from Charity Hospital in New Orleans
(Dupont and colleagues, 1978) the operations were described as subtotal gastrectomy,
radical subtotal gastrectomy and total gastrectomy, the latter having a 37% operative mortality rate and a discouragingly low survival of only 7.6%. Subtotal
gastrectomy, the predominant procedure, had an operative mortality rate of 23.7%
and a five-year survival of 14.4%. The best results were obtained by a radical
subtotal gastrectomy, an operation they described as including a 75% distal gastrectomy plus resection of the omentum and lymph nodes along the right and left
gastric arteries. In addition, in some patients, the spleen, transverse colon,
tail of the pancreas, celiac axis lymph nodes, or nodes along the porta hepatis
were included. The operative mortality for 66 patients who underwent this procedure was 16.4% and the five-year survival rate was 22.1%. This procedure, which
leaves 25% of the stomach and removes only the omentum and the lymph nodes around
the left and right gastric arteries, is not considered a radical resection by many
surgeons. When the more advanced cases were eliminated from their analysis, the
improved results from the so-called radical subtotal gastrectomy became more apparent. Subtotal gastrectomy achieved a 45% five-year survival in Hoerr group A
lesions and a 7% survival for stage B lesions, and an overall five-year survival
of 32.6%. The lesser operative mortality of the radical subtotal operation, 16.4%,
as compared to more conservative subtotal resection, 23.7%, was not commented upon.

The quality of life during the postoperative period may be almost as important as
the five-year survival rate. In the early total gastrectomy cases the distressing
symptoms of recurrent cancer were frequently attributed to the absence of the
stomach. However, experience gained from the significant number of long-term survivors after total gastrectomy performed for the Zollinger-Ellison syndrome has
demonstrated that total gastrectomy is indeed remarkably well tolerated. Zollinger
(1976) stated that two out of three patients undergoing total gastrectomy for Z-E
tumor will sustain their minimal ideal weight or above as long as they stop smoking
and avoid excessive coffee intake. Reconstructive methods that prevent reflux
esophagitis have made a most important contribution toward maintaining the general
nutritional well-being and digestive comfort of these patients. The conscientious
administration of vitamin B12 and supplemental iron will prevent the distressing
symptoms of a late-appearing anemia.

One of the largest reported series of long-term survivors following total gastrectomy is that of Koga and co-workers (1979) who reported on 27 patients surviving
longer than five years after total gastrectomy. From the standpoint of general
nutrition and rehabilitation, their patients appeared to be in satisfactory condition. However, hyperchronic anemia, serum vitamin B12 deficiency, and osteoporosis
were noted in some patients. They summarized their findings as follows:

Subjective complaints (26 patients)	No. of patients	Percent
Esophagitis	7	26.9
Dumping	2	7.6
Feeling of fullness	8	30.7
General fatigue	3	11.5
Other	6	23.0

Food intake compared with preoperative intake

< 50%	4	15.4
50%-80%	11	42.3
>80%	11	42.3

Change in body weight after operation (25 patients)

Within ± 2 kg	2	8.0
Increase > 2 kg	3	12.0
Decrease > 2 kg	20	80.0

Three patients had severe osteoporosis. All patients returned to employment.

A similar satisfactory evaluation of the quality of life after total gastrectomy was given by Lewin (1960) after his extensive studies of 26 patients surviving for over one year.

Although adaptation to the absence of the stomach varies from patient to patient, most will adjust satisfactorily, and return to a normal mode of living. A very rare patient may be classified as a "gastric cripple. The quality of life after gastrectomy is sufficiently good to support the use of total gastrectomy if it can be demonstrated that the procedure will cure the cancer in a significantly greater number of patients.

Thus, one finds today several small series of cases in which elective (en principé) radical resection of early gastric cancer has gained significant improvement in survival. When all stages of disease are grouped together, however, the improved results of the more extensive resections for early localized cancer are masked.

The somewhat limited reports from France (Lortat-Jacob and associates, 1975) and from the Memorial Hospital in New York suggest that there may be an advantage of radical resection in early cases of gastric cancer, and the New Orleans report supports the concept of "breaking out" or reviewing separately the cases of early cancer to demonstrate the value of a more extensive operation. In most other series this advantage, if indeed there is one, is lost, inasmuch as the cases are combined with a far larger group of more extensive lesions where it seems clear that total gastrectomy has no particular advantage if the gross lesion can be removed by a lesser operation.

Subtotal Gastrectomy with Extended Lymph Node Dissection

Japanese surgeons concerned with an early superficial type of gastric cancer that spreads less extensively within the stomach wall and tends to involve the serosa less frequently have turned their attention once again to the radical dissection of lymph node areas, usually in combination with subtotal gastric resection.

Majima and colleagues (1972) evaluated the effects of an extended lymph node dissection with the removal of different groups of secondary lymph nodes depending upon the location of the tumor. They found an improved (but not statistically significant) result from the removal of what they identified as group 3 lymph nodes, concluding that in cases with non- or only slight serosal invasion and with lymph node metastases, the results of resection could be improved by an extended lymph node dissection. On the other hand, if extensive serosal involvement was present, the extended dissection did not improve results.

Soga and co-workers (1979) analyzed the results of treatment in 530 cases of gastric cancer, emphasizing the extensive dissection of regional lymph nodes. They
advised the almost complete removal of at least the primary and secondary lymph
node groups draining a gastric cancer. For lesions in the upper and middle por-
tions of the stomach invading the serosa of the posterior wall, total gastrectomy,
caudal pancreatectomy and splenectomy were recommended so as to accomplish a complete en bloc removal of lymph nodes in these regions. The five-year survival rate
of their curative resections was 50.6%. Patients with negative lymph nodes had a
five-year survival rate of 63.5%; with positive nodes the survival rate fell to
29.9%.

In commenting on the presentation of Soga and associates (1979), Gilbertson (1979)
compared their results to those of gastric cancer surgery at the University of
Minnesota during the period 1936 to 1958 which he had previously analyzed. Noting
the marked improvement in survival in all stages of the disease as reported by
Soga and co-workers, he stated that the factors responsible for the improvement of
survival rates would not consist exclusively of improvement owing to lymph node
dissection. As he pointed out, patients with no lymph node involvement demonstrated an improvement in survival over his earlier series equal to those with
node involvement, a circumstance he felt not likely to occur merely because of
improved lymph node dissection. Explanation for the marked improvement would
appear to include a substantial decrease during the past several years in the virulence of the tumor, overall increase in surgical competence, significant increase
in patient resistance and improvement in biometric computation techniques.

At this point it is difficult to evaluate the potential effectiveness of extensive
lymph node dissections, but based primarily on the results of earlier vigorous
efforts at lymph node removal in this country, there would seem to be a limit
beyond which further lymph node resection would yield diminishing returns. At some
ill-defined limit, involvement of regional lymph nodes must signify systemic spread
of the disease and extensive dissection may of itself be responsible for "opening"
lymphatic channels and spreading viable cancer cells. Serosal involvement which
in itself reduces five-year survival by half (Longmire and associates, 1968) would
seem to be a contraindication to pursue an extensive lymphatic dissection. Until
further evidence is available, it seems advisable to limit the lymph node dissection to those groups around the pylorus, the hepatoduodenal ligament and the celiac
axis. Excision of additional organs for the removal of lymph nodes is rarely indicated.

SUMMARY

With the hope of improving the operative results for gastric cancer, surgeons continue to seek new and better operative techniques. In general, this effort has
resulted in the development of more extensive operations and their more frequent
use.

The limited encouragement from the use of larger operations for smaller lesions
seems worthy of further investigation and careful study but at this time the
evidence does not appear sufficient to test once again on a wide scale the elective
or en principé use of total gastrectomy. For the present, the currently accepted
indications for total gastrectomy appear to be adequate. Extensive lymph node
dissection with either total or subtotal resection also poses an important approach
for further evaluation, but again the available evidence does not justify routinely
extending the operation to radical removal of lymph nodes. Partial pancreatectomy
may in selected cases be indicated for removing a direct extension of tumor from
the gastric wall but because the procedure may be accompanied by serious postoperative complications, it cannot be recommended as a means of excising a substantial

number of lymph nodes.

Resection of the lateral segment of the liver and the transverse mesocolon or the transverse colon itself, if directly involved or devascularized, may be indicated in rare cases. Extension of the tumor through the gastric wall to involve adjacent organs is frequently associated with disseminated disease, but adjacent organ involvement alone does not preclude resection of the stomach and the involved organ.

REFERENCES

Adams, W. E., and Phemister, D. B. (1938). Carcinoma of the lower thoracic esophagus: Report of successful resection and esophagogastrostomy. J. Thorac. Surg., 7; 621.
Adashek, K., Sanger, J., and Longmire, W. P. Jr. (1979). Cancer of the stomach. Review of consecutive ten year intervals. Ann. Surg., 189, 6-10.
Allison, P. R., and Barrie, J. (1949). The treatment of malignant obstruction of the cardia. Brit. J. Surg., 37, 1.
Arhelger, S. W., Lober, P. H., and Wangensteen, O. H. (1955). Dissection of the hepatic pedicle and retropancreaticoduodenal areas for cancer of the stomach. Surgery, 38, 675.
Dupont, J. B. Jr., Lee, J. R., Burton, G. R., and Cohn, I. Jr. (1978). Adenocarcinoma of the stomach: Review of 1,497 cases. Cancer, 41, 941.
Garlock, J. H. (1948). Progress in the surgical treatment of carcinoma of the esophagus and gastric cardia. Surgery, 23, 906-911.
Gilbertson, V. A. (1969). Results of treatment of stomach cancer. An appraisal of efforts of more extensive surgery and a report of 1,983 cases. Cancer, 23, 1305.
Gilbertson, V. A. (1979). Discussion of paper by Soga et al. World J. Surg., 3, 707.
Graham, R. (1943). Total gastrectomy for carcinoma of the stomach: Symposium on gastric cancer. Arch. Surg., 46, 907-914.
Hawley, P. R., Westerholm, P., and Morson, B. C. (1970). Pathology and prognosis of carcinoma of the stomach. Brit. J. Surg., 57, 877.
Hoerr, S. O., and Hodgman, R. W. (1973). Prognosis for Carcinoma of the stomach. Surg., Gynecol. Obstet., 137, 205.
Hunt, C. J. (1952). Construction of food pouch from a segment of jejunum: A substitute for stomach in total gastrectomy. Arch. Surg., 64, 601.
Koch, N. G., Lewin, E., and Petterson, S. (1969). Partial or total gastrectomy for adenocarcinoma of the cardia. Acta. Chir. Scand., 135, 340.
Koga, S., Nishimura, O., Iwai, N., et al. (1979). Clinical evaluation of longterm survival after total gastrectomy. Am. J. Surg., 138, 635.
Lawrence, W., Jr. (1962). Reservoir construction after total gastrectomy: An instructive case. Ann. Surg., 155, 191.
Lewin, E. (1960). Gastric cancer, a clinical study with reference to total gastrectomy and microscopic grading. Acta. Chirurg. Scand., Supp. 262.
Lima-Basto, E. (1959). Functional adaptation after total gastrectomy. In Proceedings of the World Congress of Gastroenterology, Washington, D. C., 1958. The Williams and Wilkins Co., Baltimore.
Longmire, W. P. Jr. (1980). Gastric carcinoma: Is radical gastrectomy worthwhile? Assoc. Roy. Coll. Surg. Eng., 62, 25-30.
Longmire, W. P. Jr. (1977). Gewandelte Aspekte des Magenkarzinoms. Münchener Med. Wochenschrift, 119, 613-616.
Longmire, W. P. Jr., Kuzma, J. W., and Dixon, W. J. (1968). The use of triethylenethiophosphoramide as an adjunct to the surgical treatment of gastric carcinoma. Ann. Surg., 167, 293.

Longmire, W. P. Jr., and Beal, J. M. (1952). Construction of a substitute gastric reservoir following total gastrectomy. Ann. Surg., 135, 637.

Lortat-Jacob, J. J., Giuli, R., Estenne, B., and Glot, P. (1975). Interet de la gastrectomie totale pour le traitement des cancers de l'estomac. Etude de 482 interventions radicales. Chirurgie, 101, 1, 59.

Lortat-Jacob, J. L., and Richards, C. A. (1957). Ou en est la chirurgie du cancer de l'estomac? Rev. Prat., 7, 3573.

McNeer, G., Bowden, L. Booher, R. J., and McPeak, C. J. (1974). Elective total gastrectomy for cancer of the stomach. Ann. Surg., 180, 252.

Majima, S., Etani, S., Fujita, Y., and Takahashi, T. (1972). Evaluation of extended lymph node dissection for gastric cancer. Jap. J. Surg., 2, 1.

Marshal, S. G. (1957). Total versus radical partial resection for cancer of the stomach. Surg. Gynecol. Obstet., 104, 497.

Moynihan, B. (1911). A case of complete gastrectomy. Lancet, 2, 430.

Orr, T. G. (1947). A modified technique for total gastrectomy. Arch. Surg., 54, 279.

Paulino, F., and Roselli, A. (1973). Carcinoma of the stomach with special reference to total gastrectomy. Current Problems in Surgery, M. M. Ravitch, Editor. Year Book Medical Publishers, Inc., Chicago.

Phemister, D. B. (1943). Transthoracic resection for cancer of the cardiac end of the stomach. Symposium on gastric cancer. Arch. Surg., 46, 915-929.

Rush, B. F. Jr., Brown, M. W., and Ravitch, M. M. (1960). Total gastrectomy: An evaluation of its use in the treatment of gastric cancer. Cancer, 13, 643.

Rush, B. F. Jr., and Ravitch, M. M. (1962). The evolution of total gastrectomy: Collective review. Int. Abst. Surg., 114, 411.

Rutter, A. G. (1953). Ischemic necrosis of the stomach following subtotal gastrectomy. Lancet, 2, 1021.

Schlatter, C. (1898). Further observations on a case of total extirpation of the stomach in the human subject. Lancet, 2, 1314.

Schlatter, C. (1897). A unique case of complete removal of the stomach: Successful esophago-enterostomy. Med. Rec., 52, 909.

Shiu, M. H., Papacristou, D. N., Kosloff, C., and Eliopoulos, G. (In press). Selection of operative procedure for adenocarcinoma of the gastric corpus (mid-stomach): Twenty years experience with implications for future treatment strategy. Ann. Surg.

Soga, J., Lobayashi, I., Saito, J., Fujimaki, M., and Muto, T. (1979). The role of lymphadenectomy in curative surgery for gastric cancer. World J. Surg., 3, 701.

Spencer, F. C. (1956). Ischemic necrosis of remaining stomach following subtotal gastrectomy. Arch. Surg., 73, 844.

Stone, R., Rangel, D. M., Gordon, H. E., and Wilson, S. E. (1977). Carcinoma of the gastroesophageal junction. A ten year experience with esophagogastrectomy. Am. J. Surg., 134, 70.

Sweet, R. H. (1948). The treatment of carcinoma of the esophagus and cardiac end of the stomach by surgical extirpation: Two hundred three cases of extirpation. Symposium on Cancer of the Esophagus and Gastric Cardia. Surgery, 23, 952-975.

Wangensteen, O. H. (1951). Cancer of the esophagus and stomach, American Cancer Society Monograph. New York.

Zollinger, R. M., and Mazzaferri, E. L. (1976). Tumors of the islet of Langerhans. In Advances in Surgery, Vol. 10, Year Book Medical Publishers, Inc., Chicago, p. 137.

DISCUSSION

I. Häkkinen. Do you take into consideration the type of cancer?

W. Longmire. All I can comment on is that we really haven't paid much attention to the histological types. We have tried to follow the so called TNM type of classification and have not really paid much attention to the histology, which may be an error.

V. Brookes. Could we follow with the remark,'Why not?'.

W. Longmire. Well, I suppose that part of this could be determined pre-operatively by endoscopic biopsy and observation. We have been influenced by Stout and other pathologists in our country who have felt that there are such a mixture of histologies in these lesions that histology is not as important as penetration, lymph node and distant metastases as far as prognosis is concerned.

V. Brookes. Those were our conclusions.

International Variation in the Results of Treatment of Gastric Cancer

J.L. Craven

The District Hospital, York, U.K.

ABSTRACT

There is a very wide variation in the reports of the results of treatment of gastric cancer. Comparison, though hindered by the absence of standardised definitions of operative mortality, surgical treatment and pathological staging reveals that the favourable results reported from Japan owe much to their low operative mortality and high proportion of patients with 'early' gastric cancer. If the pathological stage of the tumour is taken into account there is some evidence that the Japanese results of treatment can be equalled by some Western surgeons. There is an urgent need for a more widespread adoption of a uniform classification of the disease and its treatment.

KEYWORDS

Gastric cancer; surgical treatment; operative mortality; five year survival rate; international comparison; pathological staging.

INTRODUCTION

One of the most remarkable facts in the whole field of cancer treatment is the lack of concordance between the results of treatment of stomach cancer reported by the Japanese and those reports emanating from Europe and North America and Australasia. Whilst those of the former are tinged with optimism, reporting significant improvements in resectability rate, in resections for cure and in five and ten year survival rate those of the latter remain, for the most part, mutely pessimistic. Few of the endeavours from the West can report any significant improvements in the results of treatment that could not be more fairly ascribed to the concurrent advances in anaesthesia and postoperative care. In no other cancers do the results of treatment vary so much between one country and the rest of the world. There are many clinicians who remain incurious of this fact and, whilst recognising the Japanese successes in this field, ascribe them largely to undefined differences in the nature of the neoplasm. These armchair theorists may well be right in bemoaning the bad luck of the Occident to be prey to a more fatal form of the neoplasm than is the Orient, to a neoplasm which is not only more insidious in its onset, (presenting more frequently at an advanced stage, with comparatively low operability and resectability rates) but which is less curable even when radical resection is

219

undertaken. However before these pessimistic assumptions become completely adopted by established thought it is essential that they are examined critically together with the evidence (if any) which supports them. An uncritical adoption of a defeatist attitude stifles new thoughts, and hinders new attempts to curb the ravages of a disease which is still a major cause of death in most Western countries. Whether the international variations in the results of stomach cancer treatment are real or illusory is a most important question though the data available makes comparison none too simple. The literature is vast. Reports emerge from cancer registries, from hospitals or groups of hospitals recording the results of treatment by several surgeons whose indications for treatment and surgical techniques are not defined. There are three main sources - 1. From cancer registries.
                                  2. From hospitals or groups of hospitals recording
                                     the results of treatment by several surgeons.
                                  3. From prospective multicentre studies.
These will be dealt with separately so far as is possible.

CANCER REGISTRY DATA

The publications of the several cancer registries should allow some comparison to be made of the survival rates after the treatment of stomach cancer. In Table 1 is summarised the five year survival rate of stomach cancer cases reported from cancer registries in Japan, the USA and the United Kingdom.

TABLE 1 Five Year Relative Survival Rates for Stomach Cancer Patients recorded at Cancer Registries in Japan, USA and the United Kingdom

	Males (per cent)	Females (per cent)
Japan (Osaka 1965-1968)[1]	20.0	16.6
USA (Connecticut, California etc. 1965-1969)[2]	12.0	14.0
UK (Birmingham 1960-1972)[3]	5.0	4.3

[1] Hanai and Fujimoto, 1977

[2] Axtell and Myers, 1974

[3] Brookes, Waterhouse and Powell, 1965

Initially the differences are startling and will give none of the British present any grounds for complacency but these figures repay more intensive study. Cancer registries are a relatively recent phenomenon developed out of the hope that notification of all cancer cases to a central authority would, among other benefits, provide evidence regarding the efficacy of different methods of treatment and allow comparisons such as this to occur. Such hopes are, as yet, illusory and the 'comparisons' of Table 1 are no exception. The Birmingham figures derive from a population based register with a registration efficiency of more than 95 per cent, from follow up data which is actively collected by the centre (any patient lost to follow up is regarded as dead). The American figures derive from 100 hospital based cancer registries. They thus exclude all patients who do not have hospital treatment and in addition do not include any patients diagnosed at autopsy. No data is given regarding the completeness of the follow up nor is it stated how those patients lost to follow up are categorised. The Osaka figures derive from a population based registry but one whose follow up is less complete than Birminghams for survival was assumed if no death certificate was recorded. It is doubtful if anything can be gained by comparing population based cancer registry data with that derived from hospital registries with differing, and unknown follow up rates or by comparisons between two registries one of which includes those patients diagnosed at autopsy and one which excludes them. No firm conclusions can thus be drawn from Table 1.

HOSPITAL DATA

There is a wide range in the results of treatment reported and a serious study of this group of reports leaves one somewhat perplexed. With only one or two exceptions all the reports are of an undefined retrospective nature; the indications for surgical treatment are unstandardised, as is the surgical treatment. The surgical procedures are generally undefined and the pathological staging of the cancer, if present, is incomplete and unstandardised even among the institutions which have collaborated to produce a single report. Often palliative and radical resections are not distinguished and criteria of postoperative mortality vary. Some reports exclude postoperative deaths from their assessment of five year survival rate whereas others do not. The picture is varied, perplexing and very difficult to analyse. I have included reports from Western Europe, USA and Japan and though aware of the high incidence in other central and Eastern European countries can find no reports susceptible even to this crude type of analysis. Some licence has been taken by the author in summarising the results in Table 2. Wherever possible I have abstracted data referring to a comparable time period for there has generally been some improvement in operative mortality and some increase in operability, and resection rates in recent years. Though aware of its shortcomings, wherever possible I have included the 'curative' resection rate in addition to the resection rate; the former is an expression of hope and a manifestation of surgical aggressiveness and both resection rates must be related by overall survival rate for in no reports did anything short of resection produce a five year survivor Much of the discrepancy amongst the survival rates reported from countries outside Japan lies with the variable criteria of survival rates. Whereas the survival rate after resection of the cancer is always reported, closer examination reveals that in some reports operative mortality has not been allowed for in its assessment and in others those patients not traced have been excluded from assessment. The overall survival rates are no less easy to compare; those of hospital based series exclude deaths of those not hospitalised, and others which exclude deaths of those patients not submitted to surgical treatment falsely appear more encouraging than those who include such patients. All the reports summarised in Table 2 are of cases treated in periods post 1940 and where the reports allow some distinction to be made between different time periods that has been done.

Operability Rates

These vary widely. The earlier Finnish data reported from the University Hospital of Turku by Inberg and co-workers (1975) quotes a rate of 54 per cent but both they and Remine and Priestley (1966) note a significant increase in operability rates in the second decade of their reports. The Japanese data contains uniformly high operability rates but these are approached by the later data from the Lahey Clinic (Cady and co-workers 1977), the Mayo Clinic (Remine and Priestley 1966) and by Hoerr's (1973) personal series. Though one is aware of the very variable and undefined referral practices amongst the reporting institutions and surgeons one notes an improvement in operability rate over succeeding decades and a significantly higher rate amongst the Japanese institutions.

TABLE 2 International Comparison of Surgical Treatment of Gastric Cancer

Authors	Operation rate % (& operative deaths %)		Resection rate % (& 5 yr survival %)		Curative resection rate % (& 5 yr survival %)		Overall 5 yr survival %	Early gastric cancer %
EUROPE								
Desmond	85	(14)	55	(15)	?	(?)	8	?
Zacho	86	(9)	44	(17)	?	(41)	9	?
Svennevig	71	(15)	45	(?)	35	(27)	10	?
Inberg (1946–55)	54	(8)	21	(?)	16	(21)	4	?
(1956–65)	79	(10)	45	(?)	24	(43)	11	?
USA								
Dupont	76	(26)	?	(?)	26	(22)	7	?
Cady (1940–49)	?	(9)	48	(?)	37	(15)	7	?
(1957–66)	94	(6)	58	(?)	44	(23)	11	?
Remine (1940–49)	80	(5)	44	(?)	?	?	14	?
(1950–59)	90	(4)	55	(34)	?	(46)	15	?
Hoerr*	94	(10)	56	(?)	46	(37)	15	1
JAPAN								
Mine	93	(9)	68	(23)	55	(28)	14	?
Muto	99	(9)	79	(23)	?	(?)	19	5
Kajitani (1946–50)			?	?	55	(39)	21	<1
(1956–60)	98	(3)	?	?	64	(43)	25	5
(1966–70)			?	?	76	(59)	39	22
Yamada**	100	(?)	80		65	(58)	47	18

*   PERSONAL SERIES

** ALL INOPERABLE CASES EXCLUDED

Operative Mortality

Definitions of this vary and some are undefined. The Cancer Institute in Tokyo (Kajitani and Takagi 1979) has the lowest at 3 per cent but this is almost equalled by the later data from the Mayo Clinic (Remine and Priestley 1966). Inberg and colleagues' data (1975) is alone in reporting an increase in recent years. This appears to be a consequence of the increased operability rate, involving surgical treatment of more frail and aged patients, for the mortality rate after 'curative' gastrectomy fell in successive periods reported upon.

Definitions of operative mortality may vary but these figures ranging so widely from
3 per cent to 26 per cent do suggest that patient selection, surgical technique and
patient management are not of a uniformly high standard. There appears to be inverse
correlation between operability rate and operative mortality which either suggests
that the more 'aggressive' surgeons are the best technicians or that some surgeons
are particularly unfortunate to be dealing with patients whose stomach cancers are
generally so advanced as to render the patient much more unlikely to survive any
surgical assault. These reports do not allow one to judge on this important issue.

Resection Rates

All clinicians interested in stomach cancer have come to recognise the importance
of resection in either curing or palliating stomach cancer. The reports listed in
Table 2 which distinguish between sequential time periods all report a significant
improvement in resection rates in more recent times and in each case this is
paralleled by an improvement in overall survival rates. It is clear that improvements in resection rates have been brought about in part by improvement in
anaesthesia and postoperative care but the Japanese report of Muto and colleagues
(1968) emphasises that much of the improvement in resection rates must be related
to the increased number of resectable 'early' gastric cancer cases in the more
recent periods. It appears that whereas the European and American surgeons have to
a large extent increased their resection rates following improvements in surgical
management the Japanese have improved them largely because in recent years they have
been dealing with many more resectable tumours.

Whichever time period is compared the Japanese universally report higher resection
rates than European or American workers. The highest non-Japanese resection rate
is that of Hoerr's series (1973) of personally managed patients but he, who has
long advocated surgical exploration and resection in most circumstances for both
cure and palliation, does not approach the rates reported by Mine and co-workers
(1970) Muto and colleagues (1968) or Kajitani and Takagi (1979). The question must
be posed; are the Japanese dealing with a different form of the disease, which may
present earlier, offering more frequent opportunities for resection?

'Curative' Resection Rates

Though the definition of 'curative' resection is not comparable in the series studied the favourable aspects of the Japanese reports continue. Whereas most of the
European and American data report 'curative' resection rates (generally defined as
radical subtotal or total gastrectomies) or less than 35 per cent, with only the
Lahey Clinic data (Cady and colleagues 1977) and Hoerr's personal series (1973)
recording rates above 40 per cent, the Japanese reports all contain rates of at least
55 per cent. It is interesting that Kajitani and Takagi's paper (1979) records
a 'curative' resection rate of 55 per cent in the period 1946-50 when their percentage of 'early' gastric cancer patients in their series was less than 1 per cent
and comparable to the frequency found in all the European and American papers.
During successive 5 year periods they report a most impressive improvement in
curative resection rate which, particularly in the later years, parallels the
considerable increase in the percentage of early gastric cancer cases treated. In
all the reports summarised in Table 2 there is a good correlation between operability and 'curative' resection rates; those reporting the lowest operability rates
have the lowest rate of 'curative' resection whereas those with the highest operability rate have the highest 'curative' resection rate. It is difficult to escape
the conclusion that, though some of the difference between curative resection rates
in Japan and the West is due to the increased numbers of early gastric cancer cases
in the former, there is probably an intangible contribution made by aggressiveness,

or surgical philosophy.

It has often been stated, without citing evidence that the Japanese gastric cancer
has, of itself, characteristics rendering it a more favourable subject for surgical
treatment than the Occidental variety. A study of Hoerr's (1973) and Remine and
Priestley's (1966) reports does not support that view for their survival rates after
'curative' gastrectomy are comparable to those of Mine and colleagues (1970), and
the earlier periods of Kajitani and Takagi's (1979) reports when their incidence of
early gastric cancer was low.

Overall Five Year Survival Rates

Since all the reports emanate from surgical centres their survival rates are higher
than those of the cancer registries. The European and American papers generally
report a survival rate of approximately 10 per cent after 5 years but those from the
Mayo Clinic (Remine and Priestley 1966) and those of Hoerr (1973) at about 15 per
cent do approximate to the Japanese data of Mine and others (1970) and Muto and
colleagues (1968) of 14 per cent and 19 per cent respectively. Only Kajitani and
Takagi's (1979) data from the latter periods of their study demonstrate a significant
improvement. (Yamada's data (1975) reporting almost a 50 per cent overall survival
rate are culled from a surgical series from which all inoperable cases were excluded).

It is again noted that operability rate determines outcome. Outside of Japan there
is a strong positive correlation between operability rate and overall survival;
within Japan all series have a high operability rate and a high overall survival.
Kajitani and Takagi's (1979) paper emphasises that their increasing success in
treating stomach cancer is due largely to their success at diagnosing it at a curable
stage and this fact is noted also by Muto and colleagues (1968) in a more detailed
analysis of their data which spans 20 years from 1941 to 1960.

Thus this analysis of representative reports from four European countries, the USA
and Japan demonstrates a considerable variation in the outcome of treatment. Before
attempting to answer the questions it poses it would be helpful to briefly study
three prospective studies, each based on many hospitals, yet each working to agreed
protocol and each comprised of a group of enthusiastic clinicians. Since one is
European (Lundh and colleagues 1974), one American (Kennedy 1970) and one Japanese
Miwa (1979) they present another opportunity for comparison between the Western
and Japanese experience.

                    PROSPECTIVE MULTICENTRE STUDIES

Lundh and colleagues (1974) reported data from 903 patients admitted to 7 centres
in different parts of Europe between 1966 and 1968; Kennedy's report (1970) was of
1241 patients from 7 American hospitals and Miwa reported data from 8401 patients
admitted to 103 Japanese hospitals. Whilst the European and American papers gave
considerable information on the clinical presentation of their patients, the Japanese paper gave none. The Japanese study gave a detailed pathological analysis of
their cases, each of which was categorised in terms of ground rules laid down by
the Gastric Cancer Study in Surgery and Pathology (sic); the American study also
had a very strong pathological basis and was designed to investigate the validity
of the TNM format for gastric cancer staging. However the European study gave no
pathological data, admitting the impossibility of their organising a uniform pathological assessment. 'Radical' treatment is defined histologically in the Japanese
study whereas in the European study its definition rests on the opinion of the
surgeon and is not defined histologically. Lundh and colleagues (1974) admit that
their definition of 'radical' treatment was open to several interpretations. In the

American study no attempt was made to distinguish between 'curative' and palliative gastric resections. A study of this data reveals more to contrast than to compare between them (see Table 3). Though the operability rates are comparable, resection was carried out much more frequently in the Japanese series.

TABLE 3 Comparison of Surgical Treatment, its Results and
Pathological Staging in Three Prospective Studies of Gastric
Cancer

MULTICENTRE PROSPECTIVE SERIES

Country and years of study	No. of patients	Operation rate %	Resection rate % (& operative mortality %)	Curative resection rate % (and 5 yr survival rate %)	Overall 5 yr survival
JAPAN 63-66	8401	94	72 (4)	37 (55)	25
USA 51-56	1241	95	66 (13)	? (?)	10
EUROPEAN 66-68	903	91	58 (21)	28 (23*)	9*

* FOUR YEAR SURVIVAL RATE

PATHOLOGICAL COMPARISON	JAPAN	USA	EUROPE
MEAN TUMOUR SIZE (cms)	6 x 6*	?	8 x 6
% NODE +VE	75	76	75
% HEPATIC 2°	7	⎫	25
% PERITONEAL 2°	25	⎬ 26	28
% EARLY GASTRIC CANCER	14	2.5	?

* CALCULATED

In both Japan and Europe it appears that approximately half the resections were 'curative' (though only the Japanese paper defines this histologically). There is a marked difference in operative mortality after gastric resection and the very high European operative mortality is reflected in the much lower long term survival rate both after resection and in the series overall. It is unfortunate that no careful pathological comparison can be made between the three series; though Lundh and colleagues (1974) claim that their cases were commonly so advanced as to be incurable, quoting an average tumour size of 8 x 6 cm (Table 3), involved lymph nodes 'thought' to be present in 75 per cent of patients and peritoneal metastases present in 28 per cent this data is not markedly different from either the Japanese or the American. Only the higher rate of hepatic metastases (25 per cent) in Lundh and colleagues' figures indicates a higher rate of incurability than the Japanese (7 per cent). Though one can be justifiably critical at the lack of pathological data in the European study it must be accepted, although the data is not presented, that their

proportion of favourable cancers, extending no further than the submucosa is unlikely
to be more than the usual 1-2 per cent reported by most Occidental studies and therefore much lower than the Japanese rate of 14 per cent. The American report of 2 per
cent T_1 tumours (lesions confined to the mucosa) more accurately defines this lower
rate   of favourable 'early' gastric cancers in the West.

WHY THE VARIATION?

These three prospective studies considered with the hospital data outlined in Table
2 lead one to an obvious conclusion that the only significant variations in the results
of gastric cancer treatment are between the Japanese results and those from the rest
of the World. It is clear that a large part of this variation is the result of a
very much higher rate of the favourable 'early' gastric cancer in the Japanese series.
This higher proportion of 'early' curable cancers will, in part, account for their
higher operability and resection rates, and higher 5 year survival rates both after
resection and overall but it should not overshadow the improvement due to the significantly lower operative mortality rates reported in all the Japanese series. Indeed
both Cady and colleagues (1977) and Inberg and others (1975) both make the point that
improvements in their overall survival rates in more recent times are due, in part,
to their decreased operative mortality. All the recent Japanese papers demonstrate
lower operative mortality rates.

But does the more favourable Japanese experience of gastric cancer rest only on earlier diagnosis, and safer surgery? That may not be so for such comparisons that can
be made demonstrate that the Japanese surgeon reports improved survival after resection
even when comparing his results of treatment by pathological staging with those of
Western surgeons. This improvement persists even when treatment results are compared
between Japan and the rest of the World of patients with similarly advanced cancers.
Table 4 compares figures obtained from Kennedy's paper (1970) and Miwa's very detailed
report (1979). In every comparison the Japanese data is significantly better.

TABLE 4 Treatment Results Compared by Stage of Tumour. Five
Year Survival Rates (%).

5 YEAR SURVIVAL RATES (%) OF RESECTED GASTRIC CANCER

STAGE	T1	T2	T3	T4	N0	N1	Stage I*
USA (Kennedy)	76	34	15	10	54	20	62
JAPAN (Miwa)	91	53	37	21	84	47	95

* STAGE I (JAPAN) ASSUMED EQUIVALENT TO STAGES IA + IB (TNM)

One should not place too much emphasis on comparisons of single T, N or M **stages**
since each is only one facet of tumour staging. Stage I (Japanese Reseach Society
for Gastric Cancer) is approximately equivalent to TNM stage IA and IB combined. If
this comparison is accepted it can be seen that these favourable cancers do less well
after treatment in the West than in Japan.

Comparison of data from individual institutions in the USA (Hoerr 1973) and Japan

(Kajitani 1968) can be made with some difficulty (see Table 5).

TABLE 5 Five Year Survival Rate (%) of 'Curative' Gastrectomies for Cancer*

	STAGE I	STAGE II + III COMBINED
HOERR (USA)	91	36
KAJITANI (JAPAN)	86	38

* ASSUMING	STAGE I (JAPAN) $\equiv^+$	STAGE AI (HOERR)
	STAGES II + III COMBINED $\equiv$	STAGES A-II, B-I+B-II COMBINED

The lack of uniformity of staging procedures presents problems but if it is assumed that superficial cancers with negative nodes are defined by Hoerr (1973) as stage A-I and by Kajitani as stage I and that cancers extending to the serosa or metastasising to the regional nodes are contained in Hoerr's stages A-II, B-I and B-II combined and in Kajitani's stage II and III then the calculated five year survivals tabulated in Table 4 are very comparable. (It should be emphasised that Hoerr's report is of a smaller personally treated series and Kajitani's is of the results of a surgical institution). Whilst Kajitani's overall survival rate is more than twice that of Hoerrs this may result from a decreased operative mortality (Table 2) and an increased number of 'early' gastric cancers in the Kajitani series. Nonetheless Hoerr's report is the only one of the surgical series emanating from the Western World which allows a pathological comparison to be made and shows that long term survival after a successful 'curative' gastrectomy whilst dependant on the state of advancement of the cancer is not dependant on the nationality of the surgeon and the patient.

DOES SURVIVAL DEPEND ON THE STRUCTURAL TYPE OF THE CANCER?

Hoerr's (1973) commendable results have not prevented a ground swell of Western surgical opinion developing to claim that the favourable results of treatment in Japan owe more to the biological character of the tumour than to surgical expertise. Such a statement is difficult to refute for it rests on scanty evidence. Only a few of the Western series contain any pathological data, and that is generally insufficient to allow comparison with the Japanese figures of Miwa (1979). His analysis undoubtably showed that apart from pathological staging of the cancer survival depended on:- tumour site, size, macroscopic type and degree of histological differentiation. Cancers that were proximally situated, large, infiltrative or poorly differentiated had a worse outcome after treatment than distal, small, polypoid, or well differentiated cancers. This is not inconsistent with the less complete pathological data in the Western reports. Miwa's report (1979) showed no survival potential attaching to age, sex or histological type of tumour; papillary tumours had no advantage over tubular, nor muconodular over mucocellular. Both medullary and scirrhous cancers had the same survival rate. These facts cannot be contested from the Western literature.

$\equiv^+$ Equivalent to

CONCLUSIONS

Close analysis reveals that the overall results of treatment of gastric cancer are better in Japan than in the rest of the world. Cancer registry data is difficult to compare but surgical series emanating from hospitals or individual surgeons all support this fact and prospective multicentre studies from Europe, the USA and Japan confirm it. The most apparent contributions to this difference are the decreased operative mortality and increased numbers of early gastric cancers in all Japanese reports and the cause of these differences can only be conjectural. It may be that the Japanese patient generally allows surgery to be carried out with less danger, or the Japanese surgeon is more skillful and it may be that the 'earlier' stages of Japanese gastric cancer are more frequently symptomatic than are those in Western patients but the current literature does not allow dogmatic conclusions to be drawn on these points.

Comparison of treatment between Japan and the West of gastric cancers that are equally advanced tends to indicate that the Japanese results are better, and in doing so suggests either that the Japanese cancer is more amenable to surgical resection or that the Japanese surgeon is more effective at undertaking a curative resection. There is an impression that Western surgical techniques are generally not yet as formalised as in Japan, neither margin of clearance nor extent of node resection are emphasised in the majority of Western reports whereas the more recent Japanese reports all follow the guidelines laid down by the WHO-ICC (Tsukamoto and Gaitan-Yanguas 1973). However Hoerr's (1973) personal results, are comparable to the Japanese figures when the results of treatment of equivalently staged gastric cancers are compared and this tends to suggest that carefully designed surgical techniques, as followed by him can produce the results generally reported from Japan. The Japanese have been much more successful in producing relevant pathological data on their stomach cancer patients – until the Western surgical centres can define their patients as accurately the definitive comparison of the results of treatment of gastric cancer between Japan and the West must be delayed and until then we shall discuss the causes of differing rates of early gastric cancer, operative mortality, results of resection and the overall mortality. May I make a plea now that those Western surgeons interested in gastric cancer consider registering their patients with the WHO Collaborating Centre in Tokyo. Only in this way can I see clinical, surgical and pathological data being gathered in a form which allows a proper comparison.

REFERENCES

Axtell, L. M. and Myers, M. H. (1974). Recent Trends in Survival of Cancer Patients. DHEW Publication, No. 75-767, Bethesda.

Brookes, V. S., Waterhouse, J. A. H. and Powell, D. J. (1965). Carcinoma of the stomach: a 10 year Survey of Results and of Factors Affecting Prognosis. Brit. Med. J. 1. 1577-1583

Cady, B., Ramsden, D. A., Stein, A. and Haggitt, R. G. (1977). Gastric Cancer. Amer. J. Surg., 133, 423-429.

Desmond, A. M. (1976). Radical Surgery in Treatment of Carcinoma of Stomach. Proc. Roy. Soc. Med., 69, 867-869.

Dupont, J. B., Rillens Lee, J., Burton, G. R. and Cohn, I. (1978). Adenocarcinoma of the Stomach: Review of 1,497 cases. Cancer 41, 941-947.

Hanai, A. and Fujimoto, I. (1977). Cancer Registry Statistics in Japan. In Hirayama, T. (Ed.), Epidemiology of Stomach Cancer. WHO Collaborating Centre, National Cancer Centre, Tokyo. pp. 21-33.

Hoerr, S. O. (1973). Prognosis for Carcinoma of the Stomach. Surg. Gynec. Obst., 137, 204-209.

Inberg, M. V., Heinonen, R., Rantakokklo, V. and Viikari, S. J. (1975). Surgical Treatment of Gastric Carcinoma. Arch. Surg., 110, 703-707.

Kajitani, T. (1968). Results of Surgical Treatment of Gastric Cancer. Gann Monograph on Cancer Research, 3, 245-251.

Kajitani, T. and Takagi, K. (1979). Cancer of the Stomach at Cancer Institute Hospital, Tokyo. Gann Monograph on Cancer Research, 22, 77-87.

Kennedy, B. J. (1970). TNM Classification for Stomach Cancer. Cancer 26, 971-983.

Lundh, G., Burn, J. I., Kalig, G., Richard, C. A., Thomson, J. W. W., van Elke, P. J. and Oszacki, J. (1974). A co-operative International Study of Gastric Cancer. Ann. Roy. Coll. Surg. England, 54, 219-228.

Mine, M., Majima, S., Harada, M. and Etani, S. (1970). End Results of Gastrectomy for Gastric Cancer. Surgery, 68, 753-758.

Miwa, K. (1979). Cancer of the Stomach in Japan. Gann Monograph on Cancer Research, 22, 61-75.

Muto, M., Maki, T., Majima, S. and Yamaguchi, I. (1968). Improvement in the end Results of Surgical Treatment of Gastric Cancer. Surgery, 63, 229-235.

Remine, W. H. and Priestley, J. T. (1966). Trends in Prognosis and Surgical Treatment of Cancer of the Stomach. Ann. Surg., 163, 736-745.

Svennevig, J. L. and Nysted, A. (1976). Carcinoma of the Stomach. Acta. Chir. Scand., 142, 78-81.

Tsukamoto, K. and Gaitan-Yanguas, M. (1973). A System for Registration and Classification of Stomach Cancer for WHO-International Reference Center. Jpn. J. Clin. Oncol., 12, 117-128.

Yamada, E. (1975). Surgical Results for Early Gastric Cancer. International Surgery, 60, 139-143.

Zacho, A. and Fischermann, K. (1966). The Results of Surgical Treatment of Cancer of the Stomach. Surg. Gynec. Obst., 123, 73-79.

Future Prospects for Gastric Cancer

P.S. Schein, R. Coffey and F.P. Smith

Division of Medical Oncology, Vincent T. Lombardi Cancer
Research Center, Georgetown University, Washington, D.C., U.S.A.

INTRODUCTION

Throughout this symposium, the importance of gastric cancer both internationally
and in the United Kingdom and United States has been well emphasized. The
mortality rate from stomach cancer in these two nations will approximate 15,000 per
annum. The high prevalence of this disease in Japan has led to mass-screening and
this in turn appears to have improved the percent of early cases diagnosed and
cured. Whereas this early diagnosis would unquestionably result in improved surgical
cure rates, x-ray or endoscopic screening techniques are unlikely to prove cost-
effective in the U.S. and U.K. Should a sensitive and specific tumor marker become
available mass-screening might have some application for these two countries. Such
a marker has yet to be discovered, and consequently, the vast majority of patients
will continue to present with inoperable or surgically incurable lesions. Even
where "surgical-cure" appears to have been achieved, approximately one half of such
cases will succumb from tumor recurrence. If a survival impact is to be made on
gastric cancer, more emphasis must be placed on the continued development of nonsurgical modalities of management.

DISSEMINATED GASTRIC CANCER

During the past 6 years, it has become apparent that gastric cancer represents the
most responsive malignancy of the gastro-intestinal tract. The current response
rates for patients with metastatic disease, e.g. 42% with FAM, represents an
improvement over the past use of 5-FU and the combination of 5-FU + nitrosoureas.
It is important to recognise that such effective palliative treatment can be
delivered in an out-patient setting without serious or life threatening toxicity.
Nevertheless, the duration of response and survival for patients with such advanced
disease is limited; we should not become fixated with our current treatment as had
been the case for 5-fluorouracil for over twenty years. These advances do not
lessen the need for identifying new drugs with activity for gastric cancer, to allow
for the development of future regimens with greater efficacy and reduced toxicity.

Among available new agents, cis-diammine-dichloroplatinum has been reported by
Brugolaris to produce tumor regression in 6 of 19 patients with disseminated
gastric cancer who had previously been treated with 5-FU in various combination
regimens. Additional Phase II trials of cis-platinum are being conducted. At the

Lombardi Cancer Research Center, we have developed the FAP regimen (5-FU, adriamycin and cis-platinum) and obtained partial responses in six of fourteen patients with gastric cancer. Such new studies of single agents and combinations must presently be pursued in an empirical manner. Clonogenic assays for tumor sensitivity have been reported for ovarian and multiple myeloma, and may be forthcoming for gastric cancer thus allowing for a prospective prediction of patient response.

LOCALLY ADVANCED GASTRIC CANCER

The GITSG study for this stage of disease has produced important information which should be employed in future treatment designs for locally advanced stomach cancer. In evaluating responses to chemotherapy and/or irradiation, those patients undergoing resection of the primary tumor, even though only palliative in intent, seem to have improved responses and increased survival, compared to those who go unresected. Why it appears to be a prognostic variable is unclear. Whether it enhances the effect of post-operative treatment by reducing the tumor burden or whether it lowers the evidence of local complications such as bleeding or obstruction is not known. At this point surgical resection should be encouraged whenever feasible. The overall approach to radiation therapy can be improved. The early toxicity of this modality consisted of nutritional decline and myelotoxicity. Such toxicity might be reduced by narrowing the treatment ports to the minimum required, by using tangential fields to limit normal tissue exposure and by carefully monitoring nutritional status with supplementation as indicated. The combined modality approach still conferred the best likelihood of long-term survival in the GITSG study and supports continued investigation of such therapy.

Three possible changes in the combined modality program become evident:

1. A different form or method of irradiation.
2. A change in the chemotherapy employed.
3. A change in the sequence of delivering the combined modality therapy.

Neutron therapy has generated some new excitment with its theoretic advantages over conventional irradiation. Catterall and her colleagues have reported on the treatment of thirty-nine patients with inoperable carcinoma of the stomach with 1440 neutron rads. Whereas local tumor control was felt to be good, the mean survival of such patients was only 1.5 months. We at the Lombardi Cancer Research Center have been impressed by the toxicity seen in 20 patients with locally advanced pancreatic cancer treated with neutron rads to the upper abdomen. Five of these patients developed severe hemorrhagic gastritis which required palliative gastrectomy in two. Equally distressing was the lack of survival benefit in the 20 patients when compared to others treated with conventional therapy. We therefore would caution any enthusiasm for this form of radiation to the upper gastrointestinal tract.

Intraoperative irradiation could potentially enhance the therapeutic ratio of upper abdominal irradiation since direct visualization of the tumor would allow for optimally minimizing the treatment port. Furthermore, the low penetrance of the electron beam would reduce the surrounding tissue toxicity and myelotoxicity. This treatment, as well as consideration of more effective radiation sensitizers represent potential prospects for future management.

The more effective adriamycin containing combinations might be employed either in combined modality or in a randomized comparison with combined modality therapy. The FAM combination has been domonstrated by the GITSG to be superior to 5-FU + methyl-CCNU in advanced disease; every prospect of improving the treatment results of the GITSG in locally advanced cases exists if such regimens are employed with radiation therapy.

An alteration in the sequence of delaying combined modality treatments is worthy of study. Combination chemotherapy with 5-FU + methyl CCNU appears to have a therapeutic benefit over combined modality in the first year of the GITSG supplanted by long term survivorship with the combined modality. To exploit these observations, we have initiated a "sandwich" technique. Our current trial consists of an initial 2 month course of FAM followed by 4500 rads of split course irradiation with 5-FU sensitization and subsequent return to FAM for a total treatment period of one year assuming adequate hematologic and gastrointestinal tolerance. The rationale for the initial use of chemotherapy comes from the recognition that some gastric cancers will continue to grow in the face of ongoing radiation therapy, and the period of time required to deliver the latter in such cases may be too long. Chemotherapy, if it is to be effective, should be deployed as early as possible.

ADJUVANT GASTRIC CANCER

The most important immediate future prospect of clinical investigation of gastric cancer is the evaluation of adjuvant chemotherapy in surgically curatively-resected patients at known risk for relapse. The improvement in responses achieved by diligent study of combinations in advanced stages of disease should allow for newer trials in the adjuvant phase of gastric cancer. These studies must have a prospectively randomized control arm if some conclusion is to be obtained. Currently, on-going trials include the use of 5-FU + methyl CCNU by the GITSG and 5-FU and mitomycin by the Stomach Cancer Group in Great Britain. New trials with adriamycin-containing regimens have just been initiated; a controlled trial of FAM by the CALGB and SWOG and 5-FU-Adriamycin by the North Central Cancer Treatment Group in the United States are now in progress.

DAY 2. SESSION 2. PANEL DISCUSSION

P. Wrigley. Mr. Craven, was it possible to obtain the age of the patients that were being included in the studies that you compared? Perhaps this might give an explanation for some of the differing results.

J. Craven. The mean or the median age of the Japanese patient is of the order of ten years younger than the European or American patient. There seems to be a tendency in recent figures from Europe and the UK for the gastric cancer patient becoming older.

M. Keighley. We have said a lot today about staging gastric cancer and the Conference Organisers asked me earlier whether I would present some data on intra-operative frozen sections, not so much to stage the extent of the cancer but to look at the problem of proximal extension in gastric carcinoma, and we have looked at this with the histopathology department at the General Hospital. Yesterday, Dr. Thompson talked about endoscopic cytology in diagnosis and I would just like briefly to present our findings on the value of cytology versus frozen section to define whether or not the lower oesophagus is involved with tumour. In this study we confined ourselves to patients with fundal carcinoma, because this is a group that has worried us. We cannot detect the proximal extension of tumours in this site by pre-operative radiology, or by endoscopy. We classified our 39 patients that we studied into those that had an adequate resection, that is where blocks taken from the most proximal end of the resected specimen were free of tumour. Of the 30 patients where the resection initially was adequate, our frozen section was entirely reliable, we had no false positive results, and cytology also gave us no false positive results. But in the 9 patients where we thought we had cleared the tumour macroscopically, but where eventually the blocks showed us there was tumour right up to the proximal margin, frozen sections proved positive and therefore were entirely reliable. Unfortunately cytology proved to be unreliable. So we have given up using cytology to assess the proximal extent of the disease. When we looked at the impact that this had on the clinical management and results of the patients it was quite obvious what was happening. In the time before we did frozen sections we had a proportion of patients, 7/27, who in fact had an inadequate excision because of the proximal extension of disease. Of these 7 patients we had 5 fatal leaks. Whereas during the study, and subsequently in the 52 patients in this group where we have again had an adequate excision and frozen sections have been negative, we have only had 1 fatal leak. In 13 subjects where we thought we had clearance of the tumour, but where frozen section defined that there had been inadequate clearance, we only had 5 fatal leaks. When we actually analyse that data just a little bit more carefully, where the surgeon in question actually acted upon the frozen section information and had a further proximal extension of resection we had only one fatal leak, whereas in the 4 instances where further proximal resection was not undertaken, all those patients died of anastomotic dehiscence. If you have got a patient with a fundal carcinoma, are you going to prepare that patient for a thoracotomy in the eventuality that you may have to resect a further segment of oesophagus in the chest, or should we still be doing mid-line laparotomies?

G. Slaney. Bill, would you like to comment on that? I think the thesis is that if you leave malignant cells in the oesophagael suture line, in the light of the evidence that our group have just presented to you, that seems to be a potent factor in anastomotic leak, quite apart from the effect that it will have on direct recurrence subsequently.

W. Longmire. I think that's an extremely important observation and it would certainly reinforce our attitude and approach to lesions of this kind which traditionally, or currently, have been through the upper mid-line. If we can make any evaluation preoperatively, either by X-ray or by endoscopy, and know the cell type and the degree of oesophageal involvement, we can be better prepared as to whether we are going to have to go through the chest or not. In many cases one cannot obtain that information except at operation, but we are prepared in any case to go through the upper mid-line, make our evaluation, decide on the type of procedure, then go through the right chest if it seems appropriate and check the cut margin of the oesophagus by immediate frozen section. We then would act upon what the section shows, which I think your statistics show would be extremely important. Using this approach it does allow you to either go into the chest, or not, without changing the position of the patient.

G. Slaney. With this type of lesion, do you put a man with a half left roll with the right arm up, or what?

W. Longmire. We would elevate the chest slightly with the arm in an airplane splint.

M. McMahon. I wonder if I can comment on this particular problem becuase we have been faced with this sort of situation occasionally and we find that by doing a limited median sternotomy, oesophagael mobilisation is facilitated and it is usually not necessary to enter the chest.

W. Longmire. I take it as really difficult to get through the heart and get the lower half of the oesophagus, which is frequently necessary in the cases of this kind.

G. Slaney. As some of you probably know, G.B. Ong in Hong Kong occasionally uses this sort of approach for lower oesophagael lesions. I have actually seen him get up to the aortic arch and some of the vascular surgeons are using this now for supra-renal aneurysms. I would hate to try and do it on a bulky chap. I think if you have got someone who is nice and slim, it might be worth thinking about.

W. Gillison. I would like to cast a slight doubt on Mr. Keighley's suggestion, and to ask for Professor Longmire's comments on how high he goes. Before 1977 some, if not most of the carcinoma of the cardia work was done by Professor Collis who had a superb low mortality, low leak rate, and I would have thought that practice makes perfect. I am sure Mr. Keighley is a much better oesophagael surgeon than he was three or four years ago. So I would like to throw some cold water on the frozen section theory, because we have all been embarrassed by seeing a report showing that there may be tumour at the margin of resection. Surely, practice makes perfect, and I suspect that many people would agree with that. Professor Longmire, when you have a true carcinoma of the cardia, how high do you cut across the oesophagus after you cut the vagus nerve to be sure you are usually clear?

W. Longmire. Our approach to that ordinarily would be an abdominal approach. We would try to detect grossly, by palpation, what we could and if we felt that we were getting above it, that is we felt that the primary was in the stomach and not in the lower oesophagus, we would divide the oesophagus and make a frozen section. If it was clear, we would do a total gastrectomy and a Roux-en-Y connection. If it was not clear we would go on into the chest and take more of the oesophagus.

G. Slaney. You feel, in the light of your experience, that if you have got a cardial lesion you can observe the 5 - 6 cm clearance rule and still do an adequate job from the abdomen?

W. Longmire. Yes.

R. Pichlmayr. I still do not believe that it is the infiltration of the tumour which results in leakage. Surgeons feel that they might not be radical enough and go too far from the intra-abdominal position, instead of doing a thoracic operation.

In any case of cancer in the cardia or in the fundus, I think we should take an abdomino-thoracic approach.

M. Keighley. To answer Mr. Gillison's comment, these aren't all my own cases by any means. This is a co-operative study we have been doing at the General Hospital. The patients we are operating on in this disease are usually in their seventh decade and if you can avoid having to open the chest, I think it is a great advantage. On the other hand, I don't think one should compromise your surgery and if you are setting out to do a major resection and you haven't adequately cleared the proximal line of tumour, our experience is that the results are disastrous.

I. Häkkinen. I would like to ask Dr. Smith, what is your opinion about the possibilities of immunotherapy?

F. Smith. I think you will notice the title of my first talk this morning was radiotherapy, chemotherapy and immunotherapy, and I left it out. I think that's about as much as I can say.

G. Slaney. There are many critics of the morbidity associated with chemotherapy and I think the figures you produced with your FAM regimen showed a mean survival rate of something like 9 months. That was in your treated group, with I think a range from 2 - 19 months. What you did'nt show was what the survival time was in untreated patients, who did'nt have the chemotherapy. Many studies have shown that something like 15% of patients with metastatic disease, particularly in the liver from GIT carcinoma, will survive well over intervals of that time I think there is the doubt in many clinicians' minds about whether you really are buying extra time against the morbidity unless you have a very carefully controlled study. Would you like to comment on that?

F. Smith. If you compared any treatment, particularly for gastric carcinoma, and looked at an untreated group, even with FAM, you would find that the median survival would be no different for the patients with advanced disseminated disease treated with FAM. The reason for that is that we get only a 40% response rate. To be able to demonstrate that a population of patients receiving one modality of therapy benefit substantially more than a group not receiving that therapy, one has to have at least half these individuals doing better and we don't yet have that situation in gastric carcinoma. I think, however, that if you go back to historical series, and that's fraught with every problem you want to talk about, the survival curve for our non responding group of patients is very similar to that of historical curves. There are a few who will go on and survive the 6 to 8 months but the average survival for patients with hepatic disease is about 3 - 5 months. The figures that you had, Professor Slaney, were the time of response, the duration of response. The survival in responders was about 13 months, but the duration of the response averaged from 2 to 9 months.

M. Crespi. I have a very direct question. Can you tell me of one published controlled, randomised study which gives us clear results on survival and quality of life of patients who receive the kind of chemotherapy that you are suggesting?

F. Smith. I would like to answer that in two ways, Professor Crespi. One is that no, there is not. But secondly I would venture that several years ago when digitalis was being introduced, it was considered a very dangerous drug as well. I think that second approach is quite nihilistic. In the USA we cannot do controlled studies. At our institution we feel that we have demonstrated reasonably well that there are a valuable percentage of patients who do benefit palliatively from the treatment regimen and I think, perhaps, a randomised study could be done in Rome.

M. Crespi. Perhaps. On one occasion I had the opportunity to see some women on treatment with the CMF protocol for breast carcinoma, and I would not advise anybody that I care for to have this treatment.

G. Slaney. I don't know whether Dr. Smith has got his tongue in his cheek when he mentioned digitalis, I suspect he had, but for the one or two members of the audience who don't know, Dr. William Withering who practised in this city, actually introduced the use of digitalis in the treatment of heart failure. Certainly we regard it as a pretty useful drug and have done for nearly 200 years. So we don't knock every drug on sight!

C. Newman. The implication would seem to be that only the people who respond to chemotherapy benefit from it, and equally those that don't are going to suffer added toxicity. There are other solid tumour situations when one has to exhibit chemotherapy to see whether the patient is going to be a responder. The question is how many cycles of treatment should one give, if one adopts this policy, before one puts the patient into a non-responder group and takes them off treatment?

F. Smith. I think that is an excellent question and in our FAM trial we learned that if the patient did not respond by the second cycle, which was the second month of treatment, it was very unlikely that the patient would respond. I think we would all like to have the capability of seeing prospectively that this individual is going to respond and that that individual is going to respond. Hence, treat or not treat. We have looked at all the prognostic variables. We have looked at the sites of disease, the performance status of the patients, the histologic differentiation of the disease, and we don't have that capability yet. Now possibly the clonogenic methods of identifying tumour response to anti-neoplastic agents, as is presently being developed for ovarian and multiple myloma malignancies, may become available for gastric cancer and we will have a better method of deciding whom one should treat. I tried to impress that we are not claiming FAM to be curative, we are claiming it to be well tolerated, in spite of what Professor Crespi said. I think that there are individuals here who have given FAM. Alopecia is a real problem, I recognise the difficulty with that, but there are people here who have given FAM and found it to be really quite tolerable as an out-patient regimen. Granted, there is nausea and vomiting, quite substantial in some cases during the first day of treatment when the three drugs are given together, but most of our patients, and I would invite you Professor Crespi to visit our Centre when you are in Washington some time, are able to conduct their normal business.

J. Powell. Mr. Craven gave results from three cancer registries. I think the Birmingham data must have been for all patients, in other words it was survival rate of all patients, whether they were treated or not. There could not have been a large proportion of patients who had never even had a laparotomy. I do think it illustrates an important point, that if you are quoting results it is a good idea to give them for all patients presenting and not just those who are resected, because otherwise you don't really know what the selection is.

J. Craven. Birmingham, I acknowledge, is a population based Registry and has a 95% follow-up and the American data, unfortunately, is hospital based. Yes, I distinguished them.

W. Longmire. That is not the state of Connecticut Cancer Registry?

J. Craven. No.

W. Longmire. That's one of the best cancer registries in America, which is population based and has excellent data. I am not familiar with the other one you speak of.

J. Craven. It was the only American Cancer Registry data I could find.

W. Longmire. Connecticut and California both have very excellent population based cancer registries. Connecticut has one that has been going for many years and has very excellent material and there may be in one of them a group of co-operating hospitals that I am not familiar with.

J. Waterhouse. The Sear Survey, which includes 11 or 12 cancer registries around the States, published some results and I quoted some of those yesterday. Although these cancer registries have been in existence for a long time they have generally quoted incidence rather than survival data and I believe that John Craven is right, there is not any population based survival data quoted for the whole of the Connecticut State.

W. Longmire. Well, I haven't had occasion to look it up recently, but the last time I did, survival data was in.

J. Waterhouse. For the whole State?

W. Longmire. Yes.

J. Waterhouse. Well, I did not realise that.

W. Longmire. For cancer of the stomach.

T. Hirayama. I would like to propose to Dr. Waterhouse to make an in depth comparison of the Osaka Cancer Registry and The Birmingham Cancer Registry in terms of the survival rate for gastric cancer. We know from the Osaka Cancer Registry that there are considerable variations in survival rates, medical institutions and big hospitals have better rates compared to the clinic. Such an in depth comparison would serve as a model.

J. Waterhouse. I think that is a very good idea and I know Dr. Fujimoto would be interested in that as well.

G. Slaney. Are we really seeing the same disease now in Japan that we see in the UK and the USA? The figure you produce for your stage IV cases was a 24% five year survival rate. Now that is better than we can do in the West Midlands with node negative cases. I would guess that it's about the same for the States, is it Bill?

W. Longmire. I think that is about right.

G. Slaney. For many years we felt that in colorectal cancer an A lesion was a good lesion because it was early. There is a lot of evidence now to suggest that it is a good lesion because of the biological behaviour of the tumour. Is the type of cancer you see in Japan, Dr. Takagi, with these fantastically good results, the same sort of cancer that we see in the USA and Europe?

K. Takagi. Staging is important, but gastric cancer is not one entity. A very localised cancer has a very good prognosis and the infiltrating type has the worst prognosis. Before laparotomy you must examine the patient to discover whether there are remote metastases or not.

G. Slaney. Do you think it is the same disease, or not?

T. Hirayama. No one can definitely state that we are comparing the same disease, I think that the apparent difference is strongly influenced by the fact that many cases are detected by screening. Even in the same state, cases found by screening showed a better prognosis than those found in out-patients. Hence the possible

influence of what is called lead-time bias. If we start treatment two years
earlier, then we should compare the three year survival with the five year rate.
I don't think that stomach cancer in Japan is different from stomach cancer in
other countries.

M. McMahon. Are we missing early gastric cancer because we don't see the same
incidence, or because we don't screen the patients or is it that early lesions are
not typical of cancer of the stomach in Britain?

V. Brookes. It is easy when someone does not get the same results as somebody
else to think we are dealing with a different disease. We are missing, or not yet
diagnosing, early carcinoma of the stomach, that is one point. If one excludes
that, how can one say one has been dealing with a different disease, when in 50%
of the patients in the West Midlands the diagnosis is not made until long after
the operation has been done?

G. Slaney. All of those points are taken. But on one of those slides Dr. Takagi
produced this afternoon, there was a group showing full thickness involvement of
the stomach wall, with nodal involvement, with a survival rate of 24%. Now, I
repeat, that is better than we can do in the West Midlands, or anywhere else in
the UK for node negative cases. Our figures are about 16%.

V. Brookes. They were all the resected ones, and I must stress that the resected
ones were not always radically resected. One only knows when the nodes are
negative or positive if one removes them and often in cases that are quoted as
node negative, the nodes haven't been removed.

G. Slaney. But all I am saying is that those that we have removed, and we know
they are node negative cases, the 5 year results are still worse than they are in
Japan. Even when they have got full thickness involvement and node involvement.

J. Craven. You are asking only half the question. The other half of the question
surely must be why 10%, at the minimum, of our patients die after a gastric
resection and yet the Japanese are able to get away with only 3% mortality? I also
think that our parameters of an adequate radical resection are not as well defined
as theirs. These are aspects of the same question.

G. Slaney. Part of that is the more you do, the more you see, and one the whole
the better you get at it.

I. Hakkinen. Our regional mass screening has uncovered 34 carcinomas and most of
them were silent and half of them were early. The other half contained advanced,
symptomless patients and surprisingly all of them are without recurrence at the
present time. So we have a similar phenomenon to that found in Japan but the lead-
in time can be different for even tumours of the same size.

G. Slaney. One of the many reasons that we have got interested in the biological
aspect of tumours in the West Midlands is that right through the GI tract, but
specifically in stomach, colon and rectum although the number of cases are small
in relation to the overall groups treated, the people who have the best prognosis
are the ones who have the longest duration of symptoms prior to surgery. I think
there are more factors than whether it is early or late. There is a biological
quotient in it somewhere.

J. Fielding. We have been talking about poor results in Britain but we have
investigated early gastric cancers in the West Midlands and during the sixties
there were 90 early gastric cancers. That's less than 1% but the age adjusted
five year survival in that group was 70%, so we are getting better.

PARTICIPANTS

Mr. *H.S. Abou-Zeid*, Friarage Hospital, Northallerton, North Yorkshire.
Mr. *J. Alexander-Williams*, The General Hospital, Birmingham.
Mr. *N.S. Ambrose*, Dudley Road Hospital, Birmingham.
Mr. *A. Aukland*, Queen Elizabeth Hospital, Birmingham.

Mr. *P.M. Baddeley*, The General Hospital, Birmingham.
Dr. *J. Bancewicz*, Hope Hospital, Salford, Manchester.
Dr. *P. Barker*, Selly Oak Hospital, Birmingham.
Mr. *J.R.S. Blake*, University Hospital, Queens Medical Centre, Nottingham.
Dr. *H. Bradby*, Queen Elizabeth Hospital, Birmingham.
Mr. *T.G. Brennan*, St. James's Hospital, Leeds.
Dr. *J.E. Bridger*, Oulton, Stone, Staffordshire.
Dr. *D. Brodie*, Farmitalia Carlo Erba, Barnet, Hertfordshire.
Mr. *V.S. Brookes*, Queen Elizabeth Hospital, Birmingham.
Dr. *S. Brown*, The General Hospital, Birmingham.

Mr. *G. Camelot*, Centre Hospitalier Universitaire, Besacon Cedex, France.
Dr. *J. Castro-Castro*, Hospital Provincial, Avila, Spain.
Dr. *C.P.J. Caygill*, Bacterial Metabolism Research Laboratories, London.
Mr. *L.J. Chalstrey*, Hackney Hospital, London.
Mr. *B.K. Cleary*, St. David's Hospital, Cardiff.
Dr. *D.S. Cole*, Smith, Kline and French, Welwyn Garden City, Hertfordshire.
Mr. *B. Contractor*, Sunderland District General Hospital, Sunderland.
Mr. *R. Cox*, East Birmingham Hospital, Birmingham.
Mr. *J. Craven*, York District Hospital, York.
Professor *M. Crespi*, Istituto 'Regina Elena', Rome, Italy.

Dr. *D. Day*, Royal Liverpool Hospital, Liverpool.
Mr. *De Castella*, Burton General Hospital, Burton-on-Trent, Staffordshire.
Dr. *E. Deutch*, 469, Beacon Street, Boston, Massachusetts, U.S.A.
Lt. Comm *E.P. Dewar*, Royal Naval Hospital, Gosport, Hampshire.
Dr. *A.R. Dewsbury*, Lordswood House, Lordswood Road, Harborne, Birmingham.
Dr. *R. Downing*, Queen Elizabeth Hospital, Birmingham.
Capt. *J.B. Drinkwater*, Royal Naval Hospital, Plymouth, Devon.

Mr. *J.B. Elder*, The Royal Infirmary, Oxford.
Mr. *D.J. Ellis*, North Staffs Royal Infirmary, Stoke-on-Trent, Staffordshire.
Professor *H. Ellis*, The Westminster Hospital, London.

241

Dr. T. Feizi, Clinical Research Centre, Div. of Communicable Diseases, Harrow.
Mr. J.W.L. Fielding, The Queen Elizabeth Hospital, Birmingham.
Dr. C.H.J. Ford, Surgical Immunology Unit, Queen Elizabeth Hospital, Birmingham.
Mr. J. Forrest, Queen Elizabeth Hospital, Birmingham.

Mr. D.M.J. Geewater, Queen Mary's Hospital, London.
Professor G.R. Giles, St. James's Hospital, Leeds.
Mr. W. Gillison, Kidderminster General Hospital, Kidderminster, Worcestershire.
Mr. S. Glick, Burton General Hospital, Burton-on-Trent, Staffordshire.
Dr. B. Golematis, 40, Solonos Street, Athens, Greece.
Dr. R. Gopal, The Royal Hospital, Wolverhampton.
Dr. S. Gottfried, Biorex Laboratories, London.
Mr. R. Grimley, Queen Elizabeth Hospital, Birmingham.
Mr. E. Gross, Hope Hospital, Salford, Manchester.

Dr. H. de Haas, I.C.I., Macclesfield, Cheshire.
Sister K. Haines, Wexham Park Hospital, Slough.
Professor I. Hakkinen, Department of Pathology, University of Turku, Finland.
Mr. R. Hall, York District Hospital, York.
Mr. D. Hancock, Sunderland District General Hospital, Sunderland.
Professor J.D. Hardcastle, Queens Medical Centre, Nottingham.
Mr. R. Harrison, Radiochemical Centre, Amersham, Buckinghamshire.
Mr. N. Hart, Dudley Road Hospital, Birmingham.
Dr. V. Harvey, St. Bartholomew's Hospital, London.
Mr. P. Hawker, The General Hospital, Birmingham.
Mr. I. Haynes, East Birmingham Hospital, Birmingham.
Mr. J.D. Hennessy, Sandwell District General Hospital, West Bromwich.
Mr. J.N. Hetherington, Selly Oak Hospital, Birmingham.
Dr. M. Hill, Bacterial Metabolism Research Laboratories, London.
Dr. T. Hirayama, National Cancer Centre Research Institute, Tokyo, Japan.
Mr. N.A.L. Hodges, Macarthy Laboratories, Dagenham, Essex.
Mr. A. Hooper, Queen Mary's Hospital, London.

Dr. K.S. Ibrahim, St. Stephen's Hospital, London.

Dr. J.R. Johnson, Surgical Immunology Unit, Queen Elizabeth Hospital, Birmingham.
Professor I.D.A. Johnston, Royal Victoria Infirmary, Newcastle-upon-Tyne.
Mr. B.G. Jones, Queen Elizabeth Hospital, Birmingham.
Dr. D.F. Jones, I.C.I., Macclesfield, Cheshire.

Dr. M. Karpinski, Good Hope Hospital, Birmingham.
Mr. M.R.B. Keighley, The General Hospital, Birmingham.
Dr. J. Kenny, The Christie Hospital and Holt Radium Institute, Manchester.
Dr. A.F. Keys, The Medical School, University of Manchester, Manchester.
Mr. R. Kingston, Park Hospital, Manchester.

Dr. A. Leon, Chile.
Professor K. Lewin, Department of Pathology, U.C.L.A., Los Angeles, U.S.A.
Professor W. Longmire, U.C.L.A., Los Angeles, U.S.A.
Mr. M.D. Lord, 5, Clarendon Place, Leamington Spa, Warwickshire.

Mrs. W. Maley, Park Hospital, Manchester.
Mr. M.C. Mason, Singleton Hospital, Swansea.
Mr. L. Matthews, Prince Charles Hospital, Merthyr Tydfil, South. Wales.
Dr. H. McAdam, Airedale General Hospital, Keighley, West Yorkshire.
Mr. W.A.F. McAdam, Airedale General Hospital, Keighley, West Yorkshire.
Mr. M.J. McMahon, Leeds General Infirmary, Leeds.
Dr. M.A. Melvin, Smith, Kline and French, Welyn Garden City, Hertfordshire.

Dr. S. Messina, Hackney Hospital, London.
Dr. H.J. Meyer, Hannover Medical School, Hannover, West Germany.
Dr. A. Minawa, The Cancer Registry, Queen Elizabeth Medical Centre, Birmingham.
Dr. R.C. Mitchell, Smith, Kline and French, Welwyn Garden City, Hertfordshire.
Miss J. Moore, The General Hospital, Birmingham.
Mr. M.W.E. Morgan, St. Margarets Hospital, Epping, Essex.
Mr. W.P. Morgan, University Hospital of Wales, Cardiff.
Mr. N.J.Mc. Mortensen, Royal Devon and Exeter Hospital, Exeter, Devon.
Mr. T.J. Muscroft, The General Hospital, Birmingham.

Mr. C.E. Newman, Surgical Immunology Unit, Queen Elizabeth Hospital, Birmingham.

Mr. R.W. Parker, Walsgrave Hospital, Coventry.
Dr. J. Parmar, The General Hospital, Birmingham.
Mrs. J.F. Paterson, The Cancer Registry, Queen Elizabeth Medical Centre, Birmingham.
Dr. P. Perry, Farmitalia Carlo Erba, Barnet, Hertfordshire.
Professor Dr. R. Pichlmayr, Hannover Medical School, Hannover, West Germany.
Miss J. Powell, The Cancer Registry, Queen Elizabeth Medical Centre, Birmingham.

Mr. S. Rashid, Unit for Cancer Research, Leeds University, Leeds.
Dr. P. Reid, Wexham Park Hospital, Slough.
Dr. W.H. ReMine, The Mayo Clinic, Rochester, U.S.A.
Mr. R.S. Rihan, Good Hope Hospital, Birmingham.
Mr. J.G. Roberts, Llandough Hospital, Napenarth, South Glamorgan.
Mr. A.S. Robson, Smith, Kline and French, Welwyn Garden City, Hertfordshire.
Mr. K. Rogers, Welsh National School of Medicine, Cardiff.
Mrs. C. Roginski, The Cancer Registry, Queen Elizabeth Medical Centre, Birmingham.
Mr. A.D. Rowse, 3, Fairbanks Walk, Swynnerton, Stone, Staffordshire.

Mr. R.H. Sage, Selly Oak Hospital, Birmingham.
Dr. A.B. Samii, 12, Mosntagh Street, Palestine Ave., Tehran, Iran.
Dr. A. Savage, Southmead Hospital, Bristol.
Dr. J.H. Scarffe, Christie Hospital and Holt Radium Institute, Manchester.
Dr. M.A. Simkins, Smith, Kline and French, Welwyn Garden City, Hertfordshire.
Professor G. Slaney, Queen Elizabeth Hospital, Birmingham.
Dr. F. Smith, Vincent T. Lombardi Cancer Treatment Centre, Georgetown, U.S.A.
Dr. S.R. Smith, Clinical Oncology, Queen Elizabeth Hospital, Birmingham.
Mr. Solanki, Sandwell District General Hospital, West Bromwich.
Mr. J.L. Somervell, The Manor Hospital, Walsall.
Dr. C. Starkey, The General Hospital, Birmingham.
Mr. R.D. Stedeford, Oldchurch Hospital, Romford, Essex.
Mr. D.W. Stol, Sophia Hospital, V. Heesweg, 2 Wolle, The Netherlands.
Dr. K. Summers, Wexham Park Hospital, Slough.
Dr. H. Sussman, Farmitalia Carlo Erba, Barnet, Hertfordshire.

Dr. K. Takagi, Cancer Institute Hospital, Tokyo, Japan.
Mr. R.C. Tandon, Sandwell District General Hospital, West Bromwich.
Mr. J. Temple, Queen Elizabeth Hospital, Birmingham.
Dr. H. Thompson, The General Hospital, Birmingham.
Dr. J.C. Topham, I.C.I., Macclesfield, Cheshire.
Dr. D.B. Trash, The Manor Hospital, Walsall.

Dr. C.A. Veys, Michelin Tyre Co., Ltd., Stoke-on-Trent, Staffordshire.

Dr. C.L. Walters, Leatherhead Food R.A., Leatherhead, Surrey.
Mr. A.J. Warrington, Sunderland District General Hospital, Sunderland.
Mrs. L. Ward, The Cancer Registry, Queen Elizabeth Medical Centre, Birmingham.
Dr. J. Waterhouse, The Cancer Registry, Queen Elizabeth Medical Centre, Birmingham.
Mr. J. Wellwood, Whipps Cross Hospital, London.

Dr. N. Werbin, Israel.
Mr. J.T. Williams, The Guest Hospital, Dudley, West Midlands.
Dr. R. Williams, North Staffordshire Royal Infirmary, Stoke-on-Trent, Staffordshire.
Mr. H.S. Winsey, Singleton Hospital, Swansea.
Dr. P. Wrigley, St. Bartholomew's Hospital, London.
Mr. C.S. Woodhouse, Surgical Immunology Unit, Queen Elizabeth Hospital, Birmingham.

Dr. J. Young, Queen Elizabeth Hospital, Birmingham.

SUBJECT INDEX

245